Clinical Psychology Research and Public Health

Clinical Psychology Research and Public Health

Guest Editors

Magdalena Iorga
Camelia Soponaru

MDPI

Basel • Beijing • Wuhan • Barcelona • Belgrade • Novi Sad • Cluj • Manchester

Guest Editors
Magdalena Iorga
Behavioral Sciences Department
University of Medicine and Pharmacy "Grigore T. Popa"
Iasi
Romania

Camelia Soponaru
Psychology Department
University "Alexandru Ioan Cuza" Iasi
Iasi
Romania

Editorial Office
MDPI AG
Grosspeteranlage 5
4052 Basel, Switzerland

This is a reprint of the Special Issue, published open access by the journal *Behavioral Sciences* (ISSN 2076-328X), freely accessible at: https://www.mdpi.com/journal/behavsci/special_issues/clinical_psychology.

For citation purposes, cite each article independently as indicated on the article page online and as indicated below:

Lastname, A.A.; Lastname, B.B. Article Title. *Journal Name* **Year**, *Volume Number*, Page Range.

ISBN 978-3-7258-5497-4 (Hbk)
ISBN 978-3-7258-5498-1 (PDF)
https://doi.org/10.3390/books978-3-7258-5498-1

Contents

About the Editors . . . vii

Octav-Sorin Candel
Sense of Relational Entitlement and Couple Outcomes: The Mediating Role of Couple Negotiation Tactics
Reprinted from: *Behav. Sci.* **2023**, *13*, 467, https://doi.org/10.3390/bs13060467 . . . 1

Ning Chen, Juzhe Xi and Xiwang Fan
Correlations among Psychological Resilience, Cognitive Fusion, and Depressed Emotions in Patients with Depression
Reprinted from: *Behav. Sci.* **2023**, *13*, 100, https://doi.org/10.3390/bs13020100 . . . 13

Magdalena Iorga, Lavinia Maria Pop, Irina Croitoru, Elena Hanganu and Dana-Teodora Anton-Păduraru
Exploring the Importance of Gender, Family Affluence, Parenting Style and Loneliness in Cyberbullying Victimization and Aggression among Romanian Adolescents
Reprinted from: *Behav. Sci.* **2022**, *12*, 457, https://doi.org/10.3390/bs12110457 . . . 21

Maria João Carapeto, Raquel Domingos and Guida Veiga
Attachment and Depressive Symptoms in Adolescence: The Mediatory Role of Emotion Awareness
Reprinted from: *Behav. Sci.* **2022**, *12*, 405, https://doi.org/10.3390/bs12100405 . . . 37

Sergio Salgado, Carolina González-Suhr, Gabriela Nazar, Carlos-María Alcover, Raúl Ramírez-Vielma and Claudio Bustos
Relationships between Individual and Social Resources, Anxiety and Depression in the Early Lockdown Stage by the COVID-19 in Chile
Reprinted from: *Behav. Sci.* **2022**, *12*, 357, https://doi.org/10.3390/bs12100357 . . . 49

Cristina Rivera-Picón, María Hinojal Benavente-Cuesta, María Paz Quevedo-Aguado and Pedro Manuel Rodríguez-Muñoz
The Importance of Positive Psychological Factors among People Living with HIV: A Comparative Study
Reprinted from: *Behav. Sci.* **2022**, *12*, 288, https://doi.org/10.3390/bs12080288 . . . 66

Graça Esgalhado, Henrique Pereira and Patricia Silva
Adaptation of an Emotional Stroop Test for Screening of Suicidal Ideation in Portugal
Reprinted from: *Behav. Sci.* **2022**, *12*, 281, https://doi.org/10.3390/bs12080281 . . . 78

Nurfarah Lydia Hambali, Friska Ayu, Nicholas Tze Ping Pang, Mohd Amiruddin Mohd Kassim, Hafid Algristian, Moch. Sahri, et al.
Mediating Effect of Psychological Process Variables on the Relationship between Dysfunctional Coping and Psychopathologies: A Comparative Study on Psychopathologies during COVID-19
Reprinted from: *Behav. Sci.* **2022**, *12*, 206, https://doi.org/10.3390/bs12070206 . . . 90

Qingwei Xu, Liu Han and Kaili Xu
Causal Analysis and Prevention Measures for Extreme Heavy Rainstorms in Zhengzhou to Protect Human Health
Reprinted from: *Behav. Sci.* **2022**, *12*, 176, https://doi.org/10.3390/bs12060176 . . . 101

V. Vineeth Kumar and Geetika Tankha
The Relationship between Personality Traits and COVID-19 Anxiety: A Mediating Model
Reprinted from: *Behav. Sci.* **2022**, *12*, 24, https://doi.org/10.3390/bs12020024 . . . 123

Qin Xiang Ng, Yu Liang Lim, Wayren Loke, Wee Song Yeo and Kuan Tsee Chee
Obsessive-Compulsive Disorders and Functional Urinary Disorders: A Fortuitous Association?
Reprinted from: *Behav. Sci.* **2021**, *11*, 89, https://doi.org/10.3390/bs11060089 . . . . **137**

Silvia Cimino, Eleonora Marzilli, Alessandra Babore, Carmen Trumello and Luca Cerniglia
DAT1 and Its Psychological Correlates in Children with Avoidant/Restrictive Food Intake Disorder: A Cross-Sectional Pilot Study
Reprinted from: *Behav. Sci.* **2021**, *11*, 9, https://doi.org/10.3390/bs11010009 . . . . **143**

Sin Yee Yap, Foong Leng Ng, Menaga Subramaniam, Yang Mooi Lim and Chai Nien Foo
Traditional Chinese Medicine Body Constitutions as Predictors for Depression: A Systematic Review and Meta-Analysis
Reprinted from: *Behav. Sci.* **2022**, *12*, 423, https://doi.org/10.3390/bs12110423 . . . . **157**

About the Editors

Magdalena Iorga

Magdalena Iorga, PhD is a Professor of Behavioral Sciences and Clinical Psychology at the "Grigore T. Popa" University of Medicine and Pharmacy in Iasi and supervises PhDs in Psychology. Her areas of interest are behavioral sciences, the quality of life among chronically unemployed people, bullying and cyberbullying, professional burnout, adverse childhood events and psychological lifestyles. Her research has resulted in several books and manuals, over 100 scientific articles, and she has participated in research projects as a director or team member.

Camelia Soponaru

Camelia Soponaru, PhD is a Professor of Cognitive Behavioral Therapy in the Faculty of Psychology and Educational Sciences, "Alexandru Ioan Cuza" University of Iași, Romania. She has expertise in clinical psychology, clinical assessment techniques, and psychotherapy. Her research has focused on the chronic somatic illness clinic, burnout syndrome and job satisfaction among healthcare workers, mental health and acculturative stress among international students and refugees, attitudes towards medication dispensing, and social representations.

behavioral sciences

MDPI

Article

Sense of Relational Entitlement and Couple Outcomes: The Mediating Role of Couple Negotiation Tactics

Octav-Sorin Candel

Faculty of Psychology and Educational Sciences, Alexandru Ioan Cuza University of Iaşi, 700554 Iaşi, Romania; octav.candel@uaic.ro

Abstract: Previous research shows a link between the sense of relational entitlement and various couple outcomes. However, the mechanisms linking these variables are less discussed. With this study, the aim was to test the associations between individuals' excessive and restricted sense of relational entitlement and their levels of couple satisfaction and conflict. In addition, it was tested whether the use of different negotiation tactics (cooperative and competitive) mediated the links. Six hundred and eighty-seven adults (55.2% women) participated in this study. Mediation analyses showed that a restricted sense of relational entitlement is associated with couple satisfaction and conflict through higher competitive negotiation use. Additionally, an excessive sense of relational entitlement is linked with couple satisfaction and conflict through lower cooperative negotiation use. This study has important implications for couples therapy addressing satisfaction issues, showing why and when educating couple interactions, especially those regarding negotiation, can improve relational functioning. Additionally, one's relational well-being is strongly related to one's mental health, and the applicability of the findings can be extended to all outcomes of the therapeutic process.

Keywords: sense of relational entitlement; negotiation; couple satisfaction; couple conflict

1. Introduction

Having fulfilling intimate relationships is beneficial for an individual's well-being, with couple satisfaction being related to lower depression and higher life satisfaction [1–3]. On the contrary, couple conflict correlates with higher levels of depression and negative mood [4]. Thus, studying the factors leading to changes in a couple's relational quality is crucial when discussing how to keep individuals more satisfied with their relationships and, therefore, safer from mental health issues. Among others, the sense of relational entitlement (SRE) has been proposed as a relevant personal characteristic related to relational quality [5,6]. However, the mechanisms linking it to couple satisfaction and couple conflict have not been sufficiently explored.

In this current research, I propose the use of different negotiation tactics as mediators between the sense of relational entitlement and couple satisfaction and conflict. Previous studies showed that negotiation is important for couples, both in daily interactions as well as in therapy [7–9]. In addition, entitlement was previously linked with the use of more unethical negotiation behaviors [10].

1.1. The Sense of Relational Entitlement and Couple Relationships

From a theoretical standpoint, Karney and Bradbury, in 1995, proposed the vulnerability-stress-adaption (VSA) model of couple satisfaction [11]. The authors point out that the quality of a couple's relationship can be influenced by both the stressful events encountered by the partner as well as by their existing vulnerabilities. The SRE can act as one such vulnerability.

Psychological entitlement represents the belief that one deserves more than others as well as the expectation of special treatment. While initially conceptualized as a broad dimension of narcissism, later theories proposed that individuals express various types of entitlement in various life domains [6,12,13]. The concept of SRE was developed in the context of romantic relationships, referring only to those expressions of entitlement appearing in the domain of romantic relationships. SRE can be defined as the extent to which a person expects that their needs and wishes will be fulfilled by their romantic partner, and as a person's affective and cognitive responses to a romantic partner's failure to fulfill these needs and hopes [6]. Moreover, recent studies differentiate between adaptive forms and maladaptive forms of entitlement. Among the latter, Tolmacz, in 2011, proposed excessive and restricted entitlement as forms of SRE [14]. In the context of romantic relationships, individuals with excessive entitlement have high expectations from their partners, as they demand the fulfillment of their needs and wishes. However, they are very sensitive when these expectations are violated and can experience regret regarding their relationship. On the contrary, individuals with a restricted SRE suffer from an inhibited expression of their needs and have doubts about whether is fair for them to express their wishes [13].

Tolmacz described the sense of relational entitlement as developing in the context of attachment relationships with childhood caregivers [14]. However, just like the internal working models of attachment adapt over time to different attachment figures, the sense of relational entitlement changes too. Thus, romantic relationships become the central context to study relational entitlement, since the romantic partner is the main attachment figure and source of emotional need fulfillment during adulthood. Previous studies support this perspective and show that the sense of relational entitlement is significantly linked to couple satisfaction [6,15–17]. When differentiating between the excessive and restricted types of entitlement, most studies show that both forms of relational entitlement show negative relationships with satisfaction, but these are stronger for the former compared with the latter [18,19]. In addition, other studies show the opposite link between entitlement and couple conflict. People with higher levels of entitlement (both general and relational) also report higher levels of conflict [5,20,21].

1.2. The Mediating Role of Negotiation Tactics

One key theory used in understanding the use of negotiation in couple relationships is the dual concern theory [22]. Although it originated from the organizational domain, it was later expanded to the domain of couple relationships [23]. The theory proposes that when negotiating, individuals are faced with two concerns, to defend their own interests and to foster cooperative agreement. When they intend to defend their own interest, they use more competitive negotiation tactics. On the contrary, when their shared interest is more important, they use more cooperative tactics.

Previous studies showed that using cooperative negotiation tactics is associated with higher levels of quality in one's romantic relationships, while using competitive tactics is associated with lower levels of quality [23]. Similar results were found when testing the association between effective negotiation and relational quality or equity-restoring negotiation strategies and relational satisfaction [24,25]. Moreover, competitiveness can escalate into exceedingly hostile exchanges; thus, the perpetuation of couple conflict is possible when more competitive or equity-resisting tactics are used [25–27].

While the outcomes of negotiation have been previously explored, the psychological antecedents of negotiation have received far less attention, especially in the domain of couple relationships. Past studies found that interindividual differences, such as personality traits and attachment orientation, impact negotiation behaviors [28,29]. One study that focused on the relationship between psychological entitlement and negotiation found that highly entitled individuals are more likely to use a forceful negotiation style and endorse more unethical behaviors [10]. Thus, excessively entitled individuals can fall victim to a "social trap", where one can find forcing or competitive negotiation tactics as alluring because, if successful, they allow the fulfillment of one's own needs over the partner's needs. At the same time, such tactics can have a deleterious effect on one's relationships [30]. Past literature presents scarce information about the negotiation behaviors of restrictedly entitled individuals. However, restricted entitlement is strongly associated with avoidant attachment [14]. By proxy and based on past studies showing that attachment avoidance has strong links with demanding negotiation strategies [31], one can also expect that the relationship's restricted entitlement and negotiation will show a similar pattern.

Most previous studies linked general entitlement and negotiation. However, since the level of entitlement can vary between life domains, each of these deserve attention [32]. A gap in the current couple- and family-related literature is that few studies tried to link interindividual differences, such as those in the level of entitlement, to the use of different negotiation tactics and their couple-relevant outcomes. For example, Williams and collaborators (2018) found that the sense of relational entitlement is associated with conflict resolution tactics. However, while there are similarities between conflict resolution tactics and negotiation tactics, the two processes are not the same. Moreover, the authors did not test the levels of couple conflict experienced by the participants.

1.3. The Present Study

This study takes into account the VSA model of couple satisfaction. Based on the aforementioned empirical findings, I tested whether higher levels of excessive SRE are significantly associated with lower couple satisfaction and higher couple conflict (H1). Additionally, I expected that higher levels of restricted SRE are significantly associated with lower couple satisfaction and higher couple conflict (H2). With this study, I explore one possible mechanism linking the sense of relational entitlement (both excessive and restricted), couple satisfaction and conflict. For this, I propose the use of negotiation tactics as a mediating variable. Thus, the use of competitive and cooperative negotiation tactics will mediate the link between an excessive SRE and couple satisfaction and conflict (H3). Finally, the use of competitive and cooperative negotiation tactics will mediate the relationship between a restricted SRE and couple satisfaction and conflict (H4).

2. Method

2.1. Participants

Six hundred and eighty-seven adults involved in a romantic relationship at the time of the data collection took part in this study. Among them 379 (55.2%) were women and 308 (44.8%) were men. The mean age was 22.97 years old (SD = 3.54, Min = 18, Max = 35) and the mean length of the relationship was 36.31 months (SD = 39.49, Min = 3, Max = 240). In total, 631 participants (91.8%) were not married. Additionally, 403 participants (58.7%) were cohabitating with their partner. Most participants had no children (N = 651, 94.8%), 18 participants had one child (2.6%), 15 participants had 2 children (2.2%) and three participants had 3 children (0.4%). In terms of education status, most participants had a high school degree (N = 478, 69.6%), four of them finished secondary education (0.6%), 178 had a Bachelor's degree (25.9%), 26 had a Master's degree (3.8%) and one had a Ph.D. (0.1%).

2.2. Procedure

The research was approved by the Research Ethics Committee at Alexandru Ioan Cuza University. The questionnaires were distributed to students enrolled in two undergraduate programs who also had to invite one other individual to take part in the study. The participants received an online form containing all the questionnaires used to measure the study's variables and the demographic questions. Participation was voluntary and the students received academic credits for their involvement.

2.3. Instruments

The Sense of Relational Entitlement Scale (SRE) [6]. I used the Romanian translation of the original SRE scale to assess the participants' sense of relational entitlement [15]. The instrument has 18 items and uses a Likert-type scale with answers from 1 (not at all) to 7 (very much). The questionnaire measures three types of SRE, assertive, excessive and restricted. However, previous research showed insufficient theoretical and methodological clarity for the assertive SRE domain [13]. Thus, in the present study, only the excessive (seven items, e.g., "I often feel I deserve to get more than I do in my relationship") and the restricted (three items, e.g., "I'm often preoccupied with the question of whether I deserve my partner") dimensions were retained. The scores for these dimensions were computed by averaging the items for each scale. Both subscales demonstrated good levels of internal consistency. For excessive relational entitlement, $\alpha = 0.88$; for restricted relational entitlement, $\alpha = 0.79$.

Negotiation tactics. To measure negotiation tactics, I used a scale created by Livingstone [23], who adapted De Dreu and Boles's scale [33]. This instrument contains a list of negotiation heuristics referring to retrospective accounts of negotiation tactics used by individuals in their romantic relationships. The participants had to follow the guideline "Please describe the extent to which you utilized any of the following types of tactics while you are negotiating the roles and involvement in various joint activities (e.g., household activities, free time, time spent with friends or family, etc.) with your spouse/partner" and answer to each question on a scale from 1 (never) to 5 (always). The instrument has two sub-scales, each containing eight items: competitive negotiation tactics ("Did you feel that your partner's loss was your gain", "Winner takes all") and cooperative negotiation tactics ("Were willing to compromise", "We played fair"). For both sub-scales, the total was computed by averaging the items. The scales showed adequate internal consistency. For cooperative negotiation, $\alpha = 0.65$; for competitive negotiation, $\alpha = 0.76$.

Couple Satisfaction Index 4 (CSI-4) [34]. The CSI-4 was used to assess the participants' satisfaction with their romantic relationship. The scale was previously adapted for use in Romanian [35]. Four items are included in the scale. The authors created the CSI scale by verifying the already existing measures of satisfaction and selecting the best items from them. Participants had to indicate how happy they are in their current romantic relationship using a Likert-type scale with seven points for one item ("Please indicate the degree of happiness, all things considered, of your relationship") and a Likert-type scale with six points for the others (e.g., "I have a warm and comfortable relationship with my partner"). Since the scale uses items with different measurement points, the total score was computed by summing the items. In this study, $\alpha = 0.91$, indicating a very good internal consistency.

Conflict scale [36]. The scale measured the level of conflict in the participants' romantic relationship. The instrument contained six items (e.g., "There is a lot of conflict in my relationship"). For each item, the participants had to choose an answer from 1 (strongly disagree) to 7 (strongly agree). The total score was obtained by averaging the items. The instrument demonstrated a very good internal consistency, $\alpha = 0.85$.

The scales measuring negotiation tactics and couple conflict that did not have Romanian adaptations were translated using the back-translation method.

2.4. Statistical Analyses

First, I used SPSS 21 to compute the descriptive statistics and the correlational analyses. Second, several mediation analyses were performed to verify whether the negotiation tactics used by individuals in their romantic relationship mediated the relationship between the participants' sense of relational entitlement and their couple satisfaction and conflict. Model 4 from Process, an SPSS macro, was used for this analysis [37]. Bootstrapping with 5000 re-samples was used to obtain parameter estimates of the specific indirect effects. The 95% confidence intervals (CIs) were used to determine whether these effects were statistically significant: if the 95% CI did not contain zero, then the indirect effect was considered statistically significant and mediation has been demonstrated.

3. Results

3.1. Preliminary Analyses

I assessed the normality of the distribution for each variable using the Skewness and Kurtosis measures. The values were within the limits proposed by Kim [38] when working with samples larger than 300 participants. I used Pearson product correlations to test the associations between the variables. Age and the length of the relationship were also included in the analysis. Table 1 presents these results as well as the means, standard deviations and values for Skewness and Kurtosis for the variables. Having an excessive sense of relational entitlement is significantly and negatively associated with using more competitive negotiation tactics and with more couple conflict. On the contrary, it is also significantly associated with lower couple satisfaction. A similar pattern of correlations was observed for the restricted sense of relational entitlement, but the strength of the associations was lower. Using cooperative negotiation tactics was significantly associated with higher satisfaction and lower conflict. Using competitive negotiation tactics was significantly associated with lower satisfaction and higher conflict. The length of the relationship was significantly and negatively linked with couple satisfaction. Age was significantly and positively related to the use of competitive negotiation tactics.

Table 1. Means, standard deviations and correlations between the study's variables.

	M	SD	SK	Kr	1	2	3	4	5	6	7
1. Excessive SRE	1.87	0.82	1.25	1.32	0.88						
2. Restricted SRE	2.51	1.08	0.31	−0.83	0.31 ***	0.79					
3. Cooperative NT	4.09	0.55	−0.70	0.90	−0.06	−0.01	0.65				
4. Competitive NT	1.96	0.71	0.72	0.12	0.37 ***	0.16 ***	−0.22 ***	0.76			
5. Couple satisfaction	21.95	3.15	−1.31	1.52	−0.63 ***	−0.10 **	0.23 ***	−0.26 ***	0.91		
6. Couple conflict	2.32	1.13	1.13	1.03	0.70 ***	0.19 ***	−0.18 ***	0.30 ***	−0.69 ***	0.85	
7. Age	22.97	3.54			−0.03	−0.06	−0.05	0.08 *	−0.02	−0.03	-
8. Relationship length	36.31	32.49			0.03	−0.10 **	−0.05	0.04	−0.08 *	0.01	0.43 ***

Note: SK = Skewness; Kr = Kurtosis; SRE = sense of relational entitlement; NT = negotiation tactics; *** $p < 0.001$; ** $p < 0.01$; * $p < 0.05$. Cronbach's alpha for each scale is shown on the diagonal.

A series of independent sample T tests was used to verify the differences in the variables' levels based on gender and cohabitation status. The results revealed that men, compared with women, reported significantly higher levels of couple satisfaction (t = 3.05; $p = 0.002$) and competitive negotiation tactics (t = 3.5; $p < 0.001$), as well as significantly lower levels of cooperative negotiation tactics (t = −2.70; $p = 0.007$) and restricted sense of relational entitlement (t = −5.28; $p < 0.001$). The individuals who were not cohabitating with their partners, compared with those who were, reported higher levels of couple conflict (t = 2.59; $p = 0.01$), excessive (t = 2.25; $p = 0.02$) and restricted sense of relational entitlement (t = 3.81; $p < 0.001$).

3.2. Mediation Analyses

I intended to compute a series of mediation analyses where either excessive or restricted senses of relational entitlement were introduced as predictors, cooperative and competitive negotiation tactics were used as mediators and either couple satisfaction or conflict served as outcomes. For all models, the participants' gender, their cohabitation status, their age and the length of their relationships were used as control variables.

The first model included an excessive sense of relational entitlement as the predictor, the use of competitive negotiation tactics as a mediator and couple satisfaction as the outcome. The effect of the excessive sense of relational entitlement on the use of competitive negotiation tactics was significant ($\beta = 0.41$; $p < 0.001$), as well as its effect on couple satisfaction ($\beta = -0.61$; $p < 0.001$). The effect of the mediator on the outcome was not significant ($\beta = -0.03$; $p = 0.33$). This led to a non-significant indirect effect ($\beta = -0.01$; CI (−0.04; 0.01). Thus, the mediation hypothesis was not supported. Additionally, when using couple conflict as an outcome, the effect the mediator had on it was not significant (β = 0.01; $p = 0.52$). The indirect effect was also not significant (β = 0.007; CI (−0.01; 0.03)).

The third model included a restricted sense of relational entitlement as the predictor, the use of competitive negotiation tactics as the mediator and couple satisfaction as the outcome (see Figure 1). Restricted entitlement had a significant effect on the mediator (β = 0.16; $p < 0.001$). Its total effect on the outcome was also significant (β = −0.10; $p = 0.005$). Using competitive negotiation tactics had a significant effect on couple satisfaction (β = −0.26; $p < 0.001$). The indirect effect of the sense of restricted entitlement on couple satisfaction was significant (β = −0.04; CI (−0.06; −0.02)), but its direct effect became non-significant after the introduction of the mediator (β = −0.06; $p = 0.09$). As for the control variables, some significant effects were found. The participants' gender had negative effects on the use of competitive negotiation tactics (β = −0.11; $p = 0.004$) and couple satisfaction (β = −0.16; $p < 0.001$). Additionally, their relationship duration had a negative effect on couple satisfaction (β = −0.09; $p = 0.02$), while their cohabitation status had a positive one (β = 0.11; $p = 0.006$).

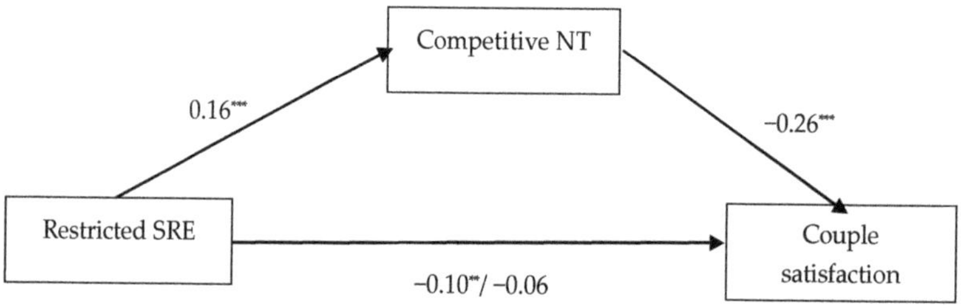

Figure 1. Total and direct effects of restricted sense of relational entitlement (SRE) on couple satisfaction, with competitive negotiation tactics (NT) as mediator. The values represent standardized regression coefficients. On the path between restricted SRE and couple satisfaction, the first value represents the total effect and the second value represents the direct effect. The effects of the controlled variables (age, gender, relationship length and cohabitation status) are not presented for brevity. ** $p < 0.01$; *** $p < 0.001$.

In the fourth model, couple conflict was used as an outcome (see Figure 2). Restricted entitlement had a significant total effect on the outcome (β = 0.19; $p < 0.001$). Using competitive negotiation tactics had a significant effect on couple conflict (β = 0.28; $p < 0.001$). The indirect effect of the sense of restricted entitlement on couple conflict was significant (β = 0.04; CI (0.02; 0.07)), as well as its direct effect after the introduction of the mediator (β = 0.14; $p < 0.001$). The participants' cohabitation status had a negative effect on couple conflict (β = −0.08; $p = 0.04$).

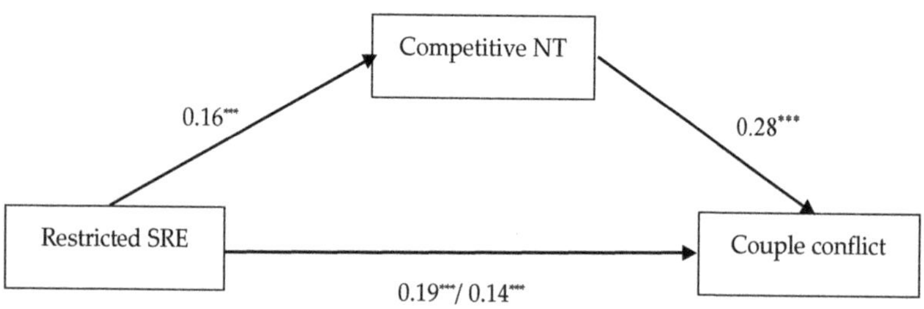

Figure 2. Total and direct effects of restricted sense of relational entitlement (SRE) on couple conflict, with competitive negotiation tactics (NT) as mediator. The values represent standardized regression coefficients. On the path between restricted SRE and couple conflict, the first value represents the total effect and the second value represents the direct effect. The effects of the controlled variables (age, gender, relationship length and cohabitation status) are not presented for brevity. *** $p < 0.001$.

The fifth model included an excessive sense of relational entitlement as the predictor, the use of cooperative negotiation tactics as the mediator and couple satisfaction as the outcome (see Figure 3). Excessive entitlement had a significant effect on the mediator (β = −0.08; p = 0.02). Its total effect on the outcome was also significant (β = −0.62; $p < 0.001$). Using cooperative negotiation tactics had a significant effect on couple satisfaction (β = 0.19; $p < 0.001$). The indirect effect of the sense of excessive entitlement on couple satisfaction was significant (β = −0.01; CI (−0.03; −0.002)), and its direct effect remained significant after the introduction of the mediator (β = −0.60; $p < 0.001$). The participants' gender had a positive effect on their use of cooperative negotiation tactics (β = 0.10; p = 0.001).

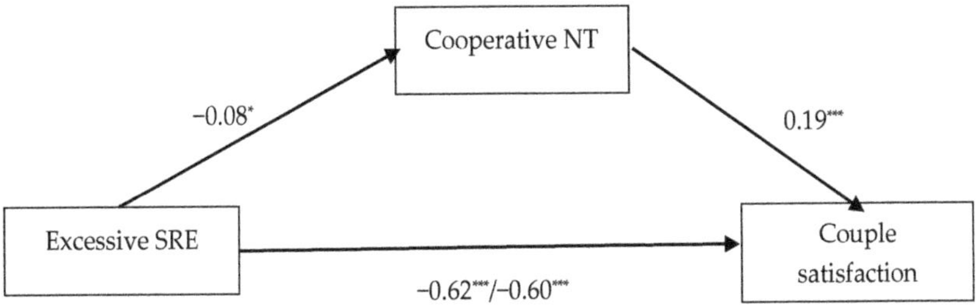

Figure 3. Total and direct effects of excessive sense of relational entitlement (SRE) on couple satisfaction, with cooperative negotiation tactics (NT) as mediator. The values represent standardized regression coefficients. On the path between excessive SRE and couple satisfaction, the first value represents the total effect and the second value represents the direct effect. The effects of the controlled variables (age, gender, relationship length and cohabitation status) are not presented for brevity. * $p < 0.05$; *** $p < 0.001$.

In the sixth model, couple conflict was used as an outcome (see Figure 4). Excessive entitlement had significant total effect on the outcome (β = 0.72; $p < 0.001$). Using cooperative negotiation tactics had a significant effect on couple conflict (β = −0.12; $p < 0.001$). The indirect effect of a sense of excessive entitlement on couple conflict was significant (β = 0.01; CI (0.001; 0.02)), as well as its direct effect after the introduction of the mediator (β = 0.71; $p < 0.001$).

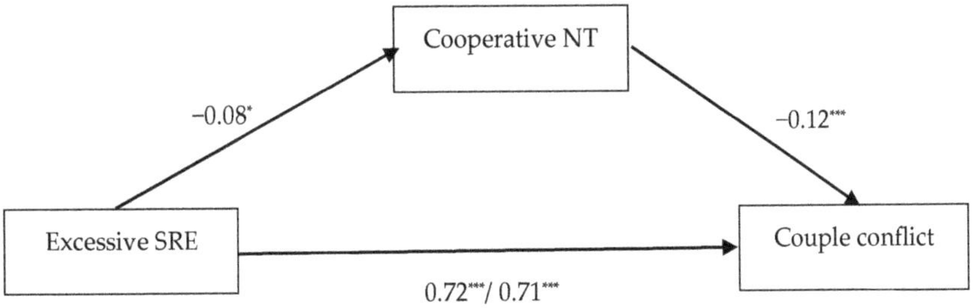

Figure 4. Total and direct effects of excessive sense of relational entitlement (SRE) on couple conflict, with cooperative negotiation tactics (NT) as mediator. The values represent standardized regression coefficients. On the path between excessive SRE and couple conflict, the first value represents the total effect and the second value represents the direct effect. The effects of the controlled variables (age, gender, relationship length and cohabitation status) are not presented for brevity. * $p < 0.05$; *** $p < 0.001$.

In models seven and eight, restricted entitlement was introduced as the predictor, the use of cooperative negotiation tactics as the mediator and either couple satisfaction (model seven) or couple conflict (model eight) as the outcomes. Restricted entitlement did not have a significant effect on the mediator ($\beta = -0.01$; $p = 61$). The indirect effects of restricted entitlement on couple satisfaction ($\beta = -0.004$; CI (-0.02; 0.01)) and couple conflict ($\beta = 0.003$; CI (-0.01; 0.01)) were not significant.

4. Discussion

This is one of the first studies to link the sense of relational entitlement, viewed here as an interpersonal difference, the negotiation tactics used in one's romantic relationship and several couple-related outcomes. I mainly aimed to test the mediating role of couple negotiation tactics (competitive and cooperative) between excessive and restricted SRE, and couple satisfaction and conflict. The results partially supported the assumptions.

For the first two hypotheses, I proposed that higher SRE (excessive or restricted) would be associated with lower levels of couple satisfaction and higher levels of couple conflict. Both hypotheses were confirmed. The relationships were stronger for excessive SRE compared with restricted SRE. All these results confirm previous findings [6,16,18,19], thus adding to the literature that presents high levels of SRE as an important inhibitor of fulfilling couple relationships. Both forms of maladaptive SRE result from unmet childhood needs, which lead to disrupting degrees of need-fulfillment seeking during adulthood [14]. Since romantic relationships are the main life domain where adults express their emotional needs, people who reported deficient close bonds in early childhood tend to also report them in later relationships. Individuals with high levels of excessive SRE exaggerate their needs and react negatively when these are not met by their partners. They are eager to observe and punish even minor transgressions from their partner. Since their partners are rarely able to adequately respond to their highly demanding needs, excessively entitled individuals become less satisfied with their relationships. Moreover, excessive entitlement can inflate self-image goals [39], and when these are not attained, the partner can be blamed, thus creating higher conflict in the relationship. Similarly, individuals with restricted SRE might feel dissatisfied and report higher conflict because they consider that their partners are not attentive to their needs [6,40]. However, their own modest and extremely cautious manner of interacting acts as a cause for such unresponsive behavior.

The mechanism linking maladaptive SRE and couple outcomes is explored more in-depth in this study. The mediation models show that excessive SRE is positively associated with the use of competitive negotiation and negatively with the use of cooperative negotiation. These results support the findings of Williams and collaborators [21], which showed that people who are more vigilant towards relationship transgression (a facet of excessive entitlement) also use more dominance and less compromise in their conflict negotiations. A novel result of this study is that restricted SRE was positively associated only with the use of competitive negotiation, which partially contradicts previous research [21]. The previous study found that individuals with restricted SRE were more likely to use compromise.

One important finding is that the use of competitive negotiation tactics mediates the relationship between restricted SRE and couple outcomes. Based on their early negative experiences with their caregivers, individuals with restricted SRE tend to see themselves as "worthless, inadequate and defective", yet they possess "masochistic characteristics" [41] (p. 226). Thus, using more competitive negotiation tactics (a negotiation style where one side must win and the other must lose) only allows the individuals, when losing, to reinforce their beliefs that something is wrong with them. Additionally, restricted SRE is positively linked with an avoidant attachment style and seems to share similar developmental conditions [6,40]. Since avoidant individuals use more non-cooperative, dominating conflict resolution strategies, one might also expect a similar response from those with high levels of restricted entitlement. However, using competitive negotiation was shown to be detrimental to one's relationship satisfaction [23,25]. Similarly, past research has shown that zero-sum beliefs are associated with lower life satisfaction [42]. Thus, people with high levels of restricted SRE presented lower levels of couple satisfaction and higher levels of couple conflict, and one linking mechanism was their use of competitive negotiation tactics. Additionally, through a decrease in the use of cooperative negotiation, higher levels of excessive SRE were associated with lower couple satisfaction and higher couple conflict. Individuals with high entitlement scores can prefer short-term personal goals over long-term development of the couple [43]. They can, as well, present an individualistic orientation, thus being more prone to use threats, bargaining and other types of unethical negotiation [10,43]. Consequently, overly concentrating on winning in any argument and choosing self-benefit instead of collective good can lead individuals to lower levels of relational happiness.

These findings have important implications for couples therapy as well as for the mental health of the individuals involved in couple relationships. Firstly, as shown by previous studies, negotiation is an important aspect of couple functioning and is relevant in various domains such as parenting, work and even technology use [23,44,45]. Moreover, negotiation can be trained in couples therapy [8]. This study shows that the negotiation tactics used by individuals can be an outcome of some internal aspects such as the sense of relational entitlement. Thus, integrating this knowledge in the field of couple and family therapy is essential to develop more comprehensive programs that account for differences in relational entitlement, especially when educating couples regarding the best ways to use negotiation. Secondly, knowing why some people are more prone to using maladaptive negotiation tactics can have larger implications beyond the well-being of the couple. Both individual case studies and empirical studies have shown that couples therapy is efficient when dealing with issues such as depression [46–48]. Moreover, since couple satisfaction acts as a predictor for depression, family therapy can be used to ensure higher levels of couple, as well as individual, functioning. Thus, educating positive couple interactions (such as using fewer competitive negotiation tactics) while also taking into account the individual issues affecting them can lead to better-suited therapeutic processes and more efficient ways to protect mental health.

On another interesting note, this study shows that SRE is an antecedent of couple conflict. Previous studies evidenced that interparental conflict is a predictor of the development of maladaptive SRE [49]. Although indirectly, these two studies present some evidence regarding the transmission of couple conflict from one generation to the other.

Despite advancing the literature and having important practical implications, this study is not without limitations. Firstly, it proposes a cross-sectional investigation using self-reported questionnaires. To truly test the mediation hypothesis, longitudinal studies are needed. Additionally, more recent studies assess the partners' behaviors by using recordings of the couples' conflicts [50,51]. With a similar methodology, future studies can investigate the negotiation tactics used by the partners during a conflictual interaction and their effects on conflict resolution. Finally, the use of negotiation seems to differ based on age and cultural characteristics. Past studies showed that younger individuals and those coming from cultures higher in individualism and masculinity tend to use more unethical or competitive tactics [52]. Since in this sample, the participants were rather homogenous in age and came from only one culture, these results need to be confirmed by research with more diverse participants.

5. Conclusions

The main aim of this study was to test the mediation role of negotiation tactics in the relationship between the sense of relational entitlement and couple satisfaction and conflict. The results showed that restricted SRE is related to higher levels of competitive negotiation use, while excessive SRE is linked to lower levels of cooperative negotiation use. Both negotiation tactics mediated the link between SRE and couple satisfaction, as well as SRE and couple conflict. The research shows that SRE is a significant antecedent of negotiation behavior and how this couple process impacts various relational outcomes.

Funding: This work was supported by a grant of the "Alexandru Ioan Cuza" University of Iasi, within the Research Grants program, Grant UAIC, code GI-UAIC-2020-01.

Institutional Review Board Statement: The study was conducted according to the guidelines of the Declaration of Helsinki and was approved by the Ethics committee for research at the Faculty of Psychology and Educational Science, Alexandru Ioan Cuza University of Iasi (code 3320bis/ 15 October 2021).

Informed Consent Statement: Informed consent was obtained from all participants involved in the study.

Data Availability Statement: The data presented in this study are available on request from the corresponding author.

Conflicts of Interest: The author declares no conflict of interest.

References

1. Gilmour, A.L.; Whisman, M.A.; Whitton, S.W. A dyadic analysis of relationship satisfaction and depressive symptoms among same-sex couples. *J. Fam. Psychol.* **2022**, *36*, 372–377. [CrossRef] [PubMed]
2. Goldfarb, M.R.; Trudel, G. Marital quality and depression: A review. *Marriage Fam. Rev.* **2019**, *55*, 737–763. [CrossRef]
3. Işık, E.; Özbiler, Ş.; Schweer-Collins, M.L.; Rodríguez-González, M. Differentiation of self predicts life satisfaction through marital adjustment. *Am. J. Fam. Ther.* **2020**, *48*, 235–249. [CrossRef]
4. McDaniel, B.T.; Drouin, M. Daily technology interruptions and emotional and relational well-being. *Comput. Hum. Behav.* **2019**, *99*, 1–8. [CrossRef] [PubMed]
5. Candel, O.S. The Link between Parenting Behaviors and Emerging Adults' Relationship Outcomes: The Mediating Role of Relational Entitlement. *Int. J. Environ. Res. Public Health* **2022**, *19*, 828. [CrossRef]
6. Tolmacz, R.; Mikulincer, M. The sense of entitlement in romantic relationships—Scale construction, factor structure, construct validity, and its associations with attachment orientations. *Psychoanal. Psychol.* **2011**, *28*, 75–94. [CrossRef]
7. Dyck, V.; Daly, K. Rising to the challenge: Fathers' role in the negotiation of couple time. *Leis. Stud.* **2006**, *25*, 201–217. [CrossRef]
8. Pizer, B.; Pizer, S.A. "The gift of an apple or the twist of an arm": Negotiation in couples and couple therapy. *Psychoanal. Dialogues* **2006**, *16*, 71–92.
9. Vowels, L.M.; Carnelley, K.B. Attachment styles, negotiation of goal conflict, and perceived partner support during COVID-19. *Personal. Individ. Differ.* **2021**, *171*, 110505. [CrossRef]
10. Neville, L.; Fisk, G.M. Getting to excess: Psychological entitlement and negotiation attitudes. *J. Bus. Psychol.* **2019**, *34*, 555–574. [CrossRef]
11. Karney, B.R.; Bradbury, T.N. The longitudinal course of marital quality and stability: A review of theory, methods, and research. *Psychol. Bull.* **1995**, *118*, 3–34. [CrossRef]
12. Exline, J.J.; Baumeister, R.F.; Bushman, B.J.; Campbell, W.K.; Finkel, E.J. Too proud to let go: Narcissistic entitlement as a barrier to forgiveness. *J. Personal. Soc. Psychol.* **2004**, *87*, 894–912. [CrossRef]
13. Tolmacz, R.; Lev-Ari, L.; Bachner-Melman, R. Refining the Assessment of Entitlement in Romantic Relationships: The Sense of Relational Entitlement Scale—Revised (SRE-R). *Front. Psychol.* **2021**, *12*, 744618. [CrossRef] [PubMed]
14. Tolmacz, R. Sense of entitlement in couple relationships: An attachment theory perspective. *Am. J. Psychoanal.* **2011**, *71*, 37–57. [CrossRef] [PubMed]
15. Candel, O.S. Sense of relational entitlement–romanian version. Factor structure and associations with romantic attachment and dyadic satisfaction. In Proceedings of the CIEA 2018 the Fifth International Conference on Adult Education. Education for Values—Continuity and Context, Iasi, Romania, 25–28 April 2018; pp. 79–86.
16. George-Levi, S.; Vilchinsky, N.; Tolmacz, R.; Liberman, G. Testing the concept of relational entitlement in the dyadic context: Further validation and associations with relationship satisfaction. *J. Fam. Psychol.* **2014**, *28*, 193–203. [CrossRef] [PubMed]
17. Tolmacz, R.; Bachner-Melman, R.; Lev-Ari, L.; Brondvine, D. Associations between pathological eating, relational attitudes and satisfaction in romantic relationships. *Eat. Weight Disord. Stud. Anorex. Bulim. Obes.* **2022**, *27*, 1385–1393. [CrossRef]
18. Candel, O.S.; Turliuc, M.N. The effect of the sense of relational entitlement on relational satisfaction, positive and negative emotions. *J. Psychol. Educ. Res.* **2019**, *27*, 46–60.
19. Candel, O.S.; Turliuc, M.N. The role of relational entitlement, self-disclosure and perceived partner responsiveness in predicting couple satisfaction: A daily-diary study. *Front. Psychol.* **2021**, *12*, 609232. [CrossRef]
20. Warrener, C.D.; Tasso, A. An empirical examination of the relationship between dating abuse and entitlement within a college population. *Partn. Abus.* **2017**, *8*, 377–394. [CrossRef]
21. Williams, D.N.; Smith, D.B.; Sukach, T.; Minaiy, C. Expecting more in relationships–implications of relational entitlement. *Am. J. Fam. Ther.* **2018**, *46*, 321–340. [CrossRef]
22. Pruitt, D.G.; Rubin, J.Z. *Social Conflict: Escalation, Stalemate, and Settlement*; McGraw-Hill: New York, NY, USA, 1986.

23. Livingston, B.A. Bargaining behind the scenes: Spousal negotiation, labor, and work–family burnout. *J. Manag.* **2014**, *40*, 949–977. [CrossRef]
24. Carroll, J.S.; Badger, S.; Yang, C. The ability to negotiate or the ability to love? Evaluating the developmental domains of marital competence. *J. Fam. Issues* **2006**, *27*, 1001–1032. [CrossRef]
25. Charbonneau, A.; Lachance-Grzela, M.; Bouchard, G. Housework allocation, negotiation strategies, and relationship satisfaction in cohabiting emerging adult heterosexual couples. *Sex Roles* **2019**, *81*, 290–305. [CrossRef]
26. De Dreu, C.K.; Van Knippenberg, D. The possessive self as a barrier to conflict resolution: Effects of mere ownership, process accountability, and self-concept clarity on competitive cognitions and behavior. *J. Personal. Soc. Psychol.* **2005**, *89*, 345–357. [CrossRef] [PubMed]
27. Gottman, J.M.; Levenson, R.W. The timing of divorce: Predicting when a couple will divorce over a 14-year period. *J. Marriage Fam.* **2000**, *62*, 737–745. [CrossRef]
28. Bakaç, C.; Kehr, H.M. Getting to the bargaining table: The role of explicit motives and traits in negotiation initiation. *Personal. Individ. Differ.* **2023**, *205*, 112099. [CrossRef]
29. Bear, J.B.; Segel-Karpas, D. Effects of attachment anxiety and avoidance on negotiation propensity and performance. *Negot. Confl. Manag. Res.* **2015**, *8*, 153–173. [CrossRef]
30. Campbell, W.K.; Buffardi, L.E. The lure of the noisy ego: Narcissism as a social trap. In *Transcending Self-Interest: Psychological Explorations of the Quiet Ego*; Wayment, H.A., Bauer, J.J., Eds.; American Psychological Association: Washington, DC, USA, 2008; pp. 23–32.
31. Ben-Ari, R.; Hirshberg, I. Attachment styles, conflict perception, and adolescents' strategies of coping with interpersonal conflict. *Negot. J.* **2009**, *25*, 59–82. [CrossRef]
32. Candel, O.S.; Turliuc, M.N. An overview of the research of psychological entitlement. Definitions and conceptual characteristics. *Rev. Psihol.* **2017**, *63*, 257–268.
33. De Dreu, C.K.; Boles, T.L. Share and share alike or winner take all? The influence of social value orientation upon choice and recall of negotiation heuristics. *Organ. Behav. Hum. Decis. Process.* **1998**, *76*, 253–276. [CrossRef]
34. Funk, J.L.; Rogge, R.D. Testing the ruler with item response theory: Increasing precision of measurement for relationship satisfaction with the Couples Satisfaction Index. *J. Fam. Psychol.* **2007**, *21*, 572–583. [CrossRef]
35. Candel, O.S. Couple satisfaction index 16. Proprietăți psihometrice și diferențe de gen în măsurarea satisfacției diadice. In *Tendințe Contemporane ale Dezvoltării Științei: Viziuni ale Tinerilor Cercetători*; Duca, M., Ed.; Universitatea de Stat Dimitrie Cantemir: Chișinău, Moldova, 2017; pp. 109–113.
36. Gordon, A.M.; Chen, S. Do you get where I'm coming from? Perceived understanding buffers against the negative impact of conflict on relationship satisfaction. *J. Personal. Soc. Psychol.* **2016**, *110*, 239–260. [CrossRef]
37. Hayes, A.F. *Introduction to Mediation, Moderation, and Conditional Process Analysis: A Regression-Based Approach*; Guilford Press: New York, NY, USA, 2013.
38. Kim, H.Y. Statistical notes for clinical researchers: Assessing normal distribution (2) using skewness and kurtosis. *Restor. Dent. Endod.* **2013**, *38*, 52–54. [CrossRef]
39. Moeller, S.J.; Crocker, J.; Bushman, B.J. Creating hostility and conflict: Effects of entitlement and self-image goals. *J. Exp. Soc. Psychol.* **2009**, *45*, 448–452. [CrossRef] [PubMed]
40. Shadach, E.; Rappaport, S.; Dollberg, D.; Tolmacz, R.; Levy, S. Relational entitlement, early recollections of parental care, and attachment orientation. *Curr. Psychol.* **2018**, *37*, 781–791. [CrossRef]
41. Meyer, W.S. A case of restricted entitlement. *Clin. Soc. Work. J.* **1991**, *19*, 223–235. [CrossRef]
42. Shin, J.E.; Kim, J.K. How a good sleep predicts life satisfaction: The role of zero-sum beliefs about happiness. *Front. Psychol.* **2018**, *9*, 1589. [CrossRef]
43. Grijalva, E.; Harms, P.D. Narcissism: An integrative synthesis and dominance complementarity model. *Acad. Manag. Perspect.* **2014**, *28*, 108–127. [CrossRef]
44. Pickens, J.C.; Whiting, J.B. Tech talk: Analyzing the negotiations and rules around technology use in intimate relationships. *Contemp. Fam. Ther.* **2020**, *42*, 175–189. [CrossRef]
45. Sheedy, A.; Gambrel, L.E. Coparenting negotiation during the transition to parenthood: A qualitative study of couples' experiences as new parents. *Am. J. Fam. Ther.* **2019**, *47*, 67–86. [CrossRef]
46. Barbato, A.; D'Avanzo, B. Efficacy of couple therapy as a treatment for depression: A meta-analysis. *Psychiatr. Q.* **2008**, *79*, 121–132. [CrossRef] [PubMed]
47. Durães, R.S.S.; Khafif, T.C.; Lotufo-Neto, F.; Serafim, A.D.P. Effectiveness of cognitive behavioral couple therapy on reducing depression and anxiety symptoms and increasing dyadic adjustment and marital social skills: An exploratory study. *Fam. J.* **2020**, *28*, 344–355. [CrossRef]
48. Whisman, M.A.; Beach, S.R. Couple therapy for depression. *J. Clin. Psychol.* **2012**, *68*, 526–535. [CrossRef] [PubMed]
49. Tolmacz, R.; Bachner-Melman, R.; Lev-Ari, L.; Almagor, K. Interparental conflict and relational attitudes within romantic relationships: The mediating role of attachment orientations. *J. Soc. Pers. Relatsh.* **2022**, *39*, 1648–1668. [CrossRef]
50. Ben-Naim, S.; Hirschberger, G.; Ein-Dor, T.; Mikulincer, M. An experimental study of emotion regulation during relationship conflict interactions: The moderating role of attachment orientations. *Emotion* **2013**, *13*, 506–519. [CrossRef] [PubMed]

51. Jakubiak, B.K.; Feeney, B.C. Hand-in-hand combat: Affectionate touch promotes relational well-being and buffers stress during conflict. *Personal. Soc. Psychol. Bull.* **2019**, *45*, 431–446. [CrossRef]
52. Volkema, R.J. Demographic, cultural, and economic predictors of perceived ethicality of negotiation behavior: A nine-country analysis. *J. Bus. Res.* **2004**, *57*, 69–78. [CrossRef]

behavioral sciences

MDPI

Article

Correlations among Psychological Resilience, Cognitive Fusion, and Depressed Emotions in Patients with Depression

Ning Chen [1,2], Juzhe Xi [3,*] and Xiwang Fan [1,*]

1 Clinical Research Center for Mental Disorders, Shanghai Pudong New Area Mental Health Center, School of Medicine, Tongji University, Shanghai 200124, China
2 College of Arts, Humanities and Social Sciences, University of Edinburgh, Edinburgh EH8 9YL, UK
3 Shanghai Key Laboratory of Mental Health and Psychological Crisis Intervention, Affiliated Mental Health Center (ECNU), School of Psychology and Cognitive Science, East China Normal University, Shanghai 200062, China
* Correspondence: jzxi@psy.ecnu.edu.cn (J.X.); fanxiwang2020@163.com (X.F.)

Abstract: *Background:* More than 300 million people worldwide suffer from depression, which is a significant contributor to the global burden of disease. This study investigated the factors influencing psychological resilience and cognitive fusion in patients with depression and the relationships of psychological resilience and cognitive fusion with depression. *Methods:* This study enrolled 172 participants (65.8% of them were female). Psychological resilience, cognitive fusion, and depression were assessed with the psychological resilience scale, the cognitive fusion questionnaire, the Hamilton Anxiety Scale (HAMA), Hamilton Depression Scale (HAMD), and Zung Self-rating Depression Scale (SDS), respectively. Furthermore, the relationships of psychological resilience and cognitive fusion with depression were investigated. *Results:* The psychological resilience and cognitive fusion scores of patients with depression varied significantly among different education levels, and HAMA, HAMD, and SDS scores were significantly negatively correlated with psychological resilience but positively correlated with cognitive fusion. *Conclusions:* Depression levels in patients with depression are closely related to psychological resilience and cognitive fusion. Therefore, anxiety and depression could be alleviated by improving the psychological resilience or reducing the cognitive fusion of patients with depression.

Keywords: psychological resilience; cognitive fusion; depressed emotions; depressive patients; depression; anxiety

1. Introduction

The World Health Organization estimates that more than 300 million people suffer from depression (major depressive disorder) worldwide, making it a significant contributor to the global burden of disease. The global average annual prevalence of depression is approximately 6%, and the lifetime prevalence of depression is 15% to 18% [1,2]. Since the COVID-19 pandemic began, the incidence of depression has more than tripled compared with the historical incidence [3]. The main clinical symptoms of depression are low mood, decreased interest, and unresponsiveness, and it is one of the most common mental disorders [4].

Despite an upsurge in research into depression in recent years, the cause and pathogenesis of depression are still unknown. Researchers generally agree that a combination of biopsychosocial and physiological factors causes depression and that cognition or thinking are also key influences on people's moods [5]. Therefore, the study of cognition [6] or thinking related to negative emotions in patients with depression is necessary to explore the pathogenesis of depression. With the rise of the third generation of cognitive-behavioral therapy represented by acceptance and commitment therapy (ACT), research on the cognitive level has expanded. This perspective focuses on patients' mental flexibility, acknowledges the universality of pain, requires patients to accept rather than resist pain and bad experiences, and emphasizes the role of mindfulness [7].

Cognitive fusion, an important theoretical model of ACT, is an essential factor in the formation and maintenance of many psychological disorders [8,9]. Cognitive fusion indicates that patients interpret their thoughts and emotions as factual and genuine, exacerbating patients' negative psychological emotions [6,10,11]. When patients experience pathological cognitive fusion, their psychological flexibility is reduced, and psychological problems occur. Many studies have confirmed the association of psychological resilience with depression. For example, in an experiment that analyzed the relationship between depression and psychological flexibility in Korean conscripts, researchers found that psychological flexibility had a negative effect on depression, particularly in the dimension of resilience [11]. Therefore, this study investigated whether improving psychological flexibility could reduce depression symptoms in patients with depression.

Research on the relationship between cognitive fusion and mental health has focused on negative affect, psychological distress, anxiety disorders, and depression. For example, it has been reported that cognitive fusion is one of the critical factors contributing to psychological disorders [12]. Scholars have reported similar results about the differences in cognitive fusion between gender and age. Nevertheless, in research related to age and gender differences, some scholars have found negligible associations between psychological flexibility, gender, and age [13]. However, studies on depression have revealed differences in the prevalence and severity of symptoms between males and females with depression, and the gender differences in depression increase with age [14–16]. Therefore, investigating whether gender and age differences exist in the psychological flexibility and cognitive fusion of patients with depression is vital to examine the correlations between depression, psychological flexibility, and cognitive fusion.

The present study used a sample of Chinese patients with depression to develop a psychopathological model exploring the relationship between psychological resilience, cognitive fusion, and depression, providing a theoretical reference for clinicians to develop practical measures to predict depression and alleviate its symptoms.

Hypotheses: (1) Demographic differences exist between cognitive fusion and psychological flexibility scores in the clinical group of depression, age, and gender; (2) Cognitive fusion and psychological flexibility are significantly correlated with depression; (3) Cognitive fusion positively predicts depression levels in patients with depression; (4) Psychological flexibility negatively predicts depression levels in patients with depression.

2. Methods

2.1. Participants

Patients with depression treated in Shanghai Pudong Mental Health Center from March 2020 to March 2022 were selected. A trained senior psychiatrist confirmed the diagnosis of major depression according to the Diagnostic and Statistical Manual of Mental Disorders, Fourth Edition (DSM-IV). The inclusion criteria were as follows: (1) no previous episodes or treatment; (2) age 10–60 years, regardless of gender; (3) Hamilton Depression Scale score (HAMD, 17 items) ≥ 8; (4) Han nationality; (5) dextral; (6) junior high school education or above; (7) willingness to voluntarily participate in the study and sign the informed consent form; and (8) ability to communicate smoothly with the study staff.

The exclusion criteria were as follows: (1) organic psychiatric disorders, schizophrenia, and mood disorders; (2) visual or auditory disorders; and (3) drug or alcohol dependence, pregnancy, or lactation.

In total, 172 participants were recruited; 16 were excluded according to the above criteria, and 156 patients with depression were enrolled after obtaining informed consent. The patients included 50 males and 106 females, with a mean age of approximately 26 years and a mean educational level of high school education.

2.2. Research Tools

Self-compiled Questionnaire of General Situation: The general situation questionnaire included age, sex, and education.

Psychological Resilience Scale (the 14-Item Resilience Scale, RS-14): The Chinese version of the psychological resilience scale developed by Ni Qianyu and Tian Jun (2013) is a 14-item short form of the RS scale with a total score of 14–98. A higher score indicates greater psychological resilience. The Cronbach's α coefficient of the scale is 0.928, showing good reliability and validity.

Cognitive Fusion Questionnaire (CFQ): The Chinese version of the cognitive fusion questionnaire (CFQ) was developed by Zhang Weichen et al. (2004). The Cronbach's α coefficient of the scale is 0.92 and the retargeting validity is 0.67. The questionnaire consists of 13 items and is divided into two sub-questionnaires: the Cognitive Fusion Questionnaire—Fusion (CFQ-F) and the Cognitive Fusion Questionnaire—Defusion (CFQ-D). The CFQ-F contains items 1, 2, 4, 5, 7, 8, 10, 11, and 13, and the CFQ-D contains items 3, 6, 9, and 12. Each item is scored on a 7-point scale: 1 = clearly does not fit; 2 = does not fit; 3 = somewhat does not fit; 4 = in the middle; 5 = somewhat fits; 6 = fits; 7 = clearly fits. Higher CFQ-F scores indicate higher degrees of cognitive integration; CFQ-D is the reverse description of cognitive integration, and higher scores indicate lower degrees of cognitive integration and higher degrees of cognitive dissociation.

Hamilton Anxiety Scale (HAMA): The Hamilton anxiety scale (HAMA), developed in 1960, is used clinically to assess the severity of the participants' anxiety disorders. The scale has 14 items, and each is scored from 0 to 4. The scale contains two factors: somatic anxiety and mental anxiety. A higher total score indicates more serious anxiety (Zimmerman et al., 2020).

Hamilton Depression Scale (HAMD): A 17-item version of the HAMD (Zimmerman et al., 2013) was adopted in this study, which is divided into five factors: anxiety/somatization, weight, cognitive impairment, block, and sleep disorders. Each item is scored from 0 to 4, and a higher score indicates more severe depression.

Self-Rating Depression Scale (SDS): The depression level of patients was assessed by the Zung self-rating depression scale (SDS). A total score $\geq$50 is classified as depression-positive. Higher scores indicate a higher degree of depression. The Cronbach's α coefficient of the scale is 0.885, the content validity is 0.826, and the internal consistency of the scale is good.

2.3. Procedures

A psychiatrist diagnosed the participants according to the DSM-IV diagnostic criteria. An assistant researcher informed the participants and the guardians of the minors about the purpose of the research. After informed consent was obtained, the assistant investigator evaluated the participants according to the HAMD, HAMA, and SDS items and instructed the participants to complete the General Demographics Questionnaire, RS-14, and CFQ to ensure that participants under 18 years of age understood the items.

2.4. Statistical Analysis

Data analysis was conducted using SPSS 26.0 software. The means and standard deviations of the RS-14 and CFQ were calculated; t-test and analysis of variance (ANOVA) were used to compare the scores of the HAMD, HAMA, SDS, CFQ, and RS-14 and its three different dimensions in patients with depression with different demographic characteristics; Pearson product–moment correlation was used to test the correlation between different variables; and cognitive fusion and psychological resilience were considered as independent variables to conduct multiple linear stepwise regression for patients' anxiety and depression levels to explore the prediction extent of psychological resilience and cognitive fusion. A two-tailed p-value of <0.05 was considered statistically significant.

3. Results

3.1. Descriptive Statistics of Variables

We use number 1 for males and number 2 for females, and this study included 50 males and 106 females. The education level of participates was coded as follows: "1" for junior high school and below; "2" for high school or equivalent-educated; "3" for undergraduate degree; and "4" for postgraduate degree or above. The mean values of each variable are shown in Table 1, and most of them maintained at a moderate level.

Table 1. Descriptive statistics of the variables (N = 156).

Variables	Mean	Standard Deviation	Variance
Gender	1.68	0.47	0.22
Age	26.76	10.55	111.28
Education	2.52	0.82	0.68
Toughness	19.28	8.24	67.83
Strength	14.24	4.74	22.48
Optimism	7.36	3.31	10.94
Psychological resilience	40.88	14.87	221.08
Cognitive fusion	47.71	10.59	112.15
HAMA	16.11	6.13	37.57
HAMD	22.67	7.10	50.39
SDS	54.03	10.58	111.86

3.2. Different Variables among Different Demographic Characteristics of Patients with Depression

In Table 2, the one-way ANOVA results showed significant differences in psychological resilience and cognitive fusion scores among patients with depression of different ages. In addition, independent sample *t*-tests revealed that the psychological resilience and cognitive fusion scores of patients with depression did not show significant differences in terms of gender. However, the ANOVA results showed significant differences in psychological resilience ($p < 0.05$) and cognitive fusion ($p < 0.01$) scores among patients with depression with different education levels.

Table 2. Comparison of the scores for psychological resilience and cognitive fusion among patients with depression with different demographic characteristics (scores, x ± s).

Variables	N	*Psychological Resilience*			*Cognitive Fusion*		
		M ± SD	t/F	P	M ± SD	t/F	P
Gender			1.028	0.305		0.044	0.965
Male	50	42.66 ± 14.98			47.76 ± 11.33		
Female	106	47.76 ± 11.33			47.68 ± 10.28		
Age			1.530	0.209		0.117	0.950
20 and below	57	37.32 ± 13.08			49.35 ± 10.09		
20–30	42	40.29 ± 15.56			48.76 ± 9.99		
30–40	37	43.32 ± 15.23			48.57 ± 9.75		
40 and above	20	47.75 ± 15.42			39.20 ± 11.46		
Education			2.981 *	0.033		5.405 **	0.001
Junior High and below	22	41.86 ± 15.13			46.45 ± 10.68		
High school Diploma	42	36.86 ± 12.06			47.88 ± 10.63		
University Diploma	81	42.16 ± 15.29			47.93 ± 10.41		
Master and above	11	44.82 ± 19.47			47.91 ± 12.82		

Note: ** significant correlation at the 1% level (two-tailed); * significant correlation at the 5% level (two-tailed).

3.3. Correlation Analysis Results of Depression, Psychological Resilience, and Cognitive Fusion

Pearson's product–moment correlations were used to calculate the relationship among psychological resilience and its three dimensions: cognitive fusion, anxiety, and depression. The results in Table 3 showed that psychological resilience was negatively correlated with HAMD, HAMA, and SDS ($p < 0.001$); by contrast, cognitive fusion was positively correlated with HAMD, HAMA, and SDS ($p < 0.001$). A significant negative correlation was found between cognitive fusion and psychological resilience ($p < 0.001$).

Table 3. Correlation analysis results of depression, anxiety, cognitive fusion, and psychological resilience and its three dimensions.

Variables	*RS-14*	*CFQ*	*HAMD*	*HAMA*	*SDS*
RS-14	1.000				
CFQ	−0.367 **	1.000			
HAMD	−0.376 **	0.414 **	1.000		
HAMA	−0.306 **	0.361 **	0.729 **	1.000	
SDS	−0.552 **	0.585 **	0.697 **	0.565 **	1.000

Note: RS-14, the 14-Item resilience scale; CFQ, cognitive fusion questionnaire; HAMD, Hamilton depression scale; HAMA, Hamilton anxiety scale; SDS, self-rating depression scale; ** significant correlation at the 1% level (two-tailed).

3.4. Results of Multiple Linear Stepwise Regression Analysis of Psychological Resilience, Cognitive Fusion, Depression, and Anxiety

The normality test was first performed and all satisfied normality. Multiple linear stepwise regression analysis was performed with HAMA, HAMD, and SDS criteria scores of the sample as dependent variables; psychological resilience and cognitive fusion scores as independent variables; and gender, age, and education level as control variables. As the results showed in Table 4, psychological resilience negatively predicted HAMA, HAMD, and SDS, while cognitive fusion positively predicted HAMA, HAMD, and SDS. The coefficient of variance inflation for each regression equation is not greater than 5, indicating that there is no multicollinearity between the independent variables within the regression equation.

Table 4. Results of regression analysis of psychological resilience, cognitive fusion, anxiety, and depression.

Dependent Variables	Predictor Variables	β	t	P	R^2	Adjust R^2
HAMA	*RS-14*	−0.083	−2.525	0.013	0.165	0.154
	CFQ	0.166	3.614	0.000		
HAMD	*RS-14*	−0.124	−3.400	0.001	0.230	0.219
	CFQ	0.214	4.178	0.000		
SDS	*RS-14*	−0.277	−6.18	0.000	0.474	0.467
	CFQ	0.441	7.003	0.000		

4. Discussion

In this study, 172 patients with clinical depression were recruited to study the relationships between psychological resilience, cognitive fusion, and depression. The results showed that different levels of education were influential factors for psychological resilience and cognitive fusion in patients with depression. People with more years of education may be able to judge what is happening more rationally and cope in a reasonable manner. Additionally, no significant differences were observed in cognitive fusion and psychological resilience in patients with depression by gender and age of onset, which is consistent with the findings of previous related studies [17,18]. Interestingly, unlike previous findings, females' average psychological resilience scores were higher than males'.

The results of the cognitive fusion and depression correlation analysis showed that cognitive fusion was significantly and positively associated with depression levels, which is consistent with the findings of Bardeen and Fergus [19]. This suggests that when negative thinking limitations influence emotions, adverse feelings may be further reinforced, leading to increased negative affect and depressive symptoms [20]. This is also largely consistent with the theoretical underpinnings of ACT, where cognitive integration is thought to exacerbate emotional distress when a person is unable to use alternatives flexibly [21,22].

By contrast, a significant negative correlation was observed between psychological resilience and depression levels. This study found that more severe depression levels were associated with lower psychological resilience scores. This may be because some patients have psychological problems such as anxiety, depression, and fear, which affect the adaptation to mental illness and lead to poor psychological resilience [23]. Additionally, the process is cyclically exacerbated, people with low psychological resilience are unable to adapt to stressful events and therefore tend to experience poorer mental health problems, like depression and anxiety [24].

In addition, cognitive fusion and psychological resilience were negatively correlated. Because of pathological cognitive fusion, patients appear to confuse thoughts with reality and dwell on negative thoughts and emotions. When 'fused', a person becomes less sensitive to immediate or genuine consequences and cognitive events begin to dominate behaviour and experience rather than other emotional or behavioral regulation [25]. Under the influence of negative thoughts, patients' self-efficacy decreases and deviates from self-worth, leading to low psychological resilience and psychological disorders. A higher degree of cognitive fusion in patients with depression is associated with lower psychological resilience and a greater likelihood of developing or exacerbating psychological problems.

This study investigated the relationships between cognitive integration, psychological resilience, and depression in patients with depression and found that cognitive integration was positively associated with symptoms of depression. By contrast, psychological resilience had a negative predictive effect on symptoms of depression, providing theoretical guidance for the diagnosis and treatment of depressed patients. However, this study has several limitations: (1) the patients included in this study were all recruited from the same psychiatric center, and thus the diversity of the sample is limited to some extent; (2) this is a cross-sectional and correlational study, which limits the ability to infer causality, and further longitudinal studies should be conducted to replicate and build on the results of this study; (3) the various dimensions of psychological resilience, such as resilience, strength, and optimism, may have different degrees of influence on depression, and this pathological model requires further refinement.

5. Conclusions

In summary, HAMA scores, HAMD scores, and SDS scores were negatively correlated with psychological resilience in this study, suggesting a close relationship between the degree of depression and psychological resilience in patients with depression. Higher levels of anxiety and depression tended to be accompanied by lower psychological resilience and a greater degree of cognitive fusion, exacerbating the level of anxiety or depression. This suggests that clinicians should improve patients' psychological resilience and provide interventions to individuals with high cognitive fusion to avoid negative cognitions, for example, Mindfulness-based Stress Reduction [26] and ACT [27], which reduces cognitive fusion and can help patients to some extent to alleviate symptoms of anxiety and depression. Measures like social support, coping self-efficacy and improving physical health [28] should also be taken to help patients with low education levels improve their psychological resilience, and decrease anxiety and depression.

Author Contributions: Methodology, N.C.; Software, N.C. Formal analysis, N.C.; Investigation, X.F.; Resources, J.X. and X.F.; Data curation, X.F.; Writing—original draft, N.C.; Supervision, J.X.; Funding acquisition, J.X. and X.F. All authors have read and agreed to the published version of the manuscript.

Funding: This study was supported by the Medical Discipline Construction Project of Pudong Health Committee of Shanghai (PWZzb2022-09), the Science and Technology Development Fund of Shanghai Pudong New Area (PKJ2020-Y34), the Research Project of Shanghai Science and Technology Commission (20dz2260300), the Medical Discipline Construction Project of Pudong Health Committee of Shanghai (PWYgy2021-02), the Shanghai Pujiang Program of China (12PJC037), and the National Social Science Foundation of China (18BSH129).

Institutional Review Board Statement: The study was conducted in accordance with the Declaration of Helsinki, and approved by the Institutional Review Board (or Ethics Committee) of Shanghai Pudong New Area Mental Health Center (protocol code: PDJWLL2020028, date of approval: May 2020).

Informed Consent Statement: Informed consent was obtained from all subjects involved in the study.

Data Availability Statement: The raw data supporting the conclusions of this article will be made available by the authors, without undue reservation.

Conflicts of Interest: The authors declare that the research was conducted without any commercial or financial relationships that could be construed as a potential conflict of interest.

References

1. Dwyer, J.B.; Aftab, A.; Radhakrishnan, R.; Widge, A.; Rodriguez, C.I.; Carpenter, L.L.; Nemeroff, C.B.; McDonald, W.M.; Kalin, N.H. Hormonal Treatments for Major Depressive Disorder: State of the Art. *Am. J. Psychiatry* **2020**, *177*, 686–705. [CrossRef] [PubMed]
2. Malhi, G.S.; Mann, J.J. Depression. *Lancet* **2018**, *392*, 2299–2312. [CrossRef] [PubMed]
3. Ettman, C.K.; Abdalla, S.M.; Cohen, G.H.; Sampson, L.; Vivier, P.M.; Galea, S. Prevalence of Depression Symptoms in US Adults Before and During the COVID-19 Pandemic. *JAMA Netw. Open* **2020**, *3*, e2019686. [CrossRef] [PubMed]
4. Wilkerson, A.; Boals, A.; Taylor, D. Sharpening our Understanding of the Consequences of Insomnia: The Relationship Between Insomnia and Everyday Cognitive Failures. *Cogn. Ther. Res.* **2011**, *36*, 134–139. [CrossRef]
5. Sander, J.B.; McCarty, C.A. Youth depression in the family context: Familial risk factors and models of treatment. *Clin. Child. Fam. Psychol. Rev.* **2005**, *8*, 203–219. [CrossRef]
6. Hayes, S.C.; Villatte, M.; Levin, M.; Hildebrandt, M. Open, aware, and active: Contextual approaches as an emerging trend in the behavioral and cognitive therapies. *Annu. Rev. Clin. Psychol.* **2011**, *7*, 141–168. [CrossRef]
7. Dindo, L.; Van Liew, J.R.; Arch, J.J. Acceptance and Commitment Therapy: A Transdiagnostic Behavioral Intervention for Mental Health and Medical Conditions. *Neurotherapeutics* **2017**, *14*, 546–553. [CrossRef]
8. Bohlmeijer, E.T.; Fledderus, M.; Rokx, T.A.; Pieterse, M.E. Efficacy of an early intervention based on acceptance and commitment therapy for adults with depressive symptomatology: Evaluation in a randomized controlled trial. *Behav. Res. Ther.* **2011**, *49*, 62–67. [CrossRef]
9. Afari, N.; Herbert, M.S.; Godfrey, K.M.; Cuneo, J.G.; Salamat, J.S.; Mostoufi, S.; Gasperi, M.; Ober, K.; Backhaus, A.; Rutledge, T.; et al. Acceptance and commitment therapy as an adjunct to the MOVE! programme: A randomized controlled trial. *Obes. Sci. Pract.* **2019**, *5*, 397–407. [CrossRef]
10. Hayes, S.C. Acceptance and Commitment Therapy, Relational Frame Theory, and the Third Wave of Behavioral and Cognitive Therapies—Republished Article. *Behav. Ther.* **2016**, *47*, 869–885. [CrossRef]
11. Lee, D.; Lee, S.J.; Park, C.S.; Kim, B.J.; Lee, C.S.; Cha, B.; Seo, J.Y.; Choi, J.W. The Mediating Effect of Impulsivity on Resilience and Depressive Symptoms In Korean Conscripts. *Psychiatry Investig.* **2019**, *16*, 773–776. [CrossRef]
12. Gholamhoseini, B.; Koolaee, A.K.; Taghvaee, D. The Effectiveness of Acceptance and Commitment Group Therapy on Depression and Body Image in Women with Obesity. *Int. J. Indian Psychol.* **2015**, *2*, 72–79. [CrossRef]
13. Gloster, A.T.; Klotsche, J.; Chaker, S.; Hummel, K.V.; Hoyer, J. Assessing psychological flexibility: What does it add above and beyond existing constructs? *Psychol. Assess.* **2011**, *23*, 970–982. [CrossRef]
14. Kessler, R.C.; McGonagle, K.A.; Swartz, M.; Blazer, D.G.; Nelson, C.B. Sex and depression in the National Comorbidity Survey. I: Lifetime prevalence, chronicity and recurrence. *J. Affect. Disord.* **1993**, *29*, 85–96. [CrossRef]
15. Jang, S.N.; Kawachi, I.; Chang, J.; Boo, K.; Shin, H.G.; Lee, H.; Cho, S.I. Marital status, gender, and depression: Analysis of the baseline survey of the Korean Longitudinal Study of Ageing (KLoSA). *Soc. Sci. Med.* **2009**, *69*, 1608–1615. [CrossRef]
16. Girgus, J.S.; Yang, K.; Ferri, C.V. The Gender Difference in Depression: Are Elderly Women at Greater Risk for Depression Than Elderly Men? *Geriatrics* **2017**, *2*, 35. [CrossRef]
17. Hulbert-Williams, N.J.; Storey, L. Psychological flexibility correlates with patient-reported outcomes independent of clinical or sociodemographic characteristics. *Support Care Cancer* **2016**, *24*, 2513–2521. [CrossRef]
18. Wicksell, R.K.; Renöfält, J.; Olsson, G.L.; Bond, F.W.; Melin, L. Avoidance and cognitive fusion–central components in pain related disability? Development and preliminary validation of the Psychological Inflexibility in Pain Scale (PIPS). *Eur. J. Pain* **2008**, *12*, 491–500. [CrossRef]
19. Bardeen, J.R.; Fergus, T.A. The interactive effect of cognitive fusion and experiential avoidance on anxiety, depression, stress and posttraumatic stress symptoms. *J. Context. Behav. Sci.* **2016**, *5*, 1–6. [CrossRef]
20. McEvoy, P.M.; Salmon, K.; Hyett, M.P.; Jose, P.E.; Gutenbrunner, C.; Bryson, K.; Dewhirst, M. Repetitive Negative Thinking as a Transdiagnostic Predictor of Depression and Anxiety Symptoms in Adolescents. *Assessment* **2019**, *26*, 324–335. [CrossRef]
21. Bond, F.W.; Hayes, S.C.; Barnes-Holmes, D. Psychological flexibility, ACT, and organizational behavior. *J. Organ. Behav. Manag.* **2006**, *26*, 25–54. [CrossRef]

22. Hayes, S.; Kirk, C.; Strosahl, D.; Kelly, G.W. *Acceptance and Commitment Therapy: The Process and Practice of Mindful Change*; Guilford press: New York, NY, USA, 2011.
23. Lau, W.K.W. The role of resilience in depression and anxiety symptoms: A three-wave cross-lagged study. *Stress Health* **2022**, *38*, 804–812. [CrossRef] [PubMed]
24. Poudel-Tandukar, K.; Chandler, G.E.; Jacelon, C.S.; Gautam, B.; Bertone-Johnson, E.R.; Hollon, S.D. Resilience and anxiety or depression among resettled Bhutanese adults in the United States. *Int. J. Soc. Psychiatry* **2019**, *65*, 496–506. [CrossRef] [PubMed]
25. Gillanders, D.T.; Bolderston, H.; Bond, F.W.; Dempster, M.; Flaxman, P.E.; Campbell, L.; Kerr, S.; Tansey, L.; Noel, P.; Ferenbach, C.; et al. The development and initial validation of the cognitive fusion questionnaire. *Behav. Ther.* **2014**, *45*, 83–101. [CrossRef] [PubMed]
26. Kabat-Zinn, J.; Hanh, T.N. *Full Catastrophe Living: Using the Wisdom of Your Body and Mind to Face Stress, Pain, and Illness*; Delta: London, UK, 2009.
27. Hayes, S.C.; Luoma, J.B.; Bond, F.W.; Masuda, A.; Lillis, J. Acceptance and commitment therapy: Model, processes and outcomes. *Behav. Res. Ther.* **2006**, *44*, 1–25. [CrossRef]
28. Southwick, S.M.; Charney, D.S. The science of resilience: Implications for the prevention and treatment of depression. *Science* **2012**, *338*, 79–82. [CrossRef]

behavioral sciences

MDPI

Article

Exploring the Importance of Gender, Family Affluence, Parenting Style and Loneliness in Cyberbullying Victimization and Aggression among Romanian Adolescents

Magdalena Iorga [1,2], Lavinia Maria Pop [2], Irina Croitoru [3,*], Elena Hanganu [4,*] and Dana-Teodora Anton-Păduraru [4]

1 Behavioral Sciences Department, "Grigore T. Popa" University of Medicine and Pharmacy, 700115 Iasi, Romania
2 Faculty of Psychology and Education Sciences, "Alexandru Ioan Cuza" University of Iasi, 700554 Iasi, Romania
3 Preventive Medicine and Interdisciplinarity Department, "Grigore T. Popa" University of Medicine and Pharmacy, 700115 Iasi, Romania
4 Pediatric Department, "Grigore T. Popa" University of Medicine and Pharmacy, 700115 Iasi, Romania
* Correspondence: irina.croitoru@umfiasi.ro (I.C.); hanganu.elena1@umfiasi.ro (E.H.)

Abstract: The increasing phenomenon of cyberbullying among adolescents needs parental, educational, and social intervention. The study aimed to identify the prevalence of cyberbullying among Romanian adolescents and the importance of gender, family-related factors, self-esteem, and parental styles in both victims and perpetrators. A total of 835 adolescents aged 10–19 years were included in the research. An online questionnaire was specially constructed for this research, gathering socio-demographic and family-related data along with information about cyberbullying as a victim, aggressor, or bystander, and strategies used in order to deal with it. Four psychological scales were used to evaluate self-esteem, loneliness, cybervictimization/cyberaggression, and parental style. (3) Results showed that the most common age for a personal smartphone is M = 10.24 ± 2.43. The main reasons why students use these networks are primarily chatting and fun and less for academic tasks. During the week, adolescents spend 5.53 ± 2.75 h on social media, while during weekends, the duration of smartphone usage almost doubles. Girls are the most common victims of cyberbullying, and less than three-quarters of students believe that aggressors can be both girls and boys, and only a quarter of them have reported an incident. Family affluence, the relationship with parents and classmates, the presence of loneliness and sociodemographic factors were found to be in a strong relationship with the presence of aggression and/or victimization among adolescents. Cyberaggression was found to be positively correlated with the aggressive parental style and negatively correlated with the compassionate and avoidant parental styles. Results are crucial for identifying cyberbullying actors and preventing the negative effects of cyberbullying on psychological, social, and academic life for students, parents, and teachers.

Keywords: cyberbullying; adolescent; loneliness; victim; perpetrator; bystander; self-esteem; parental style; family affluence; cyberaggression; cybervictimization; school

1. Introduction

The rapid advances in Information and Communication Technologies (ICT) have changed the way people interact and communicate with each other, contributing to an extremely high amount of transmitted content, the speedy exchange of ideas, a large quantity of information, and connecting people from all over the world. The positive aspects of using technologies in daily communication caused negative consequences that cannot be ignored: the rapid spread of fake information, increased time using social networks, promotion of a false image, easy way to practice aggressive behaviors and difficulties determining the identity of the sender.

Data provided by UNICEF showed that almost 98% of the population use smartphones in their daily lives [1]. One in three internet users globally is a child and usually owns a smartphone at the age of 10. The number of hours spent on the internet increases with age, along with all the associated risks. In the last decade, scientific literature continuously provided a lot of information about the consequences of the increasing use of the internet among children and young people. The more frequent use of mobile phones or the internet was associated with depression [2], self-isolation [3], anxiety [4], poor body image [5,6], and aggressive behaviors [7].

Cyberbullying (CB) has been defined as aggressive and deliberate behavior that is frequently repeated over time, carried out by a group or an individual using electronics and aimed at a victim who cannot defend himself/herself [8]. Patchin and Hinduja defined cyberbullying as being more frequent than traditional bullying and described it as deliberate and repeated harm done with technology [9,10]. Unlike adults, who can act when they are bullied online, children do not have the necessary tools to report or defend themselves. The Social Defeat Model showed that the loser of a fight among animals of the same species may show such signs as increased sleep, lowered testosterone, and less exploratory behavior [11]. In the case of young people, cyberbullying can be followed by poor academic results, absenteeism, and self and auto-aggression. Because bullying and cyberbullying are repetitive behaviors, dealing with these problems needs the presence of an adult who must act (parent, teacher, school principal, etc.). If the adult does not interfere, the victim will try to solve the problem by herself/himself, the most frequent behavior being an offensive one in order to discourage the aggressor. In its turn, the victim will become an aggressor. That is why cyberbullying has become a systemic public health issue [11,12] with a great impact on the physical, psychological, and social health of all those involved.

Recent studies have revealed an alarming increase in internet use and cyberbullying among adolescents in developed countries [13,14]. Victims and bystanders of bullying experience anxiety, poor self-esteem [15], and depressive symptoms [16] as well as frequent somatic complaints [17] suicides [18,19] and homicides [20]. Being bullied at school may be a contributing factor to the development of all mentioned consequences in adulthood. The cyberbullying experienced in adolescence is a predictor of bullying behaviors in social relations and professional lives as adults [21].

If traditional bullying develops in real settings with a real aggressor and with real witnesses, in cyberbullying, the known or unknown aggressor can follow the victim everywhere, every time, and the number of witnesses can be considerably high. That is why the consequences of cyberbullying are more severe than in the case of traditional bullying, one of the most important being self-aggressive behaviors. For example, suicide attempts were found to be a great risk in cyberbullying experiences among adolescents. A study conducted by Campisi et al., in 2019, among adolescents from ninety countries revealed that significant indicators associated with suicidal ideation or attempt included being bullied, having no close friends, being in a physical fight, and/or having had a serious injury [11].

The "EU Kids Online" study of over 25,000 children between the ages of 9 and 16 reported a prevalence of cybervictimization ranging between 2 and 14%. The highest rates were found in Estonia and Romania, and the lowest in Italy and Portugal [22]. In 2018, a study conducted by Athanasiou et al. [23] among 14–17-year-old adolescents across seven European countries, showed that the highest rate of cyber victimization was found in Romania (37.3%), and the lowest in Spain (13.3%). A previous study conducted by Grigore & Maftei [2] on 501 middle adolescents aged 12 to 15 years showed no significant associations between the participants' status, gender, or age, but participants with higher levels of state anxiety and depression were more likely to be victims. In another study, Cucos et al. [24] identified significant negative associations between intercultural sensitivity and cyber-perpetration, cybervictimization, and cyber-bystander behavior among 241 high school students, while Turliuc et al. [25] identified the relationship between cyberaggression and depressive symptoms in research including 310 adolescents.

Data about cyberbullying as an increasing phenomenon in Romania is scarce. The aim of the present research was to identify the prevalence of cybervictimization and cyber-aggression among adolescents, and to highlight the relationships between gender, family affluence, parenting styles, and loneliness. The World Health Organization defines an adolescent as a person aged 10–19, so, for the present study, only this category was considered.

2. Materials and Methods

2.1. Study Design and Study Population

The study was carried out within the project TECPC—Together Everyone Can Prevent Cyberbullying (2020-1-RO01-KA226-SCH-095269), in the framework of the Erasmus+ Programme—KA2 Strategic Partnerships Digital Education Readiness.

The study is a cross-sectional, school-based survey conducted between May-June 2022. Data collection was performed using a snowball sampling methodology focusing on the general student population from different departments from North-Eastern Romania, in rural and urban areas. Schools were informed about the objectives of the research and the questionnaires were delivered after the approval of the principals was obtained. The questionnaire was distributed online. Target participants were adolescents from secondary/gymnasium and high schools/colleges (in Romania, the mentioned study levels include students aged 10–14 and 15–19 years old). Participants were informed about the purpose of the study and the confidentiality of data, and they were informed that they could withdraw from the study whenever they wanted, without consequences. No incentives were given to participants.

The inclusion criteria were questionnaires filled in by children enrolled in private or public school, aged 10–19 years old, submitting fully filled in questionnaires. The criteria for excluding questionnaires from the research were questionnaires not fully completed and questionnaires submitted after the deadline. A total of 835 questionnaires were finally included in the research.

2.2. Study Instruments

The questionnaire was constructed using the Google Forms application (Alphabet, Mountain View, CA, USA) and was developed in order to address the prevention, recognition, and intervention of online harassment among adolescents.

The questionnaire was built following solid research of specialized literature on cyberbullying as well as discussions with teachers, school principals and students of various ages.

(a) The first part of the questionnaire gathered socio-demographic information (like age, gender, level of education of children and their parents, home environment, school environment, and members of the household). Data about family income was measured using the *Family Affluence Scale* (FAS) which was developed first in Scotland as a measure of family affluence. It was proved that, at a young age, children did not have accurate information on their family's finances, and adolescents too were not informed about the family income. Therefore, this evaluation was found to be a less intrusive and more comprehensible approach that had to be applied in order to evaluate socioeconomic status among children and teenagers [26]. The Family Affluence Scale (FAS), a four-item measure of family wealth, was developed in the WHO Health Behaviour in School-aged Children Study as an alternative measure, and in 2001–2002 the scale was composed of four items:

    1. Does your family own a car, van or truck? (No [0]; Yes, one [1]; Yes, two or more),
    2. Do you have your own bedroom for yourself? (No [0]; Yes [1]),
    3. During the past 12 months, how many times did you travel away on holiday with your family? (Not at all [0]; Once [1]; Twice [2]; More than twice [3]),
    4. How many computers do your family own? (None [0]; One [1]; Two [2]; More than two [3]).

(b) The second part includes questions about children's satisfaction with the relationships with parents, classmates, colleagues from school, friends, and teachers. Self-assessed items were constructed, and responses were assessed on a 5-point Likert scale. Other questions in this section include items about grades obtained in the previous year, as well as the relationship between mother and father from the children's perspective, children's relationships with parents, the main decision-maker in the family, self-assessment of social position (leader, popular, or lonely person), positioning in the school learning situation compared to classmates, number of best friends, and number of children in the class.

(c) The third part targeted bullying and cyberbullying behaviors, and included items that refer to children's views on the gender of people who are most often abusers or abuse others (boys or girls); if they have ever been an online abuser or a victim of physical or online bullying; if they have colleagues who terrorize others; if they have seen colleagues who are terrorized physically or online; and if they have reported the incident in those cases.

(d) The fourth part of the survey collected information about the use of mobile phones and the internet; the main reason for using the internet; the time spent on average on a usual working day and on a weekend day on the internet; the age at which children received their first phone call; how often they socialize with people they know on the internet; as well as their parents' behavior towards them regarding excessive phone use (blaming, insulting, restricting access).

(e) The final part of the questionnaire addressed several standardized scales, presented above:

- *Rosenberg self-esteem scale* consists of 10 items and it is a self-report instrument for evaluating individual self-esteem (Rosenberg, 1965). RSES is scored using four response choices, ranging from strongly agree to strongly disagree [27].
- *UCLA Loneliness scale* (ULS-8) contains the 20 items selected from the third revised version UCLA Loneliness Scale of Russell et al., in 1980. This instrument is scored on a 4-point Likert scale with values ranging from 1 (never) to 4 (always). The UCLA is a commonly used tool developed to measure one's subjective feelings of loneliness as well as feelings of social isolation [28].
- *The Cyber-aggression Scale* (CYB-AGS) constructed by Buelga & Pon in 2012 comprised 18 items rated on a 5-point Likert-type scale ranging from 1 (never) to 5 (always). These items measure the adolescent's experience as a cyberbullying perpetrator (directly or indirectly) in the past 12 months [29].
- *The Cyber victimization Questionnaire* (CYVIC) is a self-report instrument composed of 19 items, each one of which presents an aggression suffered through mobile phone or the Internet constructed by Álvarez-García et al. in 2017. The students should mark the frequency with which they were the victim of each one of these situations in the past three months, on a 4-point Likert-type scale [30].
- *The Parenting Styles and Dimensions questionnaire* (PSDQ) constructed by Batool, in 2016 has 40 items and it was designed to measure parenting styles grouping them in six typologies of supportive, controlling, compassionate, aggressive, avoidant, and orthodox [31].

2.3. Statistical Analysis

All analyses for this research were performed using IBM Statistical Package for Social Sciences (SPSS) Statistics for Windows, version 26 (SPSS Inc., Chicago, IL, USA). Results for descriptive statistics were expressed as means and standard deviations (SD).

The normality of data distribution was tested by using the Kolmogorov-Smirnoff test. Given the fact that all data points are not normally distributed, a bivariate analysis will be performed, and non-parametric tests will be applied.

The Mann–Whitney test was performed to assess comparative results considering gender, living environment, level of education, and school environment. The Kruskal–Wallis H test was used to determine if there were statistically significant differences between two groups of an independent variable on a continuous or ordinal dependent variable, considering family affluence, mothers' level of education, and fathers' level of education.

The Spearman correlation was used to test the relationship between variables. A p-value < 0.05 was considered statistically significant.

2.4. Ethical Statement

The study was conducted in accordance with the Declaration of Helsinki and approved by the Institutional Review Board No 192/30.04.2022 of EuroEd School, Iași, Romania.

3. Results

3.1. Socio-Demographic Data, Family Characteristic, Financial Status

Sociodemographic data family-related data, financial status, environmental characteristics, and household-related information were gathered.

The participants were middle school (24.8%, n = 207) and high school (75.2%, n = 628) students, and aged M = 15.84 ± 1.82 (with a minimum of 10 and a maximum of 19 years old).

Most students were female (63.0%, n = 526) and more than half of them came from rural areas (58.3%, n = 487). However, the majority stated that their school is in a city (92.6%, n = 773), and more than half of the participants stated that their school was not in the same locality as their home (52.2%, n = 436).

Children and adolescents were asked if they had at least one parent working abroad, and we identified that 1/4 of students had at least one parent working in another country (n = 205, 24.5%). Most students lived with both parents (72.6%, n = 606), few lived with only one parent—mother (13.2%, n = 110) or father (3.5%, n = 29), with grandparents and/or other relatives (10.8%, n = 90), and 18.3% (n = 153) had parents that were not living together.

In terms of parents' level of education, the analysis of responses revealed that almost half of mothers and fathers graduated high school, and a quarter of them had a higher level of education. The study also collected data about the number of children in the family. The analysis of the data showed that 18.0% (n = 150) were only children, 50.5% (n = 422) had a brother or a sister, 17.8% (n = 149) had two siblings, and 13.7% (n = 114) stated that they had more than 3 brothers or sisters. The number of children in the family was M = 2.33 ± 1.04. More details about the parents' level of education and the number of children in the family are presented in Table 1.

Table 1. Family-related data—parents' level of education [1].

Variables	M ± S.D and % *
Mothers' educational level	
Primary school	9 (1.1%)
Secondary school	106 (12.7%)
High school	404 (48.4%)
University	245 (29.3%)
I do not know	71 (8.5%)
Fathers' educational level	
Primary school	9 (1.1%)
Secondary school	98 (11.7%)
High school	426 (51.0%)
University	205 (24.6%)
I do not know	97 (11.6%)

* [1] Means and standard deviations (M ± D), frequency and percentages (%).

Family financial status was measured using a 4-item scale, the *Family Affluence Scale (FAS)*. A composite FAS score was calculated for each student based on the answers to these four items. Thus, the total scores varied between 0 points—which indicates low affluence (2.6%, n = 22), and 9 points (7.2%, n = 60)—which indicates high affluence. Scores between 3 and 5 points indicate medium affluence (37.2%, n = 310), the results showing that approximately half of the participants (49.2%, n = 411) had high family affluence. The average score was M = 5.30 ± 2.33.

3.2. Relationship with Family, Friends and Colleagues

Most students considered that the relationship between their parents was collaborative (n = 677, 81.1%) and a small number of participants declared that this relationship was conflictual (n = 62, 7.4%) or that there was no relationship between their parents (n = 96, 11.5%). Similarly, more than half of the participants considered that their parents had a normal relationship (68.6%, n = 573), but there were also cases in which disputes still occurred—sometimes (14.4%, n = 120) or quite frequently (4.7%, n = 39)—or even cases in which the parents had no relationship and did not talk to each other (12.3%, n = 103)

Students were also asked how they appreciated the relationship between their parents. On a scale of 1 (very dissatisfied) to 5 (very satisfied), about half of the students said that they were very satisfied with the relationship between their parents (48.9%, n = 408), while the rest evaluated it as being very unsatisfactory (2.5%, n = 21), unsatisfactory (6.3%, n = 53), neither satisfactory nor unsatisfactory (18.0%, n = 150) to satisfactory (24.3%, n = 203).

More than half of the children declared that there was not a single family member who made decisions, but that there was a shared decision between the members of the family (64.7%, n = 540).

The relationship between children and parents was considered to be quite peaceful usually, more than half of the students stated that their mothers (67.3%, n = 562) and fathers (68.5%, n = 572) did not offend them and never shouted at them, and the cases in which mothers (0.4%, n = 3) or fathers (0.6%, n = 5) always screamed at children were quite scarce.

Students were asked to express their satisfaction with their relationship with different categories of people on a scale of 1 (very dissatisfied) to 5 (very satisfied). In general, students were most satisfied with their relationships with friends and parents. Students stated that they had between none (7.8%, n = 65) and more than five best friends (12.7%, n = 106), with an average of M = 2.36 ± 0.80. Regarding the number of children in the class, the students stated an average of M = 27.88 ± 3.67. More self-rated items are described in Table 2.

Table 2. Self-rated items regarding satisfaction with relationship with different categories of people [1].

On a Scale of 1 to 5, How Satisfied Are You with the Relationship with	1	2	3	4	5	M ± SD
your parents	21 (2.5)	53 (6.3)	150 (18.0)	203 (24.3)	408 (48.9)	4.10 ± 1.06
your friends	7 (0.8)	35 (4.2)	91 (10.9)	327 (39.2)	375 (44.9)	4.23 ± 0.86
your classmates	31 (3.7)	77 (9.2)	247 (29.6)	294 (35.2)	186 (22.3)	3.63 ± 1.04
other students in the school	85 (10.2)	435 (52.1)	263 (31.5)	33 (4.0)	19 (2.3)	2.36 ± 0.80
teachers	34 (4.1)	78 (9.3)	253 (30.3)	300 (35.9)	170 (20.4)	3.59 ± 1.03

[1] Number of answers (N) and percentage (%), means and standard deviations (M ± SD).

3.3. Self-Evaluation of the Academic Results and Self-Positioning within the Group

On a Likert-like scale from 1 (very unsatisfied) to 5 (very satisfied), the analysis of answers showed that 1/3 of students were either satisfied with their grades (36.2%, n = 302) or indifferent (30.3%, n = 253), the average being M = 3.59 ± 1.01. In addition, more than half of the students reported achieving medium learning results compared to their classmates (59.0%, N = 493).

Additionally, using the same scale, students were asked to mention their degree of agreement/disagreement that they could be a popular person, a group leader, or, conversely, a lonely person. Thus, the results showed that students evaluated themselves as being more solitary than popular people, and fewer considered themselves to be leaders of their group. Detailed results are presented in Table 3.

Table 3. Self-rated items regarding agreement with different items [1].

Items: On a Scale of 1 to 5, I Consider That I Am A.	1	2	3	4	5	M ± SD
popular person	127 (15.2)	211 (25.3)	381 (45.6)	95 (11.4)	21 (2.5)	2.60 ± 0.96
solitaire person	62 (7.4)	99 (11.9)	303 (36.3)	314 (37.6)	57 (6.8)	3.24 ± 1.00
leader in my group	154 (18.4)	255 (30.5)	325 (38.9)	75 (9.0)	26 (3.1)	2.47 ± 0.99

[1] Number of answers (N) and percentage (%), means and standard deviations (M ± SD).

3.4. Use of Internet and Mobile Phones

The results indicated that the average age at which children had their first personal phone is M = 10.24 ± 2.43. The Mann–Whitney test (U = 70,413.00, Z = −4.203, p = 0.001) revealed that there was a significant difference at this item when considering the living environment, with children living in a city (Mdn = 10.00) receiving the first smartphone at a younger age than children living in a village (Mdn = 11).

The main reasons why students used these networks were primarily chatting (55.1%, n = 460) and for fun (35.7%, n = 298), and less so for help in solving academic tasks (9.2%, n = 77). On average, students spent 5.53 ± 2.75 h on social media during the week, while at the weekends they spent, on average, 10.82 ± 9.56.

On a scale from 1 (never) to 5 (often), students were asked how often they talked on the internet with people they knew. More than half of the students spoke at least once to an unknown person, with only 15% (n = 125) of the students being those who never spoke to someone unknown. The results indicate an average of M = 2.96 ± 1.26. However, most students (87.5%, n = 731) had blocked someone on social media at least once.

Moreover, students were asked if their parents blamed them for using their phones too much. More than half of the students admitted that their parents did this sometimes (60.2%, n = 503), while others stated that their parents never blamed their children (17.5%, n = 146) or, on the contrary, did it frequently (13.2%, n = 110), or all the time (9.1%, n = 76). However, most parents did not take action because their children spent too much time on the phone, with 73.1% (n = 610) never restricting access to the phone, and 23.0% (n = 192) doing so only occasionally.

3.5. Bullying and Cyberbullying Behaviors

Three-quarters of the students in the study (72.9%, n = 609) stated that they did not have classmates who cyberbullied others. Furthermore, in about three-quarters of the cases, students considered that girls were the most common victims of cyberbullying (73.2%, n = 611). In addition, less than three-quarters of the students (71.1%, n = 594) believed that aggressors could be both girls and boys alike.

Most students said they had never been victims of cyberbullying (81.2%, n = 678), and that they had never cyberbullied other children (86.7%, n = 724).

In terms of reporting an online bullying incident in the classroom or school, less than half of the students (38.3% n = 320) stated that they had not seen other children being bullied online in the classroom or school, and 42.0% of children did not report any incidents of a kid being bullied online (messages, social media, chatrooms) because they had not seen any messages. Detailed results are presented in Table 4.

Table 4. Reporting a cyberbullying behaviour [1].

Have You Ever Report to an Adult When You Saw a Kid Being Bullied Online (Messages, Social Media, Chatrooms, etc.)?	5.98 ± 2.62
Yes, to my parent	121 (14.5%)
Yes, to the kid's parent	32 (3.8%)
Yes, to a teacher	61 (7.3%)
Yes, to the school psychologist	6 (0.7%)
Yes, to the principal	2 (0.2%)
To other adult	44 (5.3%)
No, I did not report any incident	218 (26.1%)
I did not report ay incident because I did not see any	351 (42.0%)

[1] Means and standard deviations (M ± D), frequency and percentages (%).

3.6. Global Self-Esteem, Loneliness, Cyberbaggression, Cybervictimization and Parental Style Scales

- *Global self-esteem*

Global self-esteem scores as measured with the Rosenberg self-esteem scale (RSES) ranged from 17 up to 30 (M = 24.02 ± 1.81). Most students had a normal self-esteem (82.4%, n = 688). For the present study, Cronbach Alpha score was 0.816.

- *Loneliness*

The total score for Loneliness scale was on average M = 38.98 ± 9.88, scores ranging from 20 (0.4%, n = 3) to 71 (0.1%, n = 1). More than half of the students (54.9%, n = 458) had a moderate level of loneliness and more than a quarter had a high level of loneliness (33.3%, n = 278). Cronbach's alpha of 0.882 showed that the scale had a high level of internal consistency.

- *Cyberaggression*

The Cronbach Alpha score for Cyber-aggression was 0.911 for the total scale. For subscales, we obtained the following results: *Indirect Cyber Aggression*—M = 10.28 ± 3.65, Cronbach Alpha = 0.830, and *Direct Cyber Aggression*—M = 10.90 ± 3.02, Cronbach Alpha = 0.901.

The results proved that the respondents did not have such a high level of cyber aggression. The total CYB-AGS score was on average M = 21.18 ± 6.19, with scores ranging from 18 (40.7%, n = 340) to 71 (0.1%, n = 1).

- *Cybervictimization*

The total score for Cyber victimization was on average M = 19.84 ± 4.99, with scores ranging from 15 (12.5%, n = 104) to 47 (0.1%, n = 1). The scale had a high level of internal consistency, as determined by a Cronbach's alpha of 0.879 for the total scale.

- *Parental style*

The total score for the PSDQ scale was M = 119.19 ± 17.43, scores ranging from 39 (0.1%, n = 1) to 190 (0.2%, n = 2). The Cronbach Alpha score was 0.841.

3.7. Loneliness and School Environment

Important comparative results were identified on the Loneliness scale, in terms of the environment in which the students' schools were located (U = 19,090.50, Z = −2.668, p = 0.008), in the sense that students whose school was located in rural areas had a higher score on the loneliness scale (Mdn = 40.50), as opposed to students studying in the city (Mdn = 37.00). Participants were asked if they had classmates who assaulted other children. Thus, significant differences were identified between this variable and the Loneliness scale (U = 59,366.50, Z = −3.053, p = 0.002), in the sense that those who had aggressors among their classmates obtained a higher score on the Loneliness scale (Mdn = 40.00), compared to those who did not have such classmates (Mdn = 37.00).

Significant differences were also found on the loneliness scale in terms of family affluence (U = 15,173.50, Z = −5.762, p = 0.001), with students with a low family affluence score having a higher loneliness score (Mdn = 45.00) than those with a high family affluence score (Mdn = 35.00).

3.8. Cyberbaggression and Cybervictimization in School Environment

There are significant differences on this scale in terms of the school environment (U = 19,991.50, Z = −2.185, p = 0.029) in the sense that children studying in a city had a lower score on cyber victimization (Mdn = 18.00) compared to children studying in a village (Mdn = 19.00).

The Mann–Whitney test (U = 1632.50, Z = −3.894, p = 0.001) revealed that there were significant differences on the CYVIC scale in terms of participants' satisfaction with the relationship with their classmates, with children who were very satisfied with the relationship with their classmates having a lower score on this scale (Mdn = 17.50) compared to children who were very dissatisfied with the relationship with their colleagues having a higher score on this scale (Mdn = 20.00). Moreover, similar results were identified on the cyber victimization scale and the relationship with parents (U = 2340.50, Z = −3.536, p < 0.001) and teachers (U = 1947.00, Z = −3.026, p = 0.002), which means that students who had a very good relationship with parents (Mdn = 18.00) and teachers (Mdn = 17.00) had lower scores on this scale compared to those who were very dissatisfied with the relationship with parents (Mdn = 21.00), versus teachers (Mdn = 20.50).

Significant differences were identified regarding the variable which asked students if they had classmates who bullied other children and the cyber aggression scale (U = 51,515.50, Z = −5.804, p < 0.001), in the sense that those who had classmates that bullied others had a higher score on the cyber aggression scale (Mdn = 20.00) compared to those who did not have such classmates (Mdn = 19.00).

A Mann–Whitney test (U = 53,452.00, Z = −7.904, p = 0.001) revealed that there were significant differences on the CYB-AGS scale in terms of participants' responses when confronted with bullying behavior, with children who had seen bullying behavior scoring higher on the cyber aggression scale (Mdn = 20.00) than children who had not seen bullying behavior, who scored lower (Mdn = 18.00). Additionally, the comparative analysis (U = 44,705.50, Z = −10.305, p < 0.001) showed that children who had seen other kids being bullied had a higher score on the cyber victimization scale (Mdn = 19.00) than children who had not seen such behaviors (Mdn = 17.00). Moreover, the comparative analysis showed a significant difference in terms of reporting bullying events to an adult and the cyber aggression scale (U = 28,788.00, Z = −2.408, p = 0.016) in the sense that students who reported these events had a lower score on CYB scales (Mdn = 19.00) compared to those who did not report bullying behaviors (Mdn = 20.00).

3.9. Victim and Aggressor Roles—A Vicious Cercle

The results showed that there was a negative correlation between the CYB-AGS and children's satisfaction with their relationship with their friends (r = −0.125 **, p < 0.001), in the sense that the more dissatisfied the children were with this relationship, the more likely they were to become cyber aggressors.

A strong positive correlation was identified between the total score of CYB-AGS and the item that refers to the frequency with which children were victims of cyberbullying. Thus, the results (r = 0.486 **, p < 0.001) showed that the more often it happened that children were the victims of cyberbullying, the higher the score on the CYB-AGS scale.

The relationship between parents (r = 0.143 **, p < 0.001) and the frequency with which children happened to be victims of cyberbullying (r = 0.301 **, p < 0.001) were positively correlated with the scores obtained on the CYVIC scale, in the sense that the more conflictive the parents' relationship was and the more often the children were terrorized online, the greater the aggression suffered by children through the Internet.

Family affluence is negatively correlated with the CYVIC scale ($r = -0.068$ *, $p = 0.049$) in the sense that the higher the family affluence, the lower the score on the cyber victimization scale.

A negative correlation was also identified between the CYVIC score and students' satisfaction with their relationship with friends ($r = -0.214$ **, $p < 0.001$), meaning that the less satisfied they were with their friends' relationship, the more likely they were to become victims of cyberbullying.

A positive correlation was also identified between the responses to the item on how often children bullied others while online and the CYVIC scales ($r = 0.301$ **, $p < 0.001$), in the sense that the higher the level of cyber aggression was, the higher the scores of children on this scale.

The analysis of data showed that the higher the level of loneliness, the higher the scores on these subscales related to cyber aggression, direct or indirect, impersonation, online exclusion, visual-sexual, and written-verbal cyber victimization.

The study found that some of the parenting styles were negatively correlated with the results obtained in these subscales, which means that different types of parents predisposed children to obtain higher overall scores of cyber aggression and cyber victimization. Details regarding these significant correlations are presented in Table 5.

Table 5. Correlational results of CYB-AGS and CYVIC subscales.

Items	ICYB-AGS	DCYB-AGS	Impersonation	Visual-Sexual	Written Verbal	Online Exclusion
Have you ever been bullied online?	$r = 0.405$ ** $p = 0.000$	$r = 0.307$ *, $p = 0.000$	$r = 0.138$ ** $p = 0.000$	$r = 0.241$ ** $p = 0.000$	$r = 0.284$ ** $p = 0.000$	$r = 0.141$ ** $p = 0.000$
Have you ever bullied others while online?	$r = 0.373$ ** $p = 0.000$	$r = 0.304$ ** $p = 0.000$	$r = 0.089$ ** $p = 0.010$	$r = 0.180$ ** $p = 0.000$	$r = 0.227$ ** $p = 0.000$	$r = 0.138$ ** $p = 0.000$
UCLA scale	$r = 0.170$ ** $p = 0.000$	$r = 0.180$ ** $p = 0.000$	$r = 0.185$ ** $p = 0.000$	$r = 0.234$ ** $p = 0.000$	$r = 0.294$ ** $p = 0.000$	$r = 0.453$ ** $p =0.000$
PSDQ scale	no correlation	no correlation	no correlation	no correlation	$r = -0.069$ * $p = 0.046$	$r = -0.102$ ** $p = 0.003$

* $p < 0.05$; ** $p < 0.001$.

3.10. The Influence of the Parenting Styles

The Mann–Whitney test ($U = 56{,}161.50$, $Z = -2.937$, $p = 0.003$) revealed that there were significant differences in the PSDQ scale between children's educational levels, with middle school students scoring higher (Mdn = 120.00) than high school students.

The Mann–Whitney test ($U = 848.00$, $Z = -6.203$, $p = 0.001$) showed that there were significant differences on the PSDQ scale in terms of participants' satisfaction with the relationship with their parents, with children who were very satisfied with the relationship with their parents having a higher score at this scale (Mdn = 125.00) compared to children who were very dissatisfied with the relationship with their parents having a lower score at this scale (Mdn = 100.00).

A significant difference in terms of reporting bullying events to an adult and the PSDQ scale was revealed ($U = 28{,}561.50$, $Z = -2{,}495$, $p = 0.013$) in the sense that students who reported those events had a higher score on the PSDQ scale (Mdn = 123.00), compared to those who did not report bullying behaviors (Mdn = 118.00).

The analysis of the data showed that the mother's level of education was positively correlated only with supportive parenting styles, in the sense that the higher the mother's level of education, the more likely they were to become a supportive parent. In contrast, the relationship between parents evaluated from the children's perspective was negatively correlated with almost all parenting styles, while family affluence was negatively correlated only with aggressive parenting styles and positively correlated with supportive, compassionate, avoidant, and controlling parenting styles.

In addition, the results showed that supportive parenting styles were negatively correlated with cyber victimization scores in the sense that the better the parents fitted into this parenting style, the lower the level of cyber victimization.

The scores on the cyber aggression scale were positively correlated with the aggressive parental style and negatively correlated with the compassionate and avoidant parental styles, in the sense that the better the parents fitted into the aggressive parenting typology, the higher the level of cyber aggression. The better the parents fitted into the compassionate and avoidant parenting styles, the lower the level of cyber aggression. Details are presented in Table 6.

Table 6. Correlational results of PSDQ subscales and aggression and victimization scores *.

Items	Supportive Parents	Controlling Parents	Compassionate Parents	Aggressive Parents	Avoidant Parents	Orthodox Parents
CYB-AGS score	no correlation	no correlation	r = −0.082 * p = 0.017	r = 0.170 *, p = 0.000	r = −0.168 ** p = 0.000	no correlation
CYVIC scores	r = −0.095 ** p = 0.006	no correlation	r = −0.151 ** p = 0.000	r = 0.172 ** p = 0.000	r = −0.230 ** p = 0.000	no correlation

* $p < 0.05$; ** $p < 0.001$.

4. Discussion

The study included respondents aged 10–19, enrolled in private and public schools, from both rural and urban areas. The analysis of data showed that a quarter of the students had at least one parent working abroad.

The analysis of the answers showed that students owned a personal smartphone around the age of 10, and students living in urban areas usually had a phone at a younger age compared to respondents from rural areas. The primary reasons for using smartphones were chatting and entertainment, rather than academic tasks. During the week, adolescents spent 5.53 ± 2.75 h on social media, while at the weekends, their smartphone usage nearly doubled (10.82 ± 9.56) Almost 90% of subjects said that they blocked people who behaved aggressively online (87.5%).

We identified that students believed that girls were more prone to being victims of cyberbullying than boys, and that the aggressor could be either a girl or a boy. The literature presents different statistics regarding the prevalence of cyberbullying considering gender that seems to be a predictor of cyber-bystanding in some countries but not in others. Girls are significantly more likely than boys to be cyber-bystanders in Australia [32], the Islamic Republic of Iran [33], and Spain [34], and among Jewish adolescents in Israel [19]. However, there is no difference by gender among Arab adolescents in Israel [19] and in the Republic of Korea [35,36].

Most of the subjects considered the relationship between their parents to be collaborative (81.1%). In general, respondents declared that they were more satisfied with the relationship with their parents and friends, and less with teachers and other people in the school. More than half of the students stated that their mothers (67.3%) and fathers (68.5%) did not offend them and never shouted at them.

According to our findings, more than a quarter of the adolescents believed that the most common adults who learned about the incident were their parents, and less than half of them reported the incident to their teachers or principals. A similar percentage stated that they never reported a bullying incident to someone else. Data from the scientific literature showed that students avoided reporting incidents for different reasons: their previous experience proved that they did not receive the expected support; the victim was threatened; or, due to the presence of witnesses who did not interfere, the victim considered that this was a banned problem, accepted by the group. Corroborating the data, a good relationship with the parents made the adolescents more confident, manage their relationships better, and look for support in case of need. Higher rates of cyberbullying were reported among those whose parents' educational level was low or middle compared to high [37], and among families where there was a good relationship between children and parents.

Parental monitoring in relation to cyberbullying was found to be a protective factor for online risks. Regarding the extent of adolescent Internet and SNS use, the study of Haddon et al. [38] showed that higher levels were associated with an increased risk of cybervictimization among adolescents. We identified that the higher the mother's level of education, the more likely they were to become a supportive parent.

Similar results were reported in other studies. For example, lower levels of victimization and aggression in bullying and cyberbullying were found to be linked to the indulgent democratic or normative democratic styles, and higher levels to the authoritarian and strict styles, in a study conducted by Gómez-Ortiz et al. [39]. In a previous investigation, the same team identified that both the use of psychological control and the lack of supervision by parents were risk factors that increased the likelihood of children bullying their peers or being victimized by them [40]. The authors identified that certain parenting styles facilitated the construction of a relaxed family environment by offering affection, open communication, and encouraging minors' autonomy. By creating rules and family discipline, the parents avoid coercive practices such as physical punishment or psychological control that seem to increase the risk of aggression [41].

The literature focusing on cyberbullying is more developed regarding empathy, emotional regulation, and psychological distress in perpetrators, victims, and perpetrator-victims of cyberbullying, and not much information presents the profile of the active or passive bystander. We found that adolescents from urban areas obtained a lower score on cybervictimization. A higher score for cybervictimization was also found in subjects with low satisfaction regarding their relationship with their classmates and parents. Moreover, we found that students who had classmates that bullied others, and those who were witnesses to bullying incidents had a higher score on the cyber aggression scale. Adolescents who reported bullying events obtained a lower score on both CYB scales.

The results showed that adolescents who had aggressors among their classmates obtained a higher score on the Loneliness scale compared to those who did not have such classmates. Additionally, significant differences were identified on the scale of loneliness in terms of family affluence, showing that students whose families had a low family affluence score obtained a higher score. Family affluence was found to be negatively correlated with the CYVIC scale, in the sense that the higher the family affluence, the lower the score on the cyber victimization scale.

Cyberbullying, the "silent killer" [42] is widespread across countries [43] with rates ranged from 14.6% to 52.2% (cybervictimization) and 6.3% to 32% (cyberaggression) conforming to Zhu and his team [12].

Younger children were found to frequently report incidents than older students and studies showed that incidents increase with age, but cyberbullying reports decrease with age. Blomqvist et al. [44] found that adolescents may be less likely to disclose victimization compared to youngest ones because of their need for increased autonomy and the desire to solve the problems by themselves.

As age, gender was found to be an important variable. In many studies, more girls reported being victims of cyberbullying compared to boys, but a lot of studies showed that teenage girls are more frequent users of social networks than boys, facilitating cyber incidents [23,45,46]. Additionally, even if statistics showed that boys spend more time on using the internet, it is important to take into consideration the purpose of the use. Conforming to Cho and Yoo study [47] internet usage amount did not show significant explanatory power for cyberbullying because the effect is related to the purpose of the use. Girls are more prone to use internet for social networking while boys are more users of video games, so they are less exposed to cyberbullying incidents compared to female students. Conforming to Barlet and Coyne [48] age can moderate the relationship. The authors found that girls were more likely to report more incidents during early stages and boys during later stages of adolescence.

Some scholars identified that the relationship between cybervictimization and loneliness is bidirectional [16,18,19,23]. Adolescents with high score of loneliness were found to be less skilled for face-to-face communication and, on the one hand, to be more open to socialize and create relationships in online settings but on the second hand to be more willing to disclose private information such as personal data, photos, home address, phone number, passwords, location, etc increasing the risk of victimization [49–51].

A good relationship with parents and a positive school climate were found to be protective factors [18,51]. Apart from traditional bullying, cyberbullying is transpassing the school environment. because aggression can occur anywhere and anytime. As studies showed, victims usually disclose the incidents to their peers and less to adults, but parents and teachers have an important role in identifying cyberbullying signs. Parents' knowledge and awareness of cyberbullying signs have a significant role in the prevention of digital bullying [52]. Floros and Mylona [53] showed that security practices exercised by parents had a protective role in case of victimization but less in case of perpetration. Additionally, a survey conducted by Kowalski and his team [54] on American parents revealed that 93% of respondents believed that their children do generally good things through the Internet and 65% of them were confident that their children were at no risk while on the Internet. These results showed that the first-line guardians in case of victimizations are not always informed about the risks of online settings [55].

Our study has important implications in the school and family field because it provides insights to orient teachers' interventions and parental education training that could improve relationships with adolescents. Both the school climate (stronger and more confident relationships with teachers and a satisfactory relationship with classmates) and a better relationship with their parents will assure a healthier psychological and social life.

4.1. Strengths and Limitations of the Study

The results of the present study are important, especially because the research on cyberaggression and cybervictimization among Romanian adolescents is not abundant. The characteristics considered for the research are important so the results can be generalizable (both female and male respondents; different years of study; different ages; enrolled in public and private schools; scientific or vocational specializations; and coming from different regions of the country). The results present cyberbullying and cybervictimization in relationship with parental style, FAS [56], and sociodemographic variables, and consider the role of cyberaggression and cyberbullied students.

There are some limitations of the study. The research did not take into consideration psychological and psychiatric troubles, mental and physical deficiencies, or diagnostics of chronic diseases or behavioral-related problems. Previous studies have shown that there is an increased risk of cyberbullying for children with obesity, mental or physical diseases, or chronic illnesses. For example, it was found that children with visual impairment have an 80% higher risk of being victims of bullying [57,58]. Additionally, the study did not ask about their sexual orientation since some researchers showed that this variable could increase the risk of being bullied and cyberbullied. Therefore, considering the comparative results, the present study did not take into consideration cultural issues related to parenting styles that were proven by few researchers to be important when it comes to family rules and authoritarian parenting styles.

4.2. Reflections and Planning

In the case of cyberbullying, the approaches must transcend the school and family and must include community, parental education, health interventions, and other institutional stakeholders (policemen, counselors, psychotherapists, and lawyers) to intervene early, to prevent social marginalization and victimization, to explain the impact of cyberaggression and the social and legal consequences, and to act in cases of need.

Findings from different studies indicated a vulnerability to cyberbullying during early adolescence suggesting that early, preventive, and context-appropriate interventions may be necessary to impact this phenomenon and diminish its consequences. Adolescence represents a tumultuous and vulnerable period of transformation, and sometimes the consequences of cyberbullying transcend to adulthood and could be life-threatening.

5. Conclusions

This research confirms the major role that parenting plays in their children's involvement in bullying and cyberbullying, along with the school environment (relationships with classmates and teachers). Cyberaggression and cybervictimization were found to be related to several factors, and therefore, due to their diverse aspects (personal, familial, educational, social and psychological), the interventional programs and educational training must also be focused on adolescents, teachers and parents. The results of this study are important in order to construct appropriate approaches considering the great impact of cyberaggression and cybervictimization on the quality of life during adulthood.

Author Contributions: Conceptualization, M.I.; methodology, M.I.; formal analysis, M.I. and L.M.P.; investigation, M.I., D.-T.A.-P., I.C. and E.H.; data curation, M.I., D.-T.A.-P., I.C. and E.H.; writing—original draft preparation, M.I. and L.M.P.; writing—review and editing M.I. All authors have read and agreed to the published version of the manuscript.

Funding: This research received no external funding.

Institutional Review Board Statement: The study was conducted in accordance with the Declaration of Helsinki and approved by the Institutional Review Board No 192/30.04.2022 of EuroEd School.

Informed Consent Statement: Informed consent was obtained from all subjects involved in the study.

Data Availability Statement: Data availability upon request on corresponding author.

Acknowledgments: This study is carried out within the project TECPC—Together Everyone Can Prevent Cyberbullying (2020-1-RO01-KA226-SCH-095269), in the framework of the Erasmus+ Programme—KA2 Strategic Partnerships Digital Education Readiness.

Conflicts of Interest: The authors declare no conflict of interest.

References

1. Stoilova, M.; Livingstone, S.; Khazbak, R. *Investigating Risks and Opportunities for Children in a Digital World: A Rapid Review of the Evidence on Children's Internet Use and Outcomes*; Innocenti Discussion Paper 2020-03; UNICEF Office of Research—Innocenti: Florence, Italy, 2021.
2. Grigore, A.-N.; Maftei, A. Exploring the Mediating Roles of State and Trait Anxiety on the Relationship between Middle Adolescents' Cyberbullying and Depression. *Children* **2020**, *7*, 240. [CrossRef] [PubMed]
3. Wright, M.F.; Wachs, S. Self-Isolation and Adolescents' Friendship Quality: Moderation of Technology Use for Friendship Maintenance. *Youth Soc.* **2022**, 0044118X221080484. [CrossRef]
4. Martínez-Monteagudo, M.C.; Delgado, B.; Díaz-Herrero, Á.; García-Fernández, J.M. Relationship between suicidal thinking, anxiety, depression and stress in university students who are victims of cyberbullying. *Psychiatry Res.* **2020**, *286*, 112856. [CrossRef] [PubMed]
5. Malinowska-Cieślik, M.; Dzielska, A.; Oblacińska, A. Psychosocial Determinants of Adolescents' Cyberbullying Involvement—The Role of Body Satisfaction. *Int. J. Environ. Res. Public Health* **2022**, *19*, 1292. [CrossRef] [PubMed]
6. Pop, L.-M.; Iorga, M.; Șipoș, L.-R.; Iurcov, R. Gender Differences in Healthy Lifestyle, Body Consciousness, and the Use of Social Networks among Medical Students. *Medicina* **2021**, *57*, 648. [CrossRef] [PubMed]
7. Graf, D.; Yanagida, T.; Runions, K.; Spiel, C. Why did you do that? Differential types of aggression in offline and in cyberbullying. *Comput. Hum. Behav.* **2022**, *128*, 107107. [CrossRef]
8. Smith, P.K.; Mahdavi, J.; Carvalho, M.; Fisher, S.; Russell, S.; Tippett, N. Cyberbullying: Its nature and impact in secondary school pupils. *J. Child Psychol. Psychiatry* **2008**, *49*, 376–385. [CrossRef]
9. Patchin, J.W.; Hinduja, S. Bullies move beyond the schoolyard: A preliminary look at cyberbullying. *Youth Violence Juv. Justice* **2006**, *4*, 148–169. [CrossRef]
10. Patchin, J.W.; Hinduja, S. Measuring cyberbullying: Implications for research. *Aggress. Violent Behav.* **2015**, *23*, 69–74. [CrossRef]
11. Campisi, S.C.; Carducci, B.; Akseer, N.; Zasowski, C.; Szatmari, P.; Bhutta, Z.A. Suicidal behaviours among adolescents from 90 countries: A pooled analysis of the global school-based student health survey. *BMC Public Health* **2020**, *20*, 1–11. [CrossRef]
12. Zhu, C.; Huang, S.; Evans, R.; Zhang, W. Cyberbullying among adolescents and children: A comprehensive review of the global situation, risk factors, and preventive measures. *Front. Public Health* **2021**, *9*, 634909. [CrossRef] [PubMed]

13. Gámez-Guadix, M.; Almendros, C.; Calvete, E.; De Santisteban, P. Persuasion strategies and sexual solicitations and interactions in online sexual grooming of adolescents: Modeling direct and indirect pathways. *J. Adolesc.* **2018**, *63*, 11–18. [CrossRef] [PubMed]
14. Barón, J.O.; Vasquez, S.B.; Caballero, M.J.C. The influence of school climate and family climate among adolescents victims of cyberbullying. *Comunicar. Media Educ. Res. J.* **2016**, 24.
15. Martínez, J.; Rodríguez-Hidalgo, A.J.; Zych, I. Bullying and Cyberbullying in Adolescents from Disadvantaged Areas: Validation of Questionnaires; Prevalence Rates; and Relationship to Self-Esteem, Empathy and Social Skills. *Int. J. Environ. Res. Public Health* **2020**, *17*, 6199. [CrossRef]
16. Zhong, M.; Huang, X.; Huebner, E.S.; Tian, L. Association between bullying victimization and depressive symptoms in children: The mediating role of self-esteem. *J. Affect. Disord.* **2021**, *294*, 322–328. [CrossRef] [PubMed]
17. Rey, L.; Neto, F.; Extremera, N. Cyberbullying victimization and somatic complaints: A prospective examination of cognitive emotion regulation strategies as mediators. *Int. J. Clin. Health Psychol.* **2020**, *20*, 135–139. [CrossRef] [PubMed]
18. Nguyen, H.T.L.; Nakamura, K.; Seino, K.; Vo, V.T. Relationships among cyberbullying, parental attitudes, self-harm and suicidal behavior among adolescents: Results from a school-based survey in Vietnam. *BMC Public Health* **2020**, *20*, 476–479. [CrossRef]
19. Zaborskis, A.; Ilionsky, G.; Tesler, R.; Heinz, A. The association between cyberbullying, school bullying, and suicidality among adolescents: Findings from the cross-national study HBSC in Israel, Lithuania, and Luxembourg. *Crisis J. Crisis Interv. Suicide Prev.* **2019**, *40*, 100–114. [CrossRef]
20. Perry, R. Civil liability for cyberbullying. *UC Irvine Law Rev.* **2020**, *10*, 1219–1272. [CrossRef]
21. Yurdakul, Y.; Beyazıt, U.; Ayhan, A.B. Individual, Social, and Occupational Effects of Cyberbullying During Adolescence. In *Anthology on Combating Cyber-Aggression and Online Negativity*; University of Ankara: Ankara, Turkey, 2022; pp. 1338–1360.
22. Livingstone, S.; Haddon, L.; Görzig, A.; Ólafsson, K. Risks and safety on the internet: The perspective of European children: Full findings and policy implications from the EU Kids Online survey of 9–16-year-olds and their parents in 25 countries. 2011 European Community Safer Internet Plus Programme and Sonia Livingstone, 2011. Available online: https://www.lse.ac.uk/media-and-communications/research/research-projects/eu-kids-online (accessed on 10 August 2021).
23. Athanasiou, K.; Melegkovits, E.; Andrie, E.K.; Magoulas, C.; Tzavara, C.K.; Richardson, C.; Greydanus, D.; Tsolia, M.; Tsitsika, A.K. Cross-national aspects of cyberbullying victimization among 14–17-year-old adolescents across seven European countries. *BMC Public Health* **2018**, *18*, 800. [CrossRef]
24. Cucoș, C.; Grigore, A.N.; Maftei, A. More intercultural sensitivity, less cyberbullying: The role of religious education among high-school students. *J. Beliefs Values* **2022**, *1*, 4. [CrossRef]
25. Turliuc, M.N.; Măirean, C.; Boca-Zamfir, M. The relation between cyberbullying and depressive symptoms in adolescence. The moderating role of emotion regulation strategies. *Comput. Hum. Behav.* **2020**, *109*, 106341. [CrossRef]
26. Currie, C.E.; Elton, R.A.; Todd, J.; Platt, S. Indicators of socioeconomic status for adolescents: The WHO Health Behaviour in School-aged Children Survey. *Health Educ. Res.* **1997**, *12*, 385–397. [CrossRef] [PubMed]
27. Rosenberg, M. Rosenberg self-esteem scale (RSE). *Accept. Commit. Therapy. Meas. Package* **1965**, *61*, 18.
28. Russell, D.; Peplau, L.A.; Cutrona, C.E. The revised UCLA Loneliness Scale: Concurrent and discriminant validity evidence. *J. Personal. Soc. Psychol.* **1980**, *39*, 472–480. [CrossRef]
29. Buelga, S.; Pons, J. Agresiones entre Adolescentes a través del Teléfono Móvil y de Internet. *Psychosoc. Interv.* **2012**, *21*, 91–101. [CrossRef]
30. Álvarez-García, D.; Núñez, J.C.; Barreiro-Collazo, A.; García, T. Validation of the Cybervictimization Questionnaire (CYVIC) for adolescents. *Comput. Hum. Behav.* **2017**, *70*, 270–281. [CrossRef]
31. Batool, S.S. Construction and validation of perceived dimensions of parenting scale (PDPS). *Pak. J. Soc. Clin. Psychol.* **2016**, *14*, 15.
32. Jadambaa, A.; Thomas, H.J.; Scott, J.G.; Graves, N.; Brain, D.; Pacella, R. Prevalence of traditional bullying and cyberbullying among children and adolescents in Australia: A systematic review and meta-analysis. *Aust. N. Z. J. Psychiatry* **2019**, *53*, 878–888. [CrossRef]
33. Jaghoory, H.; Björkqvist, K.; Österman, K. Cyberbullying among adolescents: A comparison between Iran and Finland. *J. Child Adolesc. Behav.* **2015**, 3. [CrossRef]
34. Feijóo, S.; Rodríguez-Fernández, R. A Meta-Analytical Review of Gender-Based School Bullying in Spain. *Int. J. Environ. Res. Public Health* **2021**, *18*, 12687. [CrossRef] [PubMed]
35. Lee, J.Y.; Kwon, Y.; Yang, S.; Park, S.; Kim, E.M.; Na, E.Y. Differences in friendship networks and experiences of cyberbullying among Korean and Australian adolescents. *J. Genet. Psychol.* **2017**, *178*, 44–57. [CrossRef] [PubMed]
36. Choi, E.; Park, N. Can Online Education Programs Solve the Cyberbullying Problem? Educating South Korean Elementary Students in the COVID-19 Era. *Sustainability* **2021**, *13*, 11211. [CrossRef]
37. Tsitsika, A.; Janikian, M.; Wójcik, S.; Makaruk, K.; Tzavela, E.; Tzavara, C.; Greydanus, D.; Merrick, J.; Richardson, C. Cyberbullying victimization prevalence and associations with internalizing and externalizing problems among adolescents in six European countries. *Comput. Hum. Behav.* **2015**, *51*, 1–7. [CrossRef]
38. Haddon, L.; Livingstone, S. EU Kids online: National Perspectives 2012. Available online: http://www.lse.ac.uk/media@lse/research/EUKidsOnline/EU%20Kids%20III/Reports/PerspectivesReport.pdf (accessed on 17 November 2021).
39. Gómez-Ortiz, O.; Apolinario, C.; Romera, E.M.; Ortega-Ruiz, R. The role of family in bullying and cyberbullying involvement: Examining a new typology of parental education management based on adolescents' view of their parents. *Soc. Sci.* **2019**, *8*, 25. [CrossRef]

40. Gómez-Ortiz, O.; Rosario Del Rey, E.M.R.; Rosario, O.-R. Los estilos educativos paternos y maternos en la adolescencia y su relación con la resiliencia, el apego y la implicación en acoso escolar. *An. Psicol. Ann. Psychol.* **2015**, *31*, 979–989. [CrossRef]
41. Gómez-Ortiz, O.; Romera, E.M.; Ortega-Ruiz, R.; Del Rey, R. Parenting Practices as Risk or Preventive Factors for Adolescent Involvement in Cyberbullying: Contribution of Children and Parent Gender. *Int. J. Environ. Res. Public Health* **2018**, *15*, 2664. [CrossRef]
42. Paolini, A. Cyberbullying: Role of the School Counselor in Mitigating the Silent Killer Epidemic. *Int. J. Educ. Technol.* **2018**, *5*, 1–8.
43. Mikkola, M.; Ellonen, N.; Kaakinen, M.; Savolainen, I.; Sirola, A.; Zych, I.; Paek, H.-J.; Oksanen, A. Cyberharassment Victimization on Three Continents: An Integrative Approach. *Int. J. Environ. Res. Public Health* **2022**, *19*, 12138. [CrossRef]
44. Blomqvist, K.; Saarento-Zaprudin, S.; Salmivalli, C. Telling adults about one's plight as a victim of bullying: Student-and context-related factors predicting disclosure. *Scand. J. Psychol.* **2020**, *61*, 151–159. [CrossRef]
45. O'Neill, B.; Dinh, T. Mobile technologies and the incidence of cyberbullying in seven European countries: Findings from Net Children Go Mobile. *Societies* **2015**, *5*, 384–398. [CrossRef]
46. Hood, M.; Duffy, A.L. Understanding the relationship between cyber-victimisation and cyber-bullying on Social Network Sites: The role of moderating factors. *Personal. Individ. Differ.* **2018**, *133*, 103–108. [CrossRef]
47. Cho, Y.K.; Yoo, J.W. Cyberbullying, internet and SNS usage types, and perceived social support: A comparison of different age groups. *Inf. Commun. Soc.* **2017**, *20*, 1464–1481. [CrossRef]
48. Barlett, C.; Coyne, S.M. A meta-analysis of sex differences in cyber-bullying behavior: The moderating role of age. *Aggress. Behav.* **2014**, *40*, 474–488. [CrossRef]
49. Chen, L.; Ho, S.S.; Lwin, M.O. A meta-analysis of factors predicting cyberbullying perpetration and victimization: From the social cognitive and media effects approach. *New Media Soc.* **2017**, *19*, 1194–1213. [CrossRef]
50. Peluchette, J.V.; Karl, K.; Wood, C.; Williams, J. Cyberbullying victimization: Do victims' personality and risky social network behaviors contribute to the problem? *Comput. Hum. Behav.* **2015**, *52*, 424–435. [CrossRef]
51. Marciano, L.; Schulz, P.J.; Camerini, A.L. Cyberbullying perpetration and victimization in youth: A meta-analysis of longitudinal studies. *J. Comput.-Mediat. Commun.* **2020**, *25*, 163–181. [CrossRef]
52. Makri-Botsari, E.; Karagianni, G. Cyberbullying in Greek adolescents: The role of parents. *Procedia-Soc. Behav. Sci.* **2014**, *116*, 3241–3253. [CrossRef]
53. Floros, G.; Mylona, I. Association of Cyberbullying and Internet Use Disorder. *Curr. Addict. Rep.* **2022**, 1–14. [CrossRef]
54. Kowalski, R.M.; Giumetti, G.W.; Schroeder, A.N.; Lattanner, M.R. Bullying in the digital age: A critical review and meta-analysis of cyberbullying research among youth. *Psychol. Bull.* **2014**, *140*, 1073–1137. [CrossRef]
55. Whittaker, E.; Kowalski, R.M. Cyberbullying via social media. *J. Sch. Violence* **2015**, *14*, 11–29. [CrossRef]
56. Holstein, B.; Parry-Langdon, N.; Zambon, A.; Currie, C.; Roberts, C. *Socio-Economic Inequalities and Health*; Currie, C., Roberts, C., Morgan, A., Smith, R., Settertobulte, W., Samdal, O., Rasmussen, V.B., Eds.; Young Peo-ple's Health in Context; Health Behaviour in Schoolaged Children: A WHOCross-National Collaborative Study. HBSC International Report from the 2001/02 Survey; Health Policy for Children and Adolescents, No. 4; World Health Organization: Geneva, Switzerland, 2004.
57. Sentenac, M.; Arnaud, C.; Gavin, A.; Molcho, M.; Gabhainn, S.N.; Godeau, E. Peer victimization among school-aged children with chronic conditions. *Epidemiol. Rev.* **2012**, *34*, 120–128. [CrossRef] [PubMed]
58. Horwood, J.; Waylen, A.; Herrick, D.; Williams, C.; Wolke, D. Common visual defects and peer victimization in children. *Investig. Ophthalmol. Vis. Sci.* **2005**, *46*, 1177–1181. [CrossRef] [PubMed]

behavioral sciences

MDPI

Article

Attachment and Depressive Symptoms in Adolescence: The Mediatory Role of Emotion Awareness

Maria João Carapeto [1,*], Raquel Domingos [2] and Guida Veiga [2,3]

1 Departamento de Psicologia, Escola de Ciências Sociais, Universidade de Évora, 7005-345 Évora, Portugal
2 Departamento de Desporto e Saúde, Escola de Saúde e Desenvolvimento Humano, Universidade de Évora, 7005-345 Évora, Portugal
3 Comprehensive Health Research Centre (CHRC), Universidade de Évora, 7005-345 Évora, Portugal
* Correspondence: mjcarapeto@uevora.pt

Abstract: Attachment seems to influence depression through emotion regulation. However, no study has yet examined the mediatory role of emotion awareness, a particular subset of emotion regulation abilities, in the relationship between attachment and depressive problems in early and middle adolescence. The aim of this study is to examine the direct and indirect effects of attachment on depressive symptoms in adolescence, considering the mediatory role of emotion awareness dimensions. A sample of adolescents (n = 223) filled up self-report questionnaires on attachment, emotion awareness and depression. Serial mediation models suggest direct effects on depression: negative for secure attachment and positive for anxious/ambivalent attachment. Anxious/ambivalent attachment has a positive indirect effect through lower differentiation of emotions. Both secure and anxious/ambivalent attachment have indirect positive effects on depression through the sequence of bodily unawareness and differentiation of emotions. Differentiating emotions has a central role in mediating the relationship between attachment and depressive symptoms, and the lack of bodily awareness of emotions contributes to such mediation.

Keywords: internalizing; differentiation of emotions; bodily awareness; emotion regulation

1. Introduction

In current societies, depressive symptoms seriously threaten adolescents' mental health and socioemotional adjustment [1]. In this context, research about a diversity of risk factors and mechanisms for depression has been encouraged [1–4]. Therefore, this article focuses on the possible contribution of attachment and emotion awareness to depression in early to late adolescents.

The attachment theory [5,6] highlights the importance of a child's early relationships with caregivers for the child's survival, adaptive development, and mental health. Based on his/her experience with the caregiver, the child construes internal working models, which are a mental representation of the self and significant others that perdure and inspire personal behavior, cognition, affect, and emotion regulation [5]. Three main patterns of attachment that differently guide individuals' actions in times of distress, have been described [5–8]. Secure attachment representations promote a sense of security and trust in relationships and a sense of being worthy of others' attention [5,7]. Insecure anxious/ambivalent attachment representations are related to a continuous search for proximity and closeness, concerns about relationships, and fear of reject [7,8]. Insecure avoidant attachment representations focus on self-reliance and a preference for emotional distance from others [7,8].

Insecure attachment (more consistently, the anxious/ambivalent attachment) has been related to depressive symptoms [6,9,10] in both clinical and non-clinical adolescents [10]. On the other hand, secure attachment has been related to better adjustment, including fewer depressive problems [10]. This relationship between attachment and depressive symptoms seems to be mediated, at least partially, by emotion regulation [11,12], which refers to the "extrinsic and intrinsic processes responsible for monitoring, evaluating, and modifying emotional reactions, especially their intensive and temporal features, to accomplish one's goals" [13] (pp. 27–28). Emotion regulation processes are first shaped by early attachment relationships, in which the caregiver supports the child to become increasingly attuned with his/her own emotions and behaviors, decreasing the emotional arousal and improving his/her sense of comfort and safety [5,7,8]. Accordingly, insecure attachments seem to favor maladaptive emotion regulation strategies in response to distress (e.g., hyperactivating and deactivating strategies) [8,12,14]. In contrast, secure attachment is related to fewer maladaptive [8] and more adaptive emotion regulation strategies [15]. Moreover, emotion regulation difficulties are linked to adolescents' depression [16,17].

Most studies about the mediation role of emotion regulation in the relationship between attachment and depressive symptoms in adolescence [11,12] have approached emotional regulation as a process of "modifying emotional reactions" [13]. Therefore, they have neglected the "monitoring and evaluating" component, the so-called emotion awareness. Emotion awareness is an attentional process, involving interpretative and evaluative functions, that "not only enables us to monitor our emotions but also to differentiate between various emotions in a qualitative sense; to locate their antecedents; and to acknowledge the physiological correlates of the emotional experience for what they are" [18] (p. 756). Emotion awareness includes attitudinal aspects, namely the positive or negative value one attributes to emotions, the understanding of emotions as experiences more or less private to share (or to hide) and as a more or less interpersonal experience (communication of personal emotions and attention to others) [18]. Emotion awareness is, therefore, a multidimensional construct.

Emotion awareness seems to play a critical role in what concerns the development of adolescents' depressive symptoms [16,19–21]. That is, the diminished ability to identify which emotion one is feeling or what causes it hampers the ability to modify emotional reactions, leading to persistent negative emotions and increasing the likability of developing depressive problems [19,22,23]. On the other hand, some research showed that adolescents' secure attachment is related to better emotion awareness [15] and that insecure attachment is linked to difficulties in emotion awareness [8,24,25].

To date, only three studies have been conducted on the subject, and these showed that emotion awareness has a mediatory role in the positive relationship between insecure (more frequently avoidant) attachment and depression in college students [24] and adult women [26,27].

Present Study

Despite the empirical support for the relationships between attachment, emotion awareness, and depressive symptoms in adolescents, to the best of our knowledge, this is the first study to examine the mediatory role of emotion awareness in the relationship between attachment and depressive problems in early and middle adolescence. Moreover, several developmental changes occur at this stage, making it critical to understand the contribution of attachment and emotion awareness to adolescents' mental health, particularly concerning depressive symptoms: (1) The attachment system becomes more committed to emotion regulation functions as adolescents face autonomy challenges and new social contexts [28]; (2) Emotion regulation abilities seem to deteriorate [29], including emotion awareness [19,25]; (3) Depressive symptoms increase [1]. Moreover, this is also the first study to consider emotion awareness as a multidimensional construct, when examining its mediatory role in the relationship between attachment and depressive symptoms.

Thus, the present study aims to examine the direct and indirect effects of attachment patterns (secure, anxious/ambivalent, and avoidant) on depressive symptoms in early and middle adolescents, considering the mediatory role of different emotion awareness dimensions. As age and gender seem to have an influence on depression [1] and emotion awareness [19], and considering the recognized overlap and comorbidity between anxiety and depression [30], the possible effects of gender, age and anxiety will be controlled. Based on previous studies with older ages, it is expected that emotion awareness plays a mediatory role in the positive relationship between insecure attachment and depression, as well as in the negative relationship between secure attachment and depression. Giving that this is the first study to consider the multidimensionality of emotion awareness, no hypotheses are formulated regarding the role of each emotion awareness dimension.

As main contributions, we expect this work to clarify some of the mechanisms that lead to adolescents' depressive symptoms, particularly those involving attachment and emotion awareness. Moreover, we expect these findings will provide new insight to improve the prevention and treatment of adolescents' depression.

2. Materials and Methods

2.1. Participants

The sample consists of 223 participants, 96 (43%) male and 127 (57%) female, aged between 12 and 16 years old (M = 13.51, SD = 1.13), who attended the 7th grade (n = 83, 37.2%), 8th grade (n = 69, 30.9%), and 9th grade (n = 71, 31.8%) in 3 public schools in the South of Portugal. Most participants reported never having lived apart from their parent(s) (74.9%) and currently living with both their parents (76.7%) or only with their mother (20.6%). The majority reported having a single brother or sister (63.7%) and 14.8% had no brothers or sisters. Concerning educational qualifications, 26.9% reported that fathers had secondary education and 35.9% higher education; 30.5% indicated that mothers had secondary education and 46.6% higher education.

2.2. Instruments

The Childhood and Adolescence Attachment Inventory (CAAI) [31] is a self-report questionnaire that measures three attachment patterns. The secure attachment scale measures issues of trust in the other and one's abilities (e.g., I like feeling close to other people). The anxious/ambivalent scale measures apprehension and concerns about relationships (e.g., I am concerned about the possibility of being alone), while the avoidant attachment scale measures dependence and avoidance (e.g., I am concerned if I have to depend on other people) [31]. Each scale comprises 8 items to be answered on a 5-point Likert scale, from 1 (*Never*) to 5 (*Always*), and its score is obtained through the sum of each item scores. Higher scores reflect a higher level of attachment behaviors and representations on an attachment scale. The CAAI showed good psychometric qualities, such as adequate adjustment measures of the model in confirmatory factor analysis and good reliability (α = 0.83; 0.85; 0.71 for secure, insecure-anxious/ambivalent, and insecure-avoidant scales, respectively) [31]. In the present study, the reliability of the secure, insecure-anxious/ambivalent, and insecure-avoidant scales was good (α = 0.73; α = 0.84; α = 0.63, respectively).

Emotion awareness was measured using the Portuguese version [32] of the Emotion Awareness Questionnaire [18]. This self-report questionnaire comprises 30 items corresponding to six scales: differentiation of emotions (7 items; e.g., "I am often confused or puzzled about what I am feeling"), verbal sharing of emotions (3 items; e.g., "I find it difficult to explain to a friend how I feel"), not hiding emotions (5 items; e.g., "Other people don't need to know how I am feeling"), bodily unawareness of emotions (or lack of bodily awareness) (5 items; e.g., "When I am scared or nervous, I feel something in my tummy"), attending to others emotions (5 items; e.g., "It is important to know how my friends are feeling"), and analysis of own emotions (5 items; e.g., "When I am angry or upset, I try to understand why"). Items are scored on a 3-point Likert scale from 1 (*not true*) to 3 (*often true*), and the scoring is reversed for 20 items. Each scale score is the average score of its items and higher scores correspond to better emotion awareness and are associated with less negative affective states [18]. The Portuguese version showed good psychometric qualities [32]. In the present study, the reliability of the scales was good ($0.66 < \alpha < 0.74$).

The Depression Anxiety Stress Scale—21 [33,34] was used to measure depression and anxiety. In this self-report questionnaire, items are scored on a 3-point Likert scale from 0 (*did not apply to me at all*) to 3 (*applied to me very much, or most of the time*). The depression scale score is obtained through the sum of the scores of its 7 items (e.g., I couldn't seem to experience any positive feeling at all) multiplied by 2, and the anxiety score is the sum of the scores of its 7 items (e.g., "I was aware of dryness of my mouth") multiplied by 2. Higher results are associated with higher severity of symptoms. The Portuguese version showed good psychometric qualities [34]. In the present study, the reliability of the depression and anxiety scales was good ($\alpha = 0.85$ and $\alpha = 0.81$, respectively).

2.3. Procedure

This research project was approved by the Ethics Committee of the University of Évora (#18003) and the Portuguese Ministry of Education. Before conducting the study, permission to collect the data was obtained from schools' principals, and adolescents and parents provided written informed consent.

2.4. Data Analysis Strategy

The statistical analysis was carried out with the SPSS v. 24. Descriptive statistics (mean and SD) were computed for age, attachment patterns (secure, anxious/ambivalent and avoidant), emotion awareness dimensions (differentiation emotions, verbal sharing of emotions, not hiding emotions, bodily unawareness of emotions, attending to other's emotions, and analysis of own emotions), depression and anxiety, as well as gender (%). A series of *t*-tests for independent samples were computed to test gender differences and Pearson correlations were calculated between age, attachment patterns, emotion awareness dimensions, and depressive and anxiety symptoms.

Multiple mediation models were considered to test the hypotheses that attachment patterns influence depressive symptoms and that this influence is mediated by emotion awareness. Two emotion awareness dimensions, namely differentiating emotions and bodily unawareness presented the highest, medium size (>0.30) correlations with depression and were selected as mediation variables. Considering the medium size association between the two mediators ($r = 0.35$), a serial multiple mediation model was the option [35].

Analyses were performed with Hayes' Process v. 3.5 macro for SPSS [35], a software that uses a path analyses approach and is based on the regression ordinary least squares method. Based on model 6 (Figure 1) and following Hayes [35] guidelines, the serial multiple mediation models included eight predictors (three attachment patterns; two mediators, namely bodily unawareness and differentiating emotions; and three additional covariates, that is, gender, age, and anxiety) and depression as the outcome variable.

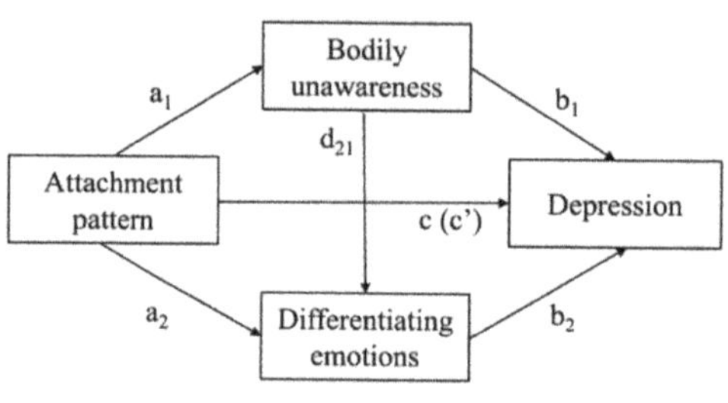

Figure 1. General serial multiple mediation model.

The analysis provided regression coefficients for each path in the models (e.g., a_1, a_2, b_1, b_2, d_{21}) including the estimates of the total (c path; mediators not included in the model) and direct (c′ path; mediators included in the model) effects of each attachment pattern on depressive symptoms and the three possible indirect effects (a_1b_1, a_2b_2, and a_1d_{21} b_2 paths) for each attachment pattern (Figure 1). To compute the direct and indirect effects of each attachment pattern, the model run three times, each one considering one specific attachment pattern as the independent variable (the other two entering as covariates). To test the significance of the coefficients of each path (including indirect paths), 95% percentile bootstrap confidence intervals and bootstrap standard errors were computed based on 10,000 bootstrap samples. In addition, a heteroscedasticity-consistent method (i.e., HC3) was used to compute standard errors to reinforce more robust inference. An effect was considered significant when the confidence interval did not include zero. Otherwise, a result was considered statistically significant when $p < 0.05$.

3. Results

Table 1 shows the mean and standard deviation values for the variables and the correlations, and Table 2 presents the descriptives by gender.

The analysis of the correlations in Table 1 suggests that secure attachment was positively related to emotion awareness dimensions, except for differentiation of emotions and bodily unawareness. Both insecure patterns were negatively associated with differentiation of emotions and verbal sharing. However, only anxious/ambivalent attachment was negatively associated with body unawareness, and avoidant attachment was negatively related to not hiding of emotions.

Depression was negatively associated with secure attachment and positively associated with both insecure attachment patterns. Moreover, depression was negatively related to emotion awareness dimensions, except for analyzing emotions. Positive associations were found between anxious/ambivalent and avoidant attachment and depression and anxiety.

As shown in Table 2, females reported higher anxious/ambivalent attachment. Males showed higher scores on differentiating emotions and bodily unawareness, whereas females scored higher on attending to others' emotions. Age was not associated with any variable.

The total, direct and indirect effects are presented in Table 3, and the coefficients for the remaining paths. Figure 2 illustrates the relationships between the variables.

The model of the total effects of attachment (age, gender, and anxiety were covariates) on depression explained 57% of the variance of depression, $F\ (6, 216) = 45.92$, $p = 0.0000$, and the model for the direct effects (mediators included) explained 60%, $F\ (8, 214) = 38.54$, $p = 0.000$.

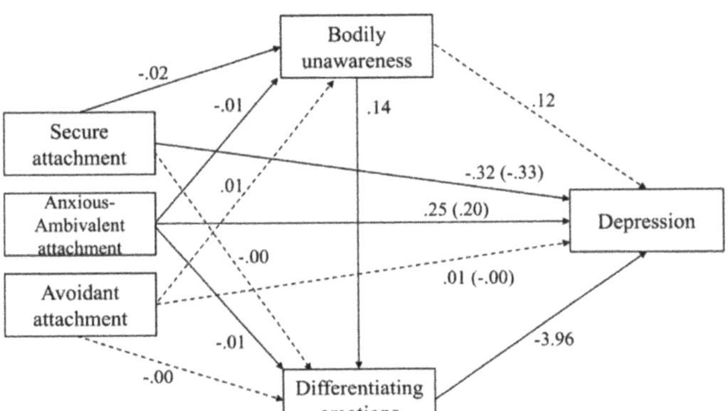

Figure 2. Serial multiple mediation models of the effects of bodily unawareness and differentiating emotions on the relationship between different patterns of attachment and depression. Unstandardized coefficients (direct effects in parentheses). Solid lines indicate significant effects (95% confidence interval does not include zero) and dashed lines illustrate non-significant effects.

The negative total (c path) and direct (c′ path) effects of secure attachment on depression indicated that more secure attachment predicted lower levels of depressive symptoms even when the emotion awareness dimensions entered the model. Besides, a positive indirect effect of secure attachment on depression via bodily unawareness and differentiating emotions ($a_1d_{21}b_2$ path) was significant.

Table 1. Descriptive statistics and Pearson's correlations between age, attachment patterns, emotion awareness dimensions, and internalizing problems (n = 223).

	M	*SD*	1	2	3	4	5	6	7	8	9	10	11
1—Age	13.51	1.13											
Attachment													
2—Secure	33.56	4.25	−0.13										
3—Anxious/Ambivalent	21.00	7.92	0.02	0.02									
4—Avoidant	24.42	10.10	0.04	−0.13	0.30 ***								
Emotion Awareness													
5—Differentiation	2.15	0.44	0.04	0.02	−0.39 ***	−0.19 **							
6—Verbal Sharing	2.00	0.53	−00.08	0.25 ***	−0.27 ***	−0.35 ***	0.32 ***						
7—Not Hiding	1.95	0.45	−0.05	0.25 ***	−0.06	−0.39 ***	0.16 *	0.43 ***					
8—Bodily Unawareness	1.88	0.54	−0.03	−0.09	−0.35 ***	−0.08	0.35 ***	0.11	−0.03				
9—Other's Emotions	2.70	0.32	0.01	0.42 **	0.05	−0.07	−0.05	0.09	0.13	−0.11			
10—Analyze Emotions	2.44	0.41	0.03	0.26 **	0.09	0.01	−0.13	0.07	0.21 **	−0.27 ***	0.40 ***		
Internalizing problems													
11—Depression	100.21	90.65	0.04	−0.27 **	0.44 ***	0.27 ***	−0.46 ***	−0.26 ***	−0.25 ***	−0.31 ***	−0.17 **	−0.02	
12—Anxiety	70.96	80.60	−0.06	−0.22 **	0.37 ***	0.31 ***	−0.38 ***	−0.21 **	−0.19 **	−0.36 ***	−0.17 *	−0.02	0.71 ***

* $p < 0.05$; ** $p < 0.01$; *** $p < 0.0010$.

Table 2. Descriptive statistics and gender differences for age, attachment patterns, emotion awareness dimensions, and internalizing problems (n = 223).

	Female		Male			
	M	SD	M	SD	t (221)	d
1—Age	13.39	1.06	13.66	1.20	−1.73	0.238
Attachment						
2—Secure	33.84	4.03	33.19	4.51	1.13	0.152
3—Anxious/Ambivalent	22.08	8.29	19.57	7.19	2.37 *	0.323
4—Avoidant	24.31	4.67	24.58	5.63	−0.39	0.052
Emotion Awareness						
5—Differentiation	2.09	0.43	2.23	0.44	−2.40 *	0.322
6—Verbal Sharing	1.99	0.51	2.01	0.55	−0.34	0.038
7—Not Hiding	1.96	0.47	1.95	0.43	0.13	0.022
8—Bodily Unawareness	1.80	0.51	1.98	0.57	−2.36 *	0.332
9—Other's Emotions	2.78	0.27	2.60	0.36	3.98 ***	0.566
10—Analyze Emotions	2.48	0.38	2.38	0.44	1.69	0.243
Internalizing problems						
11—Depression	10.57	9.58	9.72	9.77	0.64	0.088
12—Anxiety	7.57	8.49	8.47	8.76	−0.78	0.104

* $p < 0.05$; *** $p < 0.001$.

Anxious/ambivalent attachment showed positive total (c path) and direct (c′ path) effects on depression, such that more anxious/ambivalent attachment predicted higher levels of depression even when the effect of the mediators was considered. The total indirect effect of anxious/ambivalent attachment on depression was also positive, as well as two specific indirect effects, namely, through differentiating emotions (a_2b_2 path) and through bodily unawareness and differentiating emotions ($a_1d_{21}b_2$ path). The first indirect effect was more expressive than the second, b = 0.039, *boot se* = 0.021, 95% *boot CI* [0.002, 0.084]. Avoidant attachment was not significantly related to emotion awareness dimensions nor depression.

Table 3. Serial mediation analyses: Total, direct, and indirect effects of each pattern of attachment on depression, and intermediate paths.

Attachment/Path	Depression		
	Effect	SE	95% CI
Secure			
a_1	−0.019	0.008	[−0.035, −0.004]
a_2	−0.001	0.007	[−0.014, 0.013]
Total effect (c)	−0.323	0.117	[−0.554, −0.092]
Direct effect (c′)	−0.334	0.112	[−0.564, −0.097]
Indirect effects			
Total	0.011	0.033	[−0.059, 0.074]
a_1b_1	−0.002	0.019	[−0.044, 0.034]
a_2b_2	0.002	0.028	[−0.059, 0.056]
$a_1d_{21}b_2$	0.011	0.008	[0.001, 0.030]
Anxious/ambivalent			
a_1	−0.014	0.004	[−0.023, −0.006]
a_2	−0.012	0.004	[−0.020, −0.004]
Total effect (c)	0.249	0.069	[0.112, 0.386]
Direct effect (c′)	0.196	0.068	[0.066, 0.334]
Indirect effects			
Total	0.053	0.024	[0.010, 0.103]
a_1b_1	−0.002	0.013	[−0.031, 0.024]
a_2b_2	0.047	0.021	[0.011, 0.092]
$a_1d_{21}b_2$	0.008	0.005	[0.001, 0.021]

Table 3. *Cont.*

Attachment/Path	Depression		
	Effect	*SE*	95% *CI*
Avoidant			
a_1	0.008	0.007	[−0.006, 0.022]
a_2	−0.004	0.006	[−0.016, 0.007]
Total effect (c)	0.011	0.090	[−0.166, 0.188]
Direct effect (c′)	−0.003	0.087	[−0.176, 0.166]
Indirect effects			
Total	0.014	0.028	[−0.032, 0.080]
a_1b_1	0.001	0.010	[−0.018, 0.023]
a_2b_2	0.017	0.026	[−0.024, 0.081]
$a_1d_{21}b_2$	−0.005	0.005	[−0.017, 0.003]
Common paths			
b_1	0.116	0.901	[−1.611, 1.919]
b_2	−3.962	1.120	[−6.161, −1.771]
d_{21}	0.143	0.052	[0.041, 0.246]

Note. Unstandardized coefficients/estimates. Standard error and 95% confidence intervals provided by bootstrap, except for attachment total effects. An effect is significant when the confidence interval does not include zero.

Thus, secure and anxious/ambivalent attachments were negative predictors of bodily unawareness, and both anxious/ambivalent attachment and bodily unawareness were predictors (negative and positive, respectively) of differentiating emotions. The models with the attachment patterns as predictors (also gender, age, and anxiety as covariates) explained 23% of the variance of bodily unawareness, $F(6, 216) = 11.12$, $p = 0.000$, and (adding bodily unawareness to the model) 26% of differentiating emotions, $F(7, 215) = 10.58$, $p = 0.000$.

4. Discussion

The findings of the present study show that both secure and anxious/ambivalent attachment are related to depression and that bodily unawareness and differentiating emotions mediate those relationships.

In line with other studies [10], the significant direct effects in our study suggest that more secure attachment representations are linked to lower levels of depression, and more anxious/ambivalent attachment representations are related to higher levels of depression. Therefore, the influence of both secure and anxious/ambivalent attachment on depression seems to go beyond the mediated effects of the two emotion awareness dimensions (and beyond the effects of the covariates: gender, age, anxiety, and the other attachment patterns) that we discuss later. This is consistent with the proposed pervasive influence of attachment representations on the psychological organization [5,36] and with the diversity of mechanisms that have been proposed to mediate the influence of attachment on depression, such as dysfunctional attitudes, self-criticism, self-compassion, or maladaptive emotion regulation [11].

Emotion awareness seems to play a role in the pathway between attachment and adolescents' depressive symptoms. In particular, as suggested by the serial mediation analyses, more secure and anxious/ambivalent attachments both predict greater levels of depression through differentiating emotions and bodily unawareness.

First, differentiating emotions emerges as the most relevant indirect pathway from anxious/ambivalent attachment to depression. The relationship between the insecurity of attachment and differentiating emotions has been found in other studies with adolescents [25] as well as the link between differentiating emotions and depression [18,21]. Possibly, the chronic concern of being disliked and rejected by others limits the opportunities to perceive a diversity of emotional states and to understand the different causes of emotions. This hampers the possibility of coping adequately with the specificities of the emotion-evoking situations; therefore, the initial negative affect may develop into depressive symptoms [22,23]. This is especially critical because adolescents are repeatedly distressed by daily developmental challenges and interpersonal stressors [21]. On the other hand, there is some evidence that the lack of differentiation of emotions and their causes predicts maladaptive forms of emotion regulation, such as brooding rumination [37], a recognized risk factor for depression [1], especially when emotion differentiation is low [38]. Brooding rumination is also a mediator between insecure attachment and depression [11].

A second indirect pathway from anxious/ambivalent attachment to depression involves, sequentially, bodily unawareness and differentiating emotions. Accordingly, more anxious/ambivalent attachment representations might increment the focus on the physiological arousal during emotional experiences [39], which might hinder an external focus and a refined differentiation of emotional experiences based on the clues of the emotion-evoking situations [18]. Altogether, this opens the pathways to depression as mentioned above. In addition, the hypervigilant focus on body sensations might limit identifying negative emotions-evoking situations. Hence, dysfunctional attitudes and self-criticism might come into play, therefore contributing to depressive symptomatology [11,40].

Third, although the direct effect supports the hypothesis of the secure attachment's protective effect against depression [6,10], the indirect, serial path through both emotion awareness dimensions suggests a novel hypothesis that more secure attachment can also open a maladaptive pathway to depressive symptoms. Altogether, these findings suggest that trusting on own abilities and others (the core of secure attachment), and concerning about being rejected and disliked by others (the core of anxious/ambivalent attachment) are related to a higher focus on the physiological arousal throughout emotional processing and to a lower focus on the situations that evoke the emotional response. In this scenario, the entry into the scene of adaptive emotion regulation to cope with the situation seems less likely. In contrast, the maladaptive strategies (e.g., brooding rumination) seem more likely [37]. It is important to note that Rieffe and colleagues [18] had already adverted to the risk of high bodily awareness of emotions and the importance of a combined understanding of bodily awareness with other emotion regulation abilities in the process of emotional regulation. Such contradictory effects of secure attachment on depression support the idea of the complex, organismic nature of the socioemotional processes [36].

Finally, in line with other research [41], we find that avoidant attachment has no significant role in depressive symptoms. Hence, our findings do not support the relationship between avoidant attachment and greater depressive symptoms found by others [9,10,26,42], nor the hypothesis of the protective effect of avoidant attachment on depression [24] (see also [42]). Additionally, contrary to other studies [24,27], our findings do not support the influence of avoidant attachment on emotion awareness nor its indirect effect on depression through a lack of emotion awareness.

As mentioned by other authors (e.g., [42]), avoidant attachment's role on depressive symptoms needs yet to be clarified. For instance, Khan and colleagues (2020) claim the need for a finer-grain analysis of the effects of two main types of avoidant attachment (i.e., dismissive and fearful). They hypothesize that the avoidant fearful type might be a fertile ground to adolescents' depression, while the dismissive type might protect adolescents from depressive problems. Therefore, future studies should consider these two subgroups in order to disentangle the pathway from avoidant attachment to depression.

5. Conclusion

5.1. Limitations and Future Directions

Although encouraging, our findings need to be taken with caution. It is important to note that the cross-sectional design limits assertions about causality. Besides, testing the present models in other cultures would be worthwhile. Additionally, more studies are still needed to clarify the role of avoidant attachment. Our study reveals that bodily awareness of emotions, favored by both secure and anxious/ambivalent attachment representations, weakens the differentiation of emotions, thereby indirectly promoting adolescents' depressive symptoms. However, more research is needed to unfold this process.

Besides, longitudinal research is needed to further examine the role of emotion awareness dimensions, their interplay, and the intertwined with other emotion regulation strategies and cognitive-emotional processes.

5.2. Theoretical and Practical Implications

The present findings suggest that the pathways from adolescents' attachment representations to depression are multiple and that different emotion awareness abilities are involved differently. Concerning implications for practice, secure and anxious/ambivalent attachment representations and the ability to differentiate emotions and their causes are important target variables for interventions to prevent and treat adolescent depression [43].

5.3. General Conclusions

Secure and anxious/ambivalent attachment representations are related to adolescents' depressive symptoms. Emotion awareness has a partial, mediatory role in these complex relationships. In particular, the bodily awareness of emotions and the ability to differentiate emotions seem to work together to open indirect pathways from attachment to depressive symptoms. More research is needed to clarify the mechanisms involved.

Author Contributions: Conceptualization, M.J.C., R.D. and G.V.; Data curation, M.J.C. and R.D.; Formal analysis, M.J.C. and G.V.; Investigation, M.J.C., R.D. and G.V.; Methodology, M.J.C. and G.V.; Project administration, M.J.C. and G.V.; Writing—original draft, M.J.C.; Writing—review and editing, M.J.C., R.D. and G.V. All authors have read and agreed to the published version of the manuscript.

Funding: This research received no external funding.

Institutional Review Board Statement: The study was conducted in accordance with the Declaration of Helsinki and approved by the Ethics Committee of the University (#18003, 10 January 2018) and the Ministry of Education.

Informed Consent Statement: Informed consent was obtained from all subjects involved in the study.

Data Availability Statement: Not applicable.

Acknowledgments: Special thanks to the adolescents and schools who took part in this study.

Conflicts of Interest: The authors declare no conflict of interest.

References

1. Hankin, B.L. Depression during childhood and adolescence. In *The Oxford Handbook of Mood Disorders*; DeRubeis, R.J., Strunk, D.R., Eds.; Oxford University Press: New York, NY, USA, 2017; pp. 276–286.
2. Torres-Fernández, G.; Rodríguez-Valverde, M.; Reyes-Martín, S.; Hernández-Lopez, M. The Role of Psychological Inflexibility and Experiential Approach on Mental Health in Children and Adolescents: An Exploratory Study. *Behav. Sci.* **2022**, *12*, 201. [CrossRef] [PubMed]
3. Carapeto, M.J.; Domingos, R.; Veiga, G. Is the effect of body dissatisfaction on depressive symptoms dependent on weight Status? A study with early-to-middle adolescents. *Eur. J. Investig. Health Psychol. Educ.* **2020**, *10*, 1020–1034. [CrossRef]
4. Carapeto, M.J.; Feixas, G. Self-knowledge and depressive symptoms in late adolescence: A study using the repertory grid technique. *J. Constr. Psychol.* **2019**, *32*, 81–97. [CrossRef]
5. Bowlby, J. *Attachment and Loss, Vol. 1 Attachment*; Basic Books: New York, NY, USA, 1969.
6. Bowlby, J. *Attachment and Loss, Vol. 2. Separation, Anxiety and Anger*; Basic Books: New York, NY, USA, 1973.
7. Ainsworth, M.D.S.; Blehar, M.C.; Waters, E.; Wall, S. *Patterns of Attachment: A Psychological Study of the Strange Situation*; Erlbaum: Hillsdale, NJ, USA, 1978.
8. Mikulincer, M.; Shaver, P.R. Attachment orientations and emotion regulation. *Curr. Opin. Psychol.* **2019**, *25*, 6–10. [CrossRef] [PubMed]
9. Madigan, S.; Brumariu, L.E.; Villani, V.; Atkinson, L.; Lyons-Ruth, K. Representational and questionnaire measures of attachment: A meta-analysis of relations to child internalizing and externalizing problems. *Psychol. Bull.* **2016**, *142*, 367–399. [CrossRef] [PubMed]
10. Spruit, A.; Goos, L.; Weenink, N.; Rodenburg, R.; Niemeyer, H.; Stams, G.J.; Colonnesi, C. The relation between attachment and depression in children and adolescents: A multilevel meta-analysis. *Clin. Child Fam. Psychol. Rev.* **2020**, *23*, 54–69. [CrossRef]
11. Cortés-García, L.; Takkouche, B.; Rodriguez-Cano, R.; Senra, C. Mediational mechanisms involved in the relation between attachment insecurity and depression: A meta-analysis. *J. Affect. Disord.* **2020**, *277*, 706–726. [CrossRef]

12. Malik, S.; Wells, A.; Wittkowski, A. Emotion regulation as a mediator in the relationship between attachment and depressive symptomatology: A systematic review. *J. Affect. Disord.* **2015**, *172*, 428–444. [CrossRef]
13. Thompson, R.A. Emotion regulation: A theme in search of definition. *Monogr. Soc. Res. Child Dev.* **1994**, *59*, 25–52. [CrossRef]
14. Stevens, F.L. Affect regulation styles in avoidant and anxious attachment. *Individ. Differ. Res.* **2014**, *12*, 123–130.
15. Laible, D. Attachment with parents and peers in late adolescence: Links with emotional competence and social behavior. *Pers. Individ. Differ.* **2007**, *43*, 1185–1197. [CrossRef]
16. Gonçalves, S.F.; Chaplin, T.M.; Turpyn, C.C.; Niehaus, C.E.; Curby, T.W.; Sinha, R.; Ansell, E.B. Difficulties in emotion regulation predict depressive symptom trajectory from early to middle adolescence. *Child Psychiatry Hum. Dev.* **2019**, *50*, 618–630. [CrossRef] [PubMed]
17. Schäfer, J.Ö.; Naumann, E.; Holmes, E.A.; Tuschen-Caffier, B.; Samson, A.C. Emotion regulation strategies in depressive and anxiety symptoms in youth: A meta-analytic review. *J. Youth Adolesc.* **2017**, *46*, 261–276. [CrossRef] [PubMed]
18. Rieffe, C.; Oosterveld, P.; Miers, A.C.; Terwogt, M.M.; Ly, V. Emotion awareness and internalising symptoms in children and adolescents: The Emotion Awareness Questionnaire revised. *Pers. Individ. Differ.* **2008**, *45*, 756–761. [CrossRef]
19. Kranzler, A.; Young, J.F.; Hankin, B.L.; Abela, J.R.; Elias, M.J.; Selby, E.A. Emotional awareness: A transdiagnostic predictor of depression and anxiety for children and adolescents. *J. Clin. Child Adolesc. Psychol.* **2016**, *45*, 262–269. [CrossRef]
20. Sendzik, L.; Schäfer, J.Ö.; Samson, A.C.; Naumann, E.; Tuschen-Caffier, B. Emotional awareness in depressive and anxiety symptoms in youth: A meta-analytic review. *J. Youth Adolesc.* **2017**, *46*, 687–700. [CrossRef]
21. Starr, L.R.; Hershenberg, R.; Shaw, Z.A.; Li, Y.I.; Santee, A.C. The perils of murky emotions: Emotion differentiation moderates the prospective relationship between naturalistic stress exposure and adolescent depression. *Emotion* **2020**, *20*, 927–938. [CrossRef]
22. Eastabrook, J.M.; Flynn, J.J.; Hollenstein, T. Internalizing symptoms in female adolescents: Associations with emotional awareness and emotion regulation. *J. Child Fam. Stud.* **2014**, *23*, 487–496. [CrossRef]
23. Van Beveren, M.L.; Goossens, L.; Volkaert, B.; Grassmann, C.; Wante, L.; Vandeweghe, L.; Verbeken, S.; Braet, C. How do I feel right now? Emotional awareness, emotion regulation and depressive symptoms in youth. *Eur. Child Adolesc. Psychiatry* **2019**, *28*, 389–398. [CrossRef]
24. Owens, G.P.; Held, P.; Hamrick, L.; Keller, E. The indirect effects of emotion regulation on the association between attachment style, depression and meaning made among undergraduates who experienced stressful events. *Motiv. Emot.* **2018**, *42*, 429–437. [CrossRef]
25. Starr, L.R.; Shaw, Z.A.; Li, Y.I.; Santee, A.C.; Hershenberg, R. Negative emotion differentiation through a developmental lens: Associations with parental factors and age in adolescence. *Pers. Indiv. Differ.* **2020**, *152*, 109597. [CrossRef]
26. Marques, R.; Monteiro, F.; Canavarro, M.C.; Fonseca, A. The role of emotion regulation difficulties in the relationship between attachment representations and depressive and anxiety symptoms in the postpartum period. *J. Affec. Disord.* **2018**, *238*, 39–46. [CrossRef] [PubMed]
27. Monti, J.D.; Rudolph, K.D. Emotional awareness as a pathway linking adult attachment to subsequent depression. *J. Couns. Psychol.* **2014**, *61*, 374–382. [CrossRef] [PubMed]
28. Allen, J.P.; Miga, E.M. Attachment in adolescence: A move to the level of emotion regulation. *J. Soc. Pers. Relatsh.* **2010**, *27*, 181–190. [CrossRef] [PubMed]
29. Cracco, E.; Goossens, L.; Braet, C. Emotion regulation across childhood and adolescence: Evidence for a maladaptive shift in adolescence. *Eur. Child Adolesc. Psychiatry* **2017**, *26*, 909–921. [CrossRef]
30. Anderson, E.R.; Hope, D.A. A review of the tripartite model for understanding the link between anxiety and depression in youth. *Clin. Psychol. Rev.* **2008**, *28*, 275–287. [CrossRef]
31. Carvalho, M.A.D. Vinculação, Temperamento e Processamento da Informação: Implicações nas Perturbações Emocionais e Comportamentais no Início da Adolescência. Ph.D. Thesis, Universidade do Minho, Braga, Portugal, 2007. Available online: https://repositorium.sdum.uminho.pt/bitstream/1822/8410/1/vincula%C3%A7%C3%A3o%20temperamento%20e%20processamento%20de%20informa%C3%A7%C3%A3o.pdf (accessed on 19 October 2022).
32. Veiga, G.; Oosterveld, P.; Fernandes, J.; Rieffe, C. Validation of the Portuguese emotion awareness questionnaire for children and adolescents. *Eur. J. Dev. Psychol.* **2019**, *16*, 215–224. [CrossRef]
33. Lovibond, P.; Lovibond, S. The structure of negative emotional states: Comparison of the depression anxiety stress scales (DASS) with the Beck Depression and Anxiety Inventories. *Behav. Res. Ther.* **1995**, *33*, 335–343. [CrossRef]
34. Leal, I.P.; Antunes, R.; Passos, T.; Pais-Ribeiro, J.; Maroco, J. Estudo da escala de depressão, ansiedade e stresse para crianças (EADS-C). *Psicol. Saúde Doenças* **2009**, *10*, 277–284.
35. Hayes, A.F. *Introduction to Mediation, Moderation and Conditional Process Analysis: A Regression-Based Approach*, 2nd ed.; Guilford: New York, NY, USA, 2018.
36. Cicchetti, D.; Toth, S.L. The development of depression in children and adolescents. *Am. Psychol.* **1998**, *53*, 221–241. [CrossRef]
37. Eckland, N.S.; Berenbaum, H. Emotional awareness in daily life: Exploring its potential role in repetitive thinking and healthy coping. *Behav. Ther.* **2021**, *52*, 338–349. [CrossRef] [PubMed]
38. Liu, D.Y.; Gilbert, K.E.; Thompson, R.J. Emotion differentiation moderates the effects of rumination on depression: A longitudinal study. *Emotion* **2020**, *20*, 1234–1243. [CrossRef] [PubMed]
39. Oldroyd, K.; Pasupathi, M.; Wainryb, C. Social antecedents to the development of interoception: Attachment related processes are associated with interoception. *Front. Psychol.* **2019**, *10*, 712. [CrossRef] [PubMed]

40. Paulus, M.P.; Stein, M.B. Interoception in anxiety and depression. *Brain Struct. Funct.* **2010**, *214*, 451–463. [CrossRef]
41. Lacasa, F.; Mitjavila, M.; Ochoa, S.; Balluerka, N. The relationship between attachment styles and internalizing or externalizing symptoms in clinical and nonclinical adolescents. *Anal. Psicol.* **2015**, *31*, 422–432. [CrossRef]
42. Khan, F.; Fraley, R.C.; Young, J.F.; Hankin, B.L. Developmental trajectories of attachment and depressive symptoms in children and adolescents. *Attach. Hum. Dev.* **2020**, *22*, 392–408. [CrossRef]
43. Bernaras, E.; Jaureguizar, J.; Garaigordobil, M. Child and adolescent depression: A review of theories, evaluation instruments, prevention programs and treatments. *Front. Psychol.* **2019**, *10*, 543. [CrossRef]

behavioral sciences

MDPI

Article

Relationships between Individual and Social Resources, Anxiety and Depression in the Early Lockdown Stage by the COVID-19 in Chile

Sergio Salgado [1], Carolina González-Suhr [1], Gabriela Nazar [2,*], Carlos-María Alcover [3], Raúl Ramírez-Vielma [2] and Claudio Bustos [2]

1 Departamento de Administración y Economía, Universidad de La Frontera, Temuco 4811230, Chile
2 Departamento de Psicología, Universidad de Concepción, Concepción 4070386, Chile
3 Departamento de Psicología, Universidad Rey Juan Carlos, 28922 Madrid, Spain
* Correspondence: gnazar@udec.cl

Abstract: The coronavirus disease has exposed the population to psychosocial threats that could increase mental health problems. This research analyzed the relationships between emotional states (negative [−EWB] and positive [+EWB] experienced well-being), personal resources (resilient coping [RC]), dispositional resources (control beliefs about stress [BAS]), and social resources (social support [SS]), and anxiety and depressive symptoms in a sample of the Chilean population (n = 592), who answered an online questionnaire. Multiple and moderated multiple regression analyses were carried out. Depressive symptoms showed a positive relationship with −EWB ($\beta = 0.805$; $p < 0.001$) and negative relationship with +EWB ($\beta = -0.312$; $p < 0.001$), RC ($\beta = -0.089$; $p < 0.01$), BAS ($\beta = -0.183$; $p < 0.001$) and SS ($\beta = -0.082$; $p < 0.001$). Anxiety symptoms showed a positive relationship with −EWB ($\beta = 0.568$; $p < 0.001$), and a negative relationship with +EWB ($\beta = -0.101$; $p < 0.03$) and BAS ($\beta = -0.092$; $p < 0.001$). BAS moderated the relationship between experienced well-being and depression symptoms, and RC moderated the relationship between experienced well-being with both depression and anxiety symptoms. Findings confirm the buffering effect of personal and dispositional resources when facing a sanitary and social crisis. Moreover, they help to understand the role of internal psychological processes during a crisis and how to cope with life-threatening events.

Keywords: COVID-19; stress; anxiety; coping; social support; Chile

1. Introduction

The coronavirus disease (COVID-19) is recognized as one of our time's most significanthealth and humanitarian crises, registering more than 515 million confirmed cases and more than 6,240,000 deaths [1].

Different measures have been implemented as a form of control that have meant significant restrictions on daily life activities, work, and transportation, which has generated a significant vital disruption for many people. Uncertainty, changes in the work conditions, financial threats, and the loss of social support structure due to the constraint of mobility and contact expose the population to psychosocial risks, alter the daily experience of well-being, and increase vulnerability to mental health problems.

In this regard, early reports of studies carried out in countries initially affected by COVID agree on several negative psychological effects. As the pandemic spread to the west, different international [2] and local reports [3] have confirmed the impact of the pandemic on mental health, mainly anxiety and depression [4–6], but also feelings of loneliness [7], sleep disturbances [8], eating disorders [9], and substance abuse [10] among others. In Chile, where this research was carried out, a study performed on a representative sample of 13,648 Chilean people informed that 21.4% of the sample reported moderate or severe symptoms of anxiety and/or depression [3], and subsequent empirical studies have confirmed these results [11,12].

Previous research has shown that psychological well-being describes the experience of a stable, global, and deep state of well-being [13]. Thus, psychological well-being usually includes measures of the eudaimonic and hedonic aspects of well-being, with measures widely used in the scientific literature, such as positive and negative affectivity, concerning the hedonic elements [14]. However, experienced well-being has a narrower temporal referent since this construct "assesses momentary affective states and people's feelings in real-time rather than relying on the memory of these states" [13], p. 2. The momentary affective states and people's feelings in real-time can be an antecedent or even a precursor of mental health future states. These affective states are understood here as the experienced well-being, positive or negative [15], which can be considered as antecedents either improving or worsening mental health problems, such as anxiety or depressive disorders, specifically when they become persistent, disabling, or when they induce risk behaviors, such as drug or medication use. Since the experience of living in confinement was sudden and disruptive, it seems more relevant to measure immediately experienced well-being, i.e., that experienced daily, e.g., [16–18], hence the choice of a more momentary measure of affective states in this study.

As is well established in the scientific literature about stress, the relationship between psychosocial stressors and psychological and physical health is affected by the nature, number, and persistence of the contextual stressors, in interaction with the individual's biological vulnerability, psychosocial resources, and learned patterns of stress coping [19]. Coping has long been considered a crucial process in the experience and treatment of multiple emotional and physical distress events [20]. Previous research has consolidated the growing evidence that positive emotions can broaden the range of possible coping strategies available to people during times and experiences of stress, thereby enhancing people's resilience against present and future adversity [21,22]. Coping strategies influence emotional responses, and there is empirical evidence that active coping mechanisms, such as seeking active ways to solve problems or searching for help, are functional ways to deal with stress [23,24]. Resilient coping can allow people to overcome adversity from a highly stressful psychosocial event [25]. In addition, clinical researchers have also demonstrated that individual resilience can moderate the impact of stress on anxiety and depressive symptoms [22]. Recent scientific studies in a population affected by COVID-19 indicate that stress experienced is related to coping strategies [26] and that the use of coping strategies was associated with decreased anxiety and depression during the COVID-19 confinement and pandemic experiences [27,28].

Cognitive and subjective notions people have about stress, and the beliefs as to what extent control can be exerted over it [29], have been considered in scientific research as resources to deal with this experience, which in turn lead to health outcomes, particularly well-being and mental health [30]. Stress beliefs are "a form of lay belief or theory about stress held by an individual" [31], p. 595; [32]. These beliefs can be built on both theory and scientific evidence, as well as past experiences concerning experiential and vicarious situations [31]. Moreover, stress beliefs can be situation-specific or generalized [29]. Previous empirical research has found that negative stress beliefs moderate the affective response to real-life stressors [29]. Thus, when people experienced social stress, those with high negative beliefs about stress were more prone to daily high negative affect; conversely, this association was lower in those with low negative beliefs about stress. In addition, individuals who believe that stress is controllable show greater positive affect throughout daily experiences [29]. In short, the accumulated research evidence in the stress domain [33,34] suggests that both situation-specific and generalized stress beliefs could be a promising new construct in explaining health and identifying their influences on short- and long-term health.

Among other resources to face stressful life events, there is a broad range of evidence sustaining the effects of social support on well-being [35] and its buffering effect on the psychological consequences of traumatic experiences, such as pandemics and natural disasters [36,37]. Over the past decades, scientific research has found that the main evidence for the buffering model of social support (i.e., "the process of support protecting persons from potentially adverse effects of stressful events" [38] p. 310 is associated with when such social support refers to the perceived availability of interpersonal resources that enable individuals to respond to the demands caused by stressful life events [38,39]. Social support constitutes an important pool of resources provided by other people that accumulated into personal resources [40]. Thus, empirical evidence shows that social support may be a central element of health and well-being as, together with personal resources, it is related to the overall sense of identity [40]. This follows as it relates self-concept to social network and interpersonal relationships [38]. In particular, the buffering effect of social support as a resource has been found in coping with high-stress situations, such as disasters and highly disruptive life events [41,42]. For instance, Fluharty et al. (2021), in a study carried out during the first 21 weeks of the COVID-19 lockdown, found that although mental health symptoms decreased over time for all coping strategies, only socially-supportive coping was associated with an effective and faster decrease in anxiety and depressive symptoms [43]. These research results indicate a potential protective effect of social support on psychological distress associated with the lockdown experience.

In sum, to understand how the COVID-19 crisis could affect people's mental health, we take Hobfoll's well-established Conservation of Resources Theory (COR) [44,45] as a framework. This theory considers the context and the individual responses to these circumstances, which can lead to a decrease in mental health due to the loss of valuable resources (affective, personal, social). Specifically, this study set out to analyze the relationships between emotional states (experienced well-being, negative [−EWB] and positive [+EWB]), personal resources (resilient coping [RC]), dispositional resources (beliefs about stress [BAS]), and social resources (social support [SS]) and anxiety and depressive symptoms as mental health consequences of the COVID-19 pandemic in a sample of the Chilean population.

Based on the above theoretical models and empirical evidence, we proposed the following hypotheses: There is a positive relationship between −EWB and depressive (H1) and anxiety (H2) symptoms; and a negative relationship between +EWB, RC, BAS, and SS with depression (H3.1, H3.2, H3.3, and H3.4, respectively) and anxiety symptoms (H4.1, H4.2, H4.3, and H4.4, respectively). Additionally, we expect that RC, BAS, and SS, have a moderating effect on the relationship between −EWB and depression (H5.1, H5.2, and H5.3, respectively) and +EWB and depression (H6.1, H6.2, and H6.3, respectively); and, that RC, BAS, and SS have a moderating effect on the relationship between −EWB and anxiety symptoms (H7.1, H7.2, and H7.3, respectively) and +EWB and anxiety symptoms (H8.1, H8.2, and H8.3, respectively). Figure 1a,b.

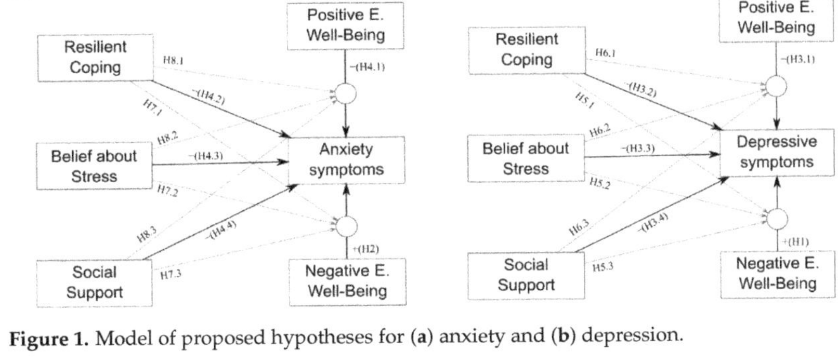

Figure 1. Model of proposed hypotheses for (**a**) anxiety and (**b**) depression.

2. Materials and Methods

2.1. Research Design and Participants

According to the purpose of the study, a cross-sectional correlational study was conducted on a non-probabilistic sample aimed at a general Chilean adult population. The sample consisted of 591 participants who took part in the study (592 responses to the online questionnaire were obtained, of which a duplicate case identified through e-mail was eliminated), with an average age of 37.63 years (SD = 12.85). 76% were female (n = 449), 23.7% were male (n = 140), and 0.3% identified as another gender (n = 2). All the participants lived in Chile. Most of the participants had a full-time day job (n = 269; 45.5%), but they also had part-time jobs (n = 43; 7.3%), were independent workers (n = 82; 13.9%), students (n = 79; 13.4%), unemployed (n = 55; 9.3%), retired (n = 30; 5.1%), homemakers (n = 24; 4.1%) and others (n = 9; 1.5%). 37.5% (n = 222) reported having postgraduate studies, 43.3% (n = 256) graduate studies, 8.3% (n = 49) technical studies, 10.7% (n = 63) had high school and 0.2% (n = 1) elementary school.

2.2. Instruments

Experienced well-being was measured by the subscale named alike from The Pemberton Happiness Index scale [13]. It is a 10-item measure, five items of +EWB (e.g., 'I did something fun with someone'), and five of −EWB (e.g., 'I was worried about personal matters'). Response options were: 'Yes, it happened to me last days' or 'No, it did not happen to me last days'. Internal consistency, as measured by Cronbach's Alpha, was above 0.89, and the results from this initial validation study provided very good support for the scale's psychometric properties (single-factor structure, and convergent and incremental validity) [13]. In this study, Cronbach's alpha was 0.73 for +EWB and 0.78 for −EWB.

Resilient Coping was measured by the Spanish version of the Brief Resilience Scale (BRS) [25,46], a four-item scale: 'I look for creative ways to alter difficult situations'. The format is a Likert response with 5 anchor points, from 0 = does not describe me at all to 6 = describes me very well. Internal consistency as measured by Cronbach's Alpha was 0.86. The scale demonstrated good psychometric properties in terms of criterion validity, homogeneity indices, and dimensional structure [25]. In this study, Cronbach's alpha was 0.83.

Beliefs about stress were measured with the Beliefs About Stress Scale (BASS) [31], subscale Control Beliefs, composed of three items: 'Stress is something I can control to some extent'. The answering format was a 4-point Likert scale: 1 completely disagree to 4: completely agree. The scales showed good to acceptable internal consistency (Cronbach's Alpha 0.73–0.87) and retest-reliability ($r_{tt6\text{-}8}$ 0.61–0.81). Correlations with optimism, pessimism, neuroticism, and somatosensory amplification (r 0.15–0.47) indicated high to medium discriminant validity. Moreover, stress beliefs appear to be multidimensional and stable over time [34]. In this study, Cronbach's alpha was 0.86.

Social support was measured with the abbreviated version of the Medical Outcome Study Social Support Survey (MOS-SSS) [47,48] composed of four items, scored on a 5-point response from 1 = never to 5 = always, sample item is (e.g., 'Do you have someone who helps you to solve your personal problems?'). The reliability of this 4-item scale was acceptable (Cronbach's Alpha was 0.83). In addition, a good fit was obtained in terms of its factorial structure [47]. In this study, Cronbach's alpha was 0.80.

Anxiety was measured by the Generalized Anxiety Disorder-7 (GAD-7) [49] in its Spanish adaptation from [50], which consists of seven items about people's experiences during the last week. An example item statement is 'Feeling nervous, anxious or on edge thinking' and the participant must respond with one of the four alternatives from 0 = never to 3 = almost every day. Cronbach's Alpha reached an excellent value (0.93). The scale was shown to be one-dimensional through factor analysis (explained variance = 72%). Likewise, the scale obtained good indices in terms of inter-rater validity, criterion validity, and discriminant validity [50]. In this study, Cronbach's alpha was 0.90.

Depression was measured by the Patient Health Questionnaire Depression Scale (PHQ-9) [51] adapted to Spanish, consisting of nine items about the frequency of a personal situation in the last week, scored on a 4-point Likert response format from 0 = never to 3 = almost every day. An example item statement is: 'Little interest or pleasure in doing things' [52]. The internal reliability of the PHQ-9 was high, with a Cronbach's Alpha of 0.89. Construct validity was established by the strong association between PHQ-9 scores and functional status, disability days, and symptom-related difficulty [51]. In this study, Cronbach's alpha was 0.90.

Both scales GAD-7 and PHQ-9 are used as screening tools in clinical contexts, however, they are also widely used for research purposes [49–51].

2.3. Procedure and Ethics

On 16 March 2020, the Chilean Government began to decree social distancing and confinement measures. They progressively increased restrictions on productive, commercial, and consumption activities as different regions detected contagions and deaths. The data were collected via an online questionnaire (Questionpro) between 24 March and 23 April. The recruitment strategy combined professional networks, social networks, professional associations, undergraduate and graduate students, and personal contacts, who were invited to participate and disseminate this invitation among their network of contacts (snowball strategy). The participants took an average of 27 min to complete all the instruments. When necessary, they could save their progress and take it up again when convenient.

First, the psychometric properties of the instruments were analyzed. Afterward, a multiple regression analysis was performed to test the relationship between the independent variables (+EWB and −EWB, RC, BAS, and SS) and the two dependent variables (depression and anxiety symptoms).

Then, a moderated multiple regression analysis was carried out to explore the potential moderating role of RC, BAS, and SS in the relationship between +EWB and −EWB and depression and anxiety symptoms. These analyses included age, gender (female = 1; male = 2; other = 3), and educational level (elementary school = 1; high school = 2; technical studies = 3; University degree = 4; Postgraduate = 5) as control variables.

To probe the moderation, two techniques were used. First, the pick-a-point approach was used, plotting the simple regression lines for three values of the moderating variable: mean, −1 sd, and +1 sd. Second, we use the J-N technique, which indicates over what range of the moderator the effect of the predictor is significant or not significant.

The project underwent assessment by the Ethics and Bioethics Committee of the Universidad de Concepción (CEBB 650-2020, March 2020), and the participants were asked to sign an informed consent. When the proposed conditions were agreed upon, the participants marked a square indicating they were over 18 years, had been informed, and understood the nature of this study and their decision to participate voluntarily.

3. Results

3.1. Psychometric Properties of the Instruments

A measurement model was tested using CFA, in which all variables with all their items were considered to verify that the scales had convergent validity (relationships between items and their factors) and discriminant validity (that the items are not strongly related to other factors, and that the factors do not have high correlations with each other). The CFA showed a good fit of the data to the model ($x2/df$ = 2.033; CFI = 0.964; TLI = 0.961; $SRMR$ = 0.06 y $RMSEA$ = 0.042 [0.038, 0.045]), which also supports discriminant validity of the measures. Table 1 shows the descriptive values, internal consistency (polychoric), and Pearson correlations.

Table 1. Mean, standard deviation, internal consistency, and Pearson's correlations for the variables under study.

Variable	n	Mean	SD	αord	Pearson's Correlations						
					(1)	(2)	(3)	(4)	(5)	(6)	(7)
1. Depression symptoms	591	1.846	0.6377	0.9042	1	0.72 **	−0.23 **	−0.48 **	−0.43 **	−0.33 **	0.53 **
2. Anxiety	591	2.106	0.7244	0.9041		1	−0.12 **	−0.40 **	−0.33 **	−0.26 **	0.52 **
3. SS	591	3.752	0.9038	0.8044			1	0.12 **	0.18 **	0.21 **	−0.10 *
4. BAS	591	2.949	0.7788	0.8682				1	0.56 **	0.28 **	−0.29 **
5. RC	591	3.719	0.7557	0.8369					1	0.32 **	−0.27 **
6. +EWB	591	0.6968	0.2799	0.7381						1	−0.17 **
7. −EWB	591	0.5739	0.2849	0.7866							1

Note: αor: Cronbach's alpha based on polychoric correlation. SS: Social Support; BAS: Beliefs about stress; REC: Resilient Coping; +EW: Positive experienced well-being; −EW: Negative Experienced well-being. * $p < 0.05$; ** $p < 0.01$.

The model for depression symptoms as a dependent variable presented a slight increase in the variance of the residuals when the predicted value increased. In contrast, the model for anxiety as a dependent was homoscedastic, observing in a first analysis that the residuals had positive skewness, controlled using the logarithm of anxiety. The moderation models meet the assumptions of linearity and normality of residuals.

3.2. Multiple Regression Analysis

Regarding the dependent variable depression, the regression model explained 47.6% of the variance (F (12, 578) = 45.77, $p < 0.001$, adjusted $R^2 = 0.476$).

In line with the hypotheses H1, H3.1, H3.2, H3.3, and H3.4 (see Table 2, non-moderated) a positive significant coefficient was obtained for the −EWB and significant negative coefficients for +EWB, RC, BAS, and SS. No control variables showed a significant relationship with depression symptoms.

Table 2. Non-moderated and Moderated regression analysis summary for the interaction between SS (Social Support), BAS (Beliefs about stress), and RC (Resilient Coping); and +EWB (Positive experienced well-being), and −EWB (Negative experienced well-being) predicting depression symptoms.

Variable	Non-Moderated		Moderated	
	B	CI 95%	B	CI 95%
(Intercept)	3.281 **	[2.331, 4.231]	1.944 **	[0.769, 3.119]
SS	−0.082 **	[−0.126, −0.038]	−0.025	[−0.177, 0.126]
BAS	−0.183 **	[−0.243, −0.123]	−0.194	[−0.393, 0.003]
RC	−0.089 **	[−0.152, −0.028]	0.219 *	[0.006, 0.434]
+EWB	−0.312 **	[−0.460, −0.165]	0.158	[−0.594, 0.910]
−EWB	0.805 **	[0.661, 0.949]	2.463 **	[1.669, 3.257]
Gender = Male	−0.069	[−0.159, 0.019]	−0.048	[−0.135, 0.040]
Gender = Other	0.317	[−0.329, 0.963]	0.463	[−0.172, 1.098]
Education = High School	−0.100	[−1.017, 0.817]	−0.097	[−0.997, 0.802]
Education = Technical studies	−0.303	[−1.225, 0.620]	−0.341	[−1.246, 0.563]
Education = University Degree	−0.334	[−1.248, 0.580]	−0.337	[−1.233, 0.559]
Education = Postgraduate	−0.470	[−1.385, 0.445]	−0.462	[−1.359, 0.434]
Age(years)	−0.003	[−0.007, 0.000]	−0.003 *	[−0.007, −0.000]
SS x +EWB			−0.003	[−0.153, 0.148]
SS x −EWB			−0.083	[−0.229, 0.064]
BAS x +EWB			0.273 **	[0.070, 0.476]
BAS x −EWB			−0.280 **	[−0.492, −0.068]
RC x +EWB			−0.345 **	[−0.561, −0.129]
RC x −EWB			−0.140	[−0.359, 0.078]

Table 2. *Cont.*

Variable	Non-Moderated		Moderated	
	B	CI 95%	*B*	CI 95%
Adjusted R^2	0.476		0.514	
F	45.766 **		33.651 **	
ΔR^2			0.027	
ΔF			5.318 **	

Note: * $p < 0.05$; ** $p < 0.01$. All numeric predictor variables are centered to the mean.

Regarding anxiety, the regression model explained 37.9% of the variance (F (12, 578) = 31.09, $p < 0.001$, adjusted $R^2 = 0.379$). In line with the hypotheses H2, H4.1, and H4.4 (see Table 3, non-moderated), significant weights in a positive direction were shown with −EWB, and in a negative direction with +EWB and BAS. The control variable gender showed a significant regression weight, which indicated that men showed a lower level of anxiety compared to women. Hypotheses H4.2 and H4.3 were not supported.

Table 3. Non-moderated and Moderated analysis summary for SS (Social Support), BAS (Beliefs about stress), RC (Resilient Coping), +EWB (Positive experienced well-being), and −EWB (Negative experienced well-being) predicting anxiety symptoms.

Variable	Non-Moderated		Moderated	
	B	CI 95%	*B*	CI 95%
(Intercept)	0.904 **	[0.342, 1.465]	0.239	[−0.847, 1.325]
SS	0.002	[−0.024, 0.028]	0.051	[−0.043, 0.144]
BAS	−0.092 **	[−0.128, −0.057]	−0.555	[−1.188, 0.079]
BAS2			0.082	[−0.030, 0.194]
RC	−0.027	[−0.064, 0.010]	0.44	[−0.225, 1.105]
RC2			−0.049	[−0.147, 0.049]
+EWB	−0.101 *	[−0.189, −0.015]	−1.207 *	[−2.307, −0.107]
−EWB	0.568 **	[0.484, 0.654]	2.167 **	[1.069, 3.264]
Gender = Male	−0.081 **	[−0.133, −0.028]	−0.082 **	[−0.135, −0.029]
Gender = Other	0.065	[−0.317, 0.447]	0.085	[−0.295, 0.466]
Education = High School	−0.106	[−0.648, 0.436]	−0.037	[−0.574, 0.501]
Education = Technical studies	−0.121	[−0.666, 0.425]	−0.047	[−0.588, 0.495]
Education = University Degree	−0.152	[−0.692, 0.388]	−0.085	[−0.620, 0.451]
Education = Postgraduate	−0.143	[−0.684, 0.398]	−0.076	[−0.612, 0.460]
Age 2 (years)	0.001	[−0.001, 0.003]	0.001	[−0.001, 0.003]
SS x +EWB			−0.056	[−0.149, 0.037]
SS x −EWB			−0.024	[−0.114, 0.065]
BAS x +EWB			0.852 **	[0.232, 1.472]
BAS x −EWB			0.059	[−0.626, 0.746]
BAS2 x +EWB			−0.147 **	[−0.258, −0.035]
BAS2 x −EWB			−0.013	[−0.134, 0.108]
RC x +EWB			0.219	[−0.476, 0.914]
RC x −EWB			−0.858 *	[−1.569, −0.147]
RC2 x +EWB			−0.046	[−0.147, 0.055]
RC2 x −EWB			0.113 *	[0.011, 0.215]
Adjusted R^2	0.379		0.419	
F	31.094 **		16,991 **	
ΔR^2			0.026	
ΔF			2.148 *	

Note: Regression calculated on logarithmic transformation of anxiety symptoms scale. * $p < 0.05$; ** $p < 0.01$.

3.3. Moderated Multiple Regression Analysis

Subsequently, a moderated multiple regression analysis was carried out to explore the potential moderating role of RC, BAS, and SS in the relationship between +EWB and −EWB, and depressive and anxious symptoms. Regarding depression symptoms, when comparing the moderated regression model with the original (non-moderated) model, a significant difference was observed that supports the significance of the moderation (F (6, 572) = 5.318, $p < 0.001$).

As shown in Table 2 (moderated), BAS significantly moderated the relationship between −EWB and depression symptoms. In this case, the relationship was positive for all BAS values, so as control beliefs increased, decreased the relationship between −EWB and depression symptoms (see Figure 2). On the other hand, BAS and RC significantly moderated the relationship between +EWB and depression symptoms. Here, for all BAS values, the relationship between +EWB and depression symptoms was inverse; that is, as BAS increased, the strength of that relationship decreased (see Figure 3). Additionally, when RC was low (less than one SD), the effect of +EWB on depression symptoms was near zero; as RC increased, the reverse relationship became progressively stronger (see Figure 4). The moderating effect on the relationship between −EWB and +EWB, and depression symptoms, support the hypotheses H5.2, H6.1, and H6.2, whereas hypotheses H5.1, H5.3, and H6.3 were not supported.

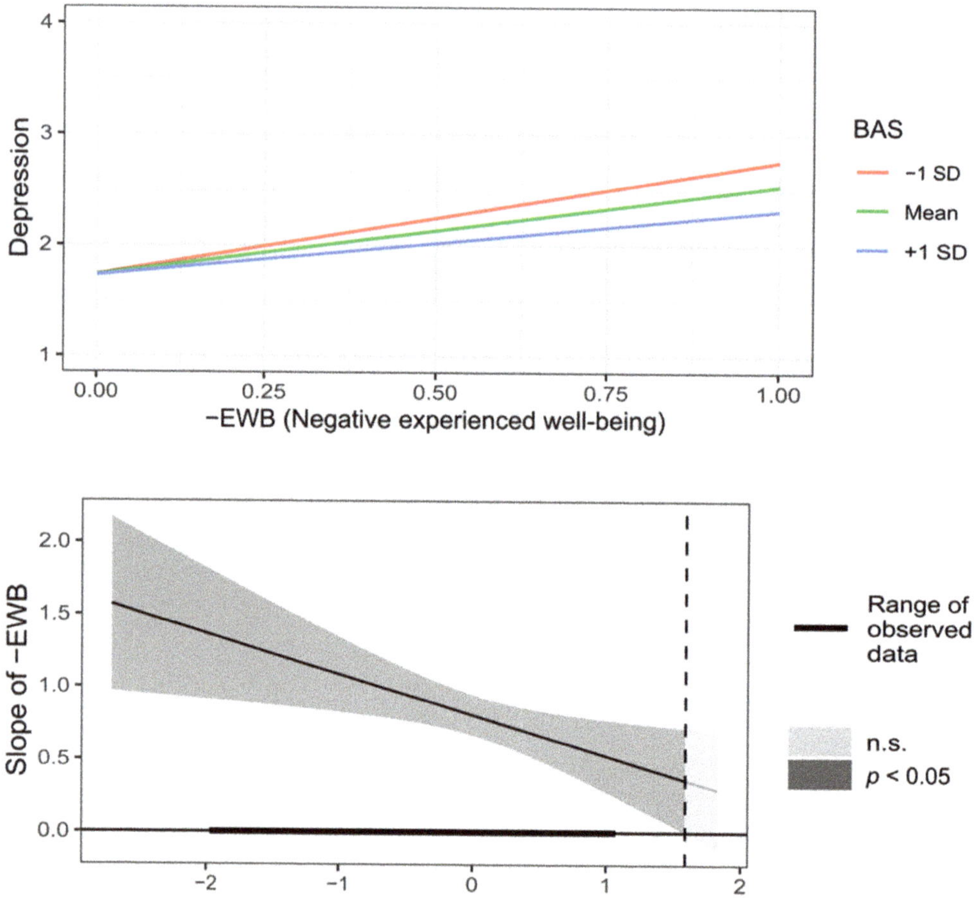

Figure 2. Graphic representation of BAS (Beliefs about stress) moderation on the relationship between −EWB (Negative experienced well-being) and depression symptoms.

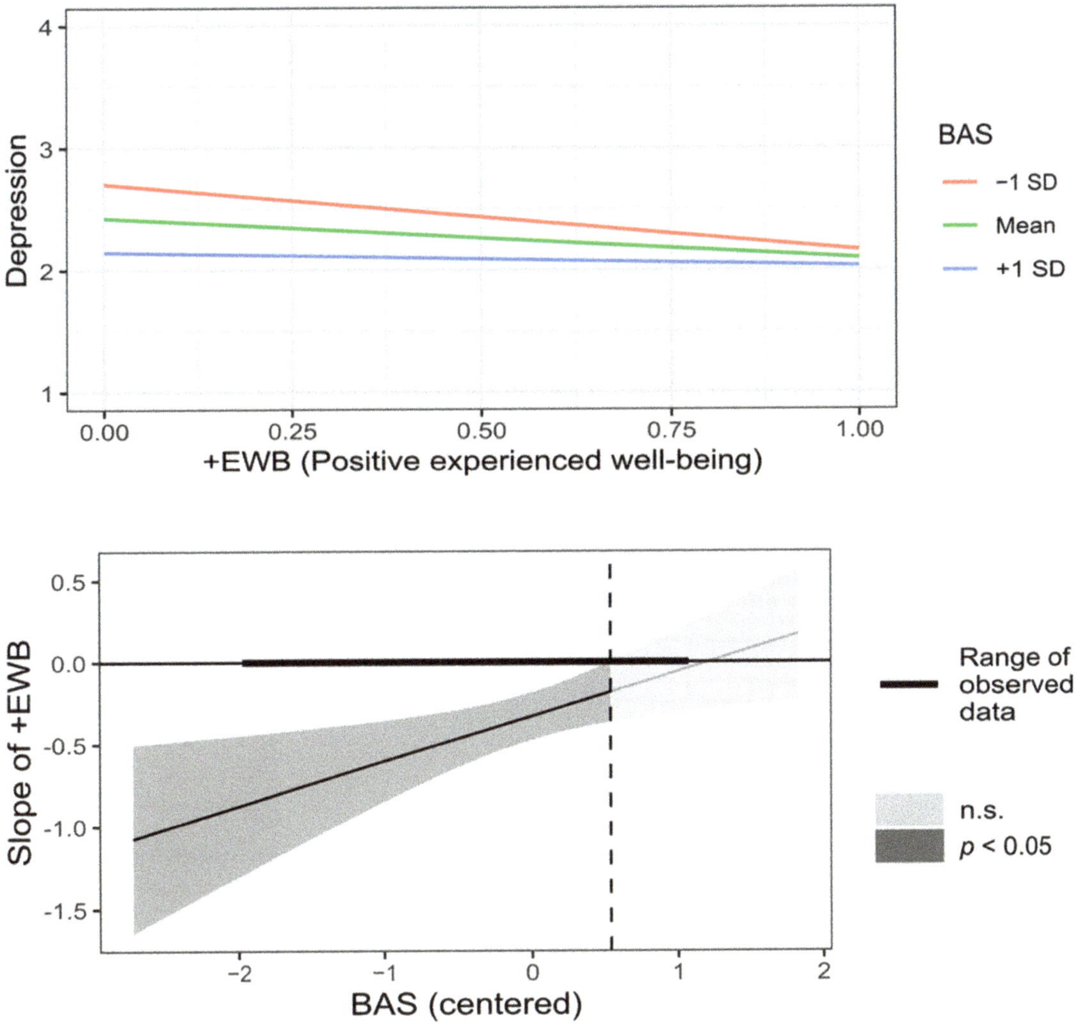

Figure 3. Graphic representation of BAS (Beliefs about stress) moderation on the relationship between +EWB (Positive experienced well-being) and depression symptoms.

Regarding the moderation of the relationship between +EWB and −EWB, and anxiety, when comparing the linear moderated regression model with the original model, there was no significant difference (F (6, 572) = 1.018, p = 0.41). Then, it was taken into account that the graphic exploration of these effects revealed that the moderation of BAS and RC was not linear: A distinctive U-shaped curve was detected in the effect of RC in the relation between −EWB on anxiety, and an inverted U-shaped curve in the effect of BAS in the relation between +EWB on anxiety. Therefore, the polynomial in degree two (quadratic) for BAS and RC was added to the moderated regression model, and this model did show a significant change compared to the model with linear moderation (F (6, 566) = 3.277, p = 0.003). As shown in Figure 5, for all viable RC values, the direct relationship between −EWB and anxiety is significant. When RC decreases below the mean, the relation between −EWB and anxiety becomes stronger, but the relation between −EWB and anxiety is nearly the same for values of RC near and higher than the mean. In the case of BAS, as shown in

Figure 6, the region of no significance starts at 1.83 and ends at 4.39; so, for BAS lower than 1.83 (8.12% of the sample), there is a significant inverse relation between +EWB and anxiety; between 1.83 and the mean of BAS (2.94), the relation tends to zero and for values higher than the mean, the relation becomes stronger, but not enough to be outside the region of no significance. Therefore, regarding the moderating effect on the relationship between −EWB and +EWB, and anxiety, the hypotheses H7.1 and H8.2 were supported, and the hypotheses H7.2, H7.3, H8.1, and H8.3 were not supported.

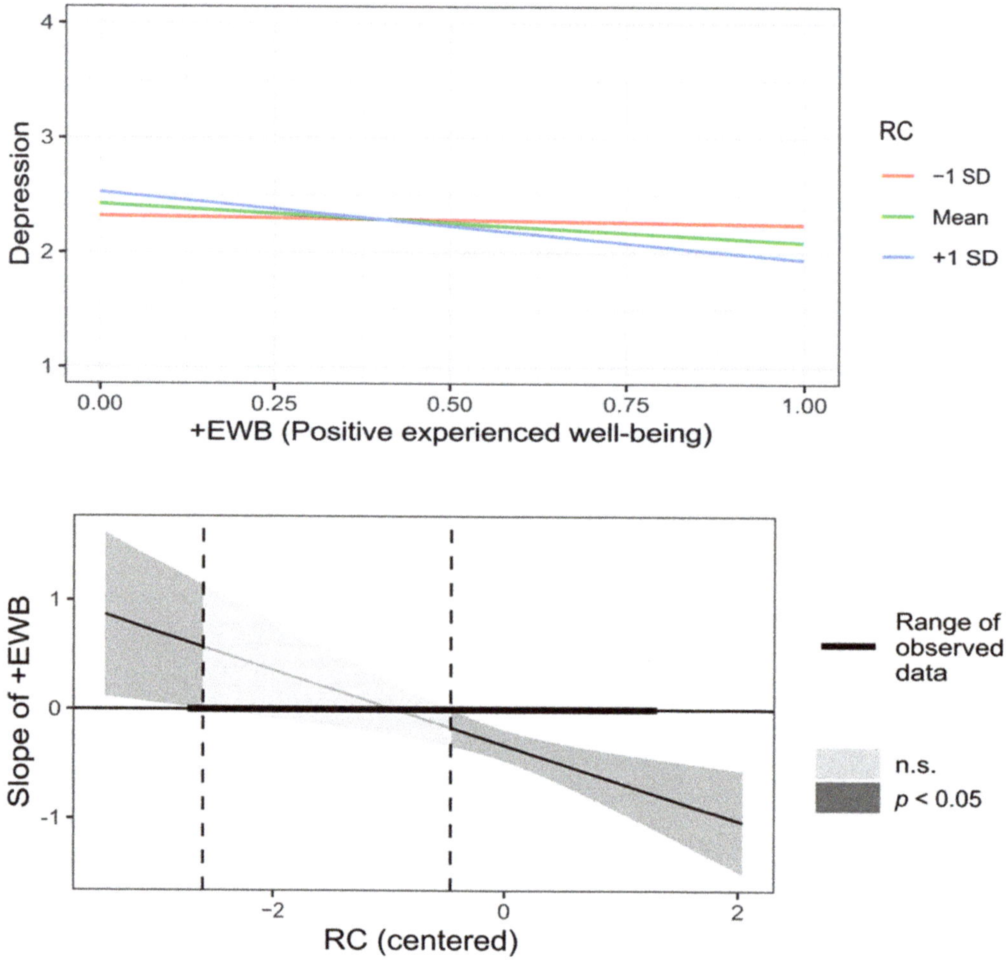

Figure 4. Graphic representation of BC (Resilient coping) moderation on the relationship between +EWB (Positive experienced well-being) and depression symptoms.

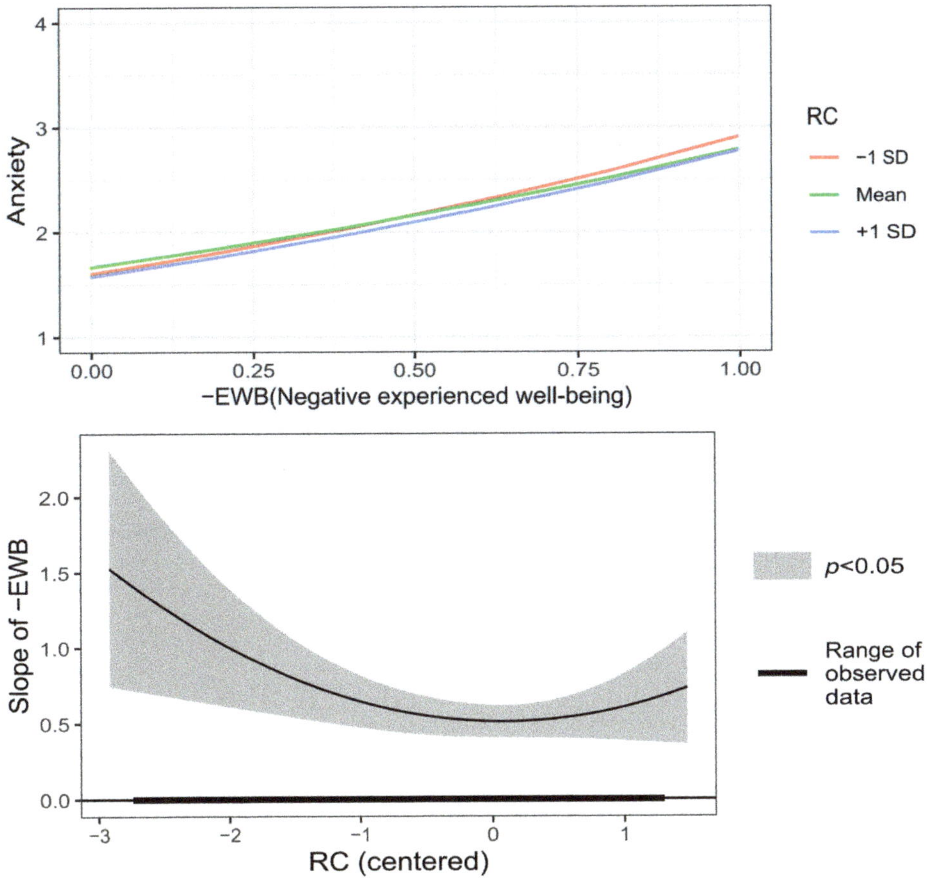

Figure 5. Graphic representation of RC (Resilient coping) moderation on the relationship between −EWB (Negative experienced well-being) and anxiety symptoms.

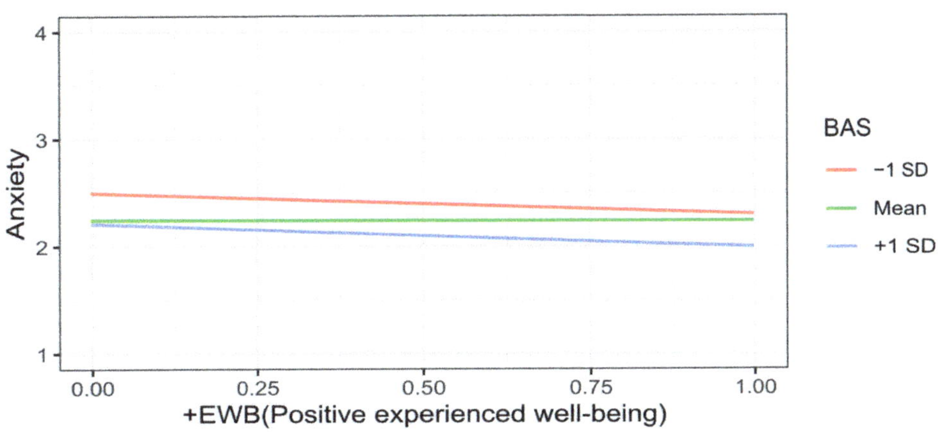

Figure 6. *Cont.*

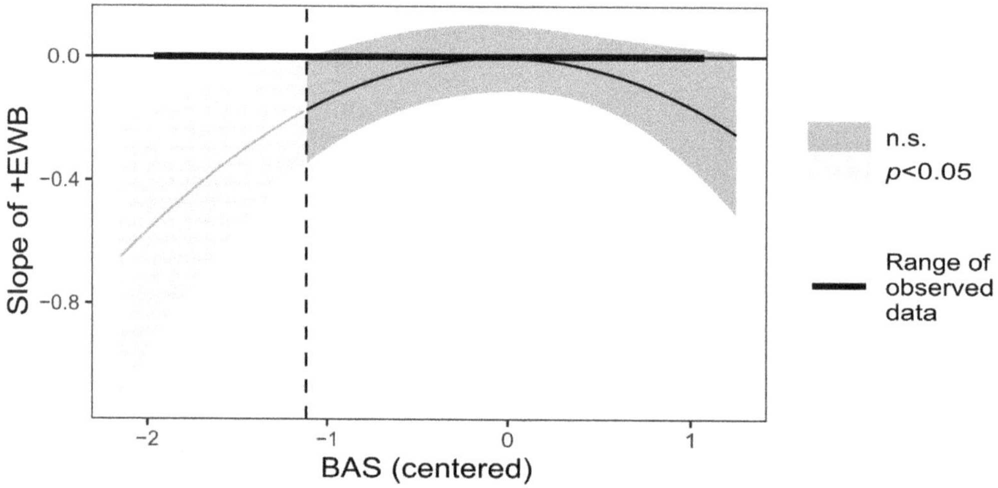

Figure 6. Graphic representation of BAS (Beliefs about stress) moderation on the relationship between +EWB (Positive experienced well-being) and anxiety symptoms.

4. Discussion

Following the conservation of resources theory (COR) [44,45], the purpose of this work was to test the relationships between emotional states (experienced well-being, negative [−EWB] and positive [+EWB]), personal resources (i.e., resilient coping [RC]), dispositional resources (i.e., beliefs about stress [BAS]), social resources (i.e., social support [SS]), and anxiety and depressive symptoms as mental health consequences of the COVID-19 pandemic in a sample of the Chilean population. According to COR theory, lower levels of personal, social, and material resources are important determinants of poorer psychological adaptation to adverse situations. Specifically, the COR theory postulates that the loss of resources not only is more powerful than resource gain in magnitude, but also it tends to affect people more quickly and at an increasing rate over time, which is relevant in the context of the COVID -19 crisis.

Meta-analytic results on the prevalence of depression in the general population during the COVID -19 outbreak [53] show that the pooled prevalence of depression was 25% (95% CI: 18–33%), which appears to be seven times higher than the global estimated prevalence of depression in the general population in 2017 (3.44%) [54]. Additionally, in previous empirical studies, it has been found that during the initial stages of lockdown, Chile showed high levels of stress, which is expected in a country with a low level of social protection, thus the approach of this study seems particularly relevant [55,56]. These results, showing increased levels of stress, anxiety, and depressive symptoms, have been confirmed in both cross-sectional and longitudinal studies with data obtained during the first year of the pandemic and even in subsequent years, e.g., [53,57–59]. Moreover, these empirical results are confirmed cross-culturally, as empirical evidence shows similar indicators of worse mental health across geographic areas, e.g., [60–63].

Our findings revealed that variables related to personal resources (coping strategies), dispositional resources (beliefs about stress) and affective states (experienced positive well-being), and social resources (social support) are negatively related to depression symptoms in confinement, whereas experienced negative well-being is positively related. Our results allow a first approximation to the identification of the factors associated with the presence of depressive symptomatology in lockdown, such as EWB, and add RC, BAS, and SS, to other personal and social factors inversely related to depression in confinement, such as group membership, personal identity strength, and perceived personal control [64], or psychological flexibility [65].

Regarding anxiety, results show a negative relationship between control belief of stress and positive well-being, and positive with negative well-being. Once again, our results not only note the increased anxiety due to confinement, a general phenomenon across countries during the pandemic [36,66,67] and a proven increase in comparison with pre-pandemic anxiety levels (e.g., [68]) but identify possible associated factors that mitigate its incidence, adding into the knowledge of other effective coping behaviors [27].

Furthermore, our study has found interesting differences in the moderating effects of personal, dispositional, and social resources in the relationship between dominant affective states and depressive and anxiety symptomatology. Thus, while the effects are linear for +EWB and RC in the relationship between +EWB and depression symptoms, and for BAS in the relationship between −EWB and depression symptoms, that moderating effect of both variables is quadratic for the relationships between +EWB and anxiety (but just BAS was significant).

Contrary to expectations, we did not find any direct or moderating effect of SS on the study variables. Although this contradicts much of the research carried out during the COVID-19 pandemic [26,64–69], there is also evidence that government-imposed stay-at-home and personal distancing were independently associated with higher symptoms of depression and generalized anxiety disorder, beyond the potential protective effects of available social resources, such as SS and social network size [55]. This may be as a result of isolation and social distance being imposed suddenly and our data came from the first weeks of confinement, all of which could have limited the relations and communication with social networks and perceived SS. Future longitudinal studies should check whether, in subsequent weeks, the role of SS was maintained or altered, and if so, in which direction.

The results obtained allow us to go beyond the mere confirmation of the worsening of mental health during confinement and represent an additional step in identifying factors that can suffer the consequences of current and future lockdowns and severe confinements (for instance, currently in several regions of China). This practical value of our study will have to be corroborated by data from longitudinal designs that allow confirmation of the possible existence of causal relationships between variables, as well as the moderation effects detected.

4.1. Strengths and Limitations

Although time has passed since these data were collected, the results obtained are timely and relevant for various reasons. First, they show that some psychological variables do not develop linear effects, which is commonly reported in the literature, so their scientific novelty does not rely solely on the situation caused by the COVID-19 pandemic. Second, we believe that the initial reaction of people in a situation of abrupt limitation of social routines, as it was at early lockdown, is not exhausted in this event, and it can be extrapolated to other hard and inadvertent situations. These findings help us to better understand internal psychological processes during a crisis and to be prepared for other public health crises, natural disasters, or armed conflicts, that profoundly affect our lives.

As a consequence of the sampling process, based on the snowball technique, the participants are a non-probabilistic sample of the population. Future studies in this research domain should include concentrating on specific people or contexts (professional groups, vulnerable groups, youth, or older people among others) or representative samples to identify more accurately the differential effects in each setting. Although the sample is unbalanced in terms of gender, it was possible to analyze its effect, concluding what is already known in the literature regarding a higher prevalence of anxiety for females. Additionally, the cross-sectional nature of the design only allows the identification of associations between variables, and future research could be based on experimental, quasi-experimental, or longitudinal designs. In any case, the relationships found are largely supported, albeit in other settings, by previous literature. However, respondents were not tested before for mental or physical disease, and mental and physical chronic diseases were not considered for the present research. In addition, some other sociodemographic variables or family/work/financial data that have been shown to be relevant to people's mental and physical lives during the pandemic outbreak were not considered and should be included in future studies, using other techniques such as diary data collection or in-depth interviews.

4.2. Practical Implications

The results obtained allow us to go beyond the mere confirmation of the worsening of mental health during confinement and represent an additional step in identifying factors that can suffer the consequences of current and future lockdowns and severe confinements (for instance, currently in several regions of China). This practical value of our study will have to be corroborated by data from longitudinal designs that allow confirmation of the possible existence of causal relationships between variables, as well as the moderation effects detected. Additionally, some other practical recommendations arise. First, to improve personal resources conservation, it is important to promote the ability to focus on positive experiences and intensify and prolong these positive feelings. Resilience training and self-esteem development in educational curricula, together with pedagogical practices such as systematic positive feedback, can be strategies to enhance personal resources. Second, in terms of social support and protection, it is relevant to use social networks and new digital technologies to train and reinforce social resources that favor personal growth and mutual care.

5. Conclusions

The coronavirus disease (COVID-19) has disrupted the daily experience and exposed the population to psychosocial threats that alter well-being and increase vulnerability to mental health problems. These findings support the relationship between affective states and immediate emotional experience, namely experienced well-being, with depressive and anxiety symptoms during confinement. Additionally, it highlights the protective role of personal and social resources. Specifically, someone's resilience, control beliefs of stress, and social support were found as relevant assets with a buffer effect that can impede that experiences of distress under a crisis turned into mental health problems.

Author Contributions: Conceptualization: S.S., C.G.-S., G.N., C.-M.A. and R.R.-V.; Data analysis: S.S., C.G.-S. and C.B.; writing—original draft preparation; S.S., C.G.-S., G.N., C.-M.A. and R.R.-V.; writing—review and editing: S.S., C.G.-S., G.N., C.-M.A., R.R.-V. and C.B. All authors have read and agreed to the published version of the manuscript.

Funding: This research has been partially supported by the project DIUFRO DI20-0080 (Universidad de La Frontera, Chile) and the Agencia Nacional de Investigación y Desarrollo, ANID, MEC80190085.

Institutional Review Board Statement: The study was conducted following the Declaration of Helsinki and approved by the Institutional Review Board (or Ethics Committee) of the Ethics and Bioethics Committee of the Universidad de Concepción (CEBB 650-2020, March 2020) for studies involving humans.

Informed Consent Statement: Informed consent was obtained from all subjects involved in the study.

Data Availability Statement: Not applicable.

Conflicts of Interest: The authors declare no conflict of interest.

References

1. Johns Hopkins University & Medicine Coronavirus Resources Center. Available online: https://coronavirus.jhu.edu/map.html (accessed on 10 May 2022).
2. World Health Organization. Considerations for Quarantine of Individuals in the Context of Containment for Coronavirus Disease (COVID-19): Interim Guidance. March 2020. Available online: https://apps.who.int/iris/handle/10665/331497 (accessed on 15 September 2021).
3. MDS Chile, Ministerio de Desarrollo Social de Chile. Encuesta Social COVID-19 [Social Survey COVID-19]. Available online: http://observatorio.ministeriodesarrollosocial.gob.cl/noticias/not1.php# (accessed on 15 September 2021).

4. Brooks, S.K.; Webster, R.K.; Smith, L.E.; Woodland, L.; Wessely, S.; Greenberg, N.; Rubin, G.J. The psychological impact of quarantine and how to reduce it: Rapid review of the evidence. *Lancet* **2020**, *395*, 912–920. [CrossRef]
5. Cao, W.; Fang, Z.; Hou, G.; Han, M.; Xu, X.; Dong, J.; Zheng, J. The psychological impact of the COVID-19 epidemic on college students in China. *Psychiatry Res.* **2020**, *287*, 112934. [CrossRef] [PubMed]
6. Wang, Y.; Di, Y.; Ye, J.; Wei, W. Study on the public psychological states and its related factors during the outbreak of coronavirus disease 2019 (COVID-19) in some regions of China. *Psychol. Health Med.* **2021**, *26*, 13–22. [CrossRef]
7. Pai, N.; Vella, S.L. COVID-19 and loneliness: A rapid systematic review. *Aust. N. Z. J. Psychiatry* **2021**, *55*, 1144–1156. [CrossRef] [PubMed]
8. Partinen, M.; Holzinger, B.; Morin, C.M.; Espie, C.; Chung, F.; Penzel, T.; Benedict, C.; Bolstad, C.J.; Cedernaes, J.; Chan, R.N.Y.; et al. Sleep and daytime problems during the COVID-19 pandemic and effects of coronavirus infection, confinement and financial suffering: A multinational survey using a harmonised questionnaire. *BMJ Open* **2021**, *11*, e050672.
9. Gao, Y.; Bagheri, N.; Furuya-Kanamori, L. Has the COVID-19 pandemic lockdown worsened eating disorders symptoms among patients with eating disorders? A systematic review. *J. Public Health* **2022**, 1–10. [CrossRef]
10. Avena, N.M.; Simkus, J.; Lewandowski, A.; Gold, M.S.; Potenza, M.N. Substance use disorders and behavioral addictions during the COVID-19 pandemic and COVID-19-related restrictions. *Front. Psychiatry* **2021**, *12*, 653674. [CrossRef]
11. Caqueo-Urízar, A.; Urzúa, A.; Aragón-Caqueo, D.; Charles, C.H.; El-Khatib, Z.; Otu, A.; Yaya, S. Mental health and the COVID-19 pandemic in Chile. *Psychol. Trauma Theory Res. Pract. Policy.* **2020**, *12*, 521–523. [CrossRef]
12. Duarte, F.; Jiménez-Molina, A. Psychological distress during the COVID-19 epidemic in Chile: The role of economic uncertainty. *PLoS ONE* **2021**, *16*, e0251683. [CrossRef]
13. Hervás, G.; Vázquez, C. Construction and validation of a measure of integrative well-being in seven languages: The Pemberton Happiness Index. *Health Qual. Life Outcomes* **2013**, *11*, 66. [CrossRef]
14. Watson, D.; Clark, L.A.; Carey, G. Positive and negative affectivity and their relation to anxiety and depressive disorders. *J. Abnorm. Psychol.* **1988**, *97*, 346–353. [CrossRef] [PubMed]
15. Diener, E.; Sandvik, E.; Pavot, W.; Gallagher, D. Response artifacts in the measurement of subjective well-being. *Soc. Indic. Res.* **1991**, *24*, 35–56. [CrossRef]
16. Brose, A.; Blanke, E.S.; Schmiedek, F.; Kramer, A.C.; Schmidt, A.; Neubauer, A.B. Change in mental health symptoms during the COVID-19 pandemic: The role of appraisals and daily life experiences. *J. Pers.* **2021**, *89*, 468–482. [CrossRef] [PubMed]
17. Cunningham, T.J.; Fields, E.C.; Kensinger, E.A. Boston College daily sleep and well-being survey data during the early phase of the COVID-19 pandemic. *Sci. Data* **2021**, *8*, 110. [CrossRef] [PubMed]
18. Lades, L.K.; Laffan, K.; Daly, M.; Delaney, L. Daily emotional well-being during the COVID-19 pandemic. *Br. J. Health Psychol.* **2020**, *25*, 902–911. [CrossRef]
19. Schneiderman, N.; Ironson, G.; Siegel, S.D. Stress and health: Psychological, behavioral, and biological determinants. *Annu. Rev. Clin. Psychol.* **2005**, *1*, 607–628. [CrossRef] [PubMed]
20. Lazarus, R.S. Coping theory and research: Past, present, and future. *Psychosom. Med.* **1993**, *55*, 234–247. [CrossRef]
21. Folkman, S.; Moskowitz, J.T. Stress, positive emotion, and coping. *Curr. Dir. Psychol. Sci.* **2000**, *9*, 115–118. [CrossRef]
22. Gloria, C.T.; Steinhardt, M.A. Relationships among positive emotions, coping, resilience and mental health. *Stress Health* **2016**, *32*, 145–156. [CrossRef]
23. Carver, C.S.; Connor-Smith, J. Personality and coping. *Annu. Rev. Psychol.* **2010**, *61*, 679–704. [CrossRef]
24. Taylor, S.E.; Stanton, A.L. Coping resources, coping processes, and mental health. *Annu. Rev. Clin. Psychol.* **2007**, *3*, 377–401. [CrossRef] [PubMed]
25. Moret-Tatay, C.; Fernández-Muñoz, J.J.; Civera-Mollá, C.; Navarro-Pardo, E.; Alcover, C.M. Psychometric properties and Factor structure of the BRCS in an elderly Spanish sample. *An. Psychol.* **2015**, *31*, 1030–1034. [CrossRef]
26. Ye, Z.; Yang, X.; Zeng, C.; Wang, Y.; Shen, Z.; Li, X.; Lin, D. Resilience, Social Support, and Coping as Mediators between COVID-19-related Stressful Experiences and Acute Stress Disorder among College Students in China. *Appl. Psychol. Health Well-Being* **2020**, *12*, 1074–1094. [CrossRef]
27. Fullana, M.A.; Hidalgo-Mazzei, D.; Vieta, E.; Radua, J. Coping behaviors associated with decreased anxiety and depressive symptoms during the COVID-19 pandemic and lockdown. *J. Affect. Disord.* **2020**, *275*, 80–81. [CrossRef] [PubMed]
28. Traunmüller, C.; Stefitz, R.; Schneider, M.; Schwerdtfeger, A. Resilience moderates the relationship between the psychological impact of COVID-19 and anxiety. *Psychol. Health Med.* **2021**, *28*, 1–12. [CrossRef]
29. Laferton, J.A.C.; Stenzel, N.M.; Fischer, S. The Beliefs About Stress Scale (BASS): Development, reliability, and validity. *Int. J. Stress Manag.* **2018**, *25*, 72–83. [CrossRef]
30. Keller, A.; Litzelman, K.; Wisk, L.E.; Maddox, T.; Cheng, E.R.; Creswell, P.D.; Witt, W.P. Does the perception that stress affects health matter? The association with health and mortality. *Health Psychol.* **2012**, *31*, 677–684. [CrossRef]
31. Kilby, C.J.; Sherman, K.A.; Wuthrich, V.M. A Scoping Review of Stress Beliefs: Literature Integration, Measurement Issues, and Theoretical Concerns. *Anna. Behav. Med.* **2020**, *54*, 595–610. [CrossRef]
32. Furnham, A. Lay theories of work stress. *Work Stress* **1997**, *11*, 68–78. [CrossRef]
33. Crum, A.J.; Salovey, P.; Achor, S. Rethinking stress: The role of mindsets in determining the stress response. *J. Pers. Soc. Psychol.* **2013**, *104*, 716–733. [CrossRef]

34. Laferton, J.; Fischer, S.; Ebert, D.D.; Stenzel, N.M.; Zimmermann, J. The Effects of Stress Beliefs on Daily Affective Stress Responses. *Anna. Behav. Med.* **2020**, *54*, 258–267. [CrossRef] [PubMed]
35. Thoits, P.A. Mechanisms linking social ties and support to physical and mental health. *J. Health Soc. Behav.* **2011**, *52*, 145–161. [CrossRef] [PubMed]
36. Li, F.; Luo, S.; Mu, W.; Li, Y.; Ye, L.; Zheng, X.; Xu, B.; Ding, Y.; Ling, P.; Zhou, M.; et al. Effects of sources of social support and resilience on the mental health of different age groups during the COVID-19 pandemic. *BMC Psychiatry* **2021**, *21*, 16. [CrossRef] [PubMed]
37. Sippel, L.M.; Pietrzak, R.H.; Charney, D.S.; Mayes, L.C.; Southwick, S.M. How does social support enhance resilience in the trauma-exposed individual? *Ecol. Soc.* **2015**, *20*, 10. [CrossRef]
38. Cohen, S.; Wills, T.A. Stress, social support, and the buffering hypothesis. *Psychol. Bull.* **1985**, *98*, 310–357. [CrossRef] [PubMed]
39. Hobfoll, S.E. Social support: Will you be there when I need you? In *A Lifetime of Relationships*; Vanzetti, N., Duck, S., Eds.; Thomson Brooks/Cole Publishing Co.: Pacific Grove, CA, USA, 1996; pp. 46–74.
40. Hobfoll, S.E.; Freedy, J.; Lane, C.; Geller, P. Conservation of social resources: Social support resource theory. *J. Soc. Pers. Relat.* **1990**, *7*, 465–478. [CrossRef]
41. Arnberg, F.K.; Hultman, C.M.; Michel, P.O.; Lundin, T. Social support moderates posttraumatic stress and general distress after disaster. *J. Trauma Stress.* **2012**, *25*, 721–727. [CrossRef]
42. Hobfoll, S.E.; Walfisch, S. Coping with a threat to life: A longitudinal study of self-concept, social support, and psychological distress. *Am. J. Community Psychol.* **1984**, *12*, 87–100. [CrossRef]
43. Fluharty, M.; Bu, F.; Steptoe, A.; Fancourt, D. Coping strategies and mental health trajectories during the first 21 weeks of COVID-19 lockdown in the United Kingdom. *Soc. Sci. Med.* **2021**, *279*, 113958. [CrossRef]
44. Hobfoll, S.E. Conservation of resources: A new attempt at conceptualizing stress. *Am. Psychol.* **1989**, *44*, 513–524. [CrossRef]
45. Hobfoll, S.E. The influence of culture, community, and the nested-self in the stress process: Advancing conservation of resources theory. *Appl. Psychol.* **2001**, *50*, 337–421. [CrossRef]
46. Sinclair, V.G.; Wallston, K.A. The development and psychometric evaluation of the Brief Resilient Coping Scale. *Assessment* **2004**, *11*, 94–101. [CrossRef] [PubMed]
47. Gjesfjeld, C.D.; Greeno, C.G.; Kim, K.H. A confirmatory factor analysis of an abbreviated social support instrument: The MOS-SSS. *Res. Soc. Work Pract.* **2008**, *18*, 231–237. [CrossRef]
48. Sherbourne, C.D.; Stewart, A.L. The MOS social support survey. *Soc. Sci. Med.* **1991**, *32*, 705–714. [CrossRef]
49. Spitzer, R.L.; Kroenke, K.; Williams, J.B.W.; Löwe, B. A Brief Measure for Assessing Generalized Anxiety Disorder: The GAD-7. *Arch. Intern. Med.* **2006**, *166*, 1092–1097. [CrossRef]
50. Garcia-Campayo, J.; Zamorano, E.; Ruiz, M.A.; Pardo, A.; Perez-Paramo, M.; Lopez-Gomez, V.; Freire, O.; Rejas, J. Cultural adaptation into Spanish of the generalized anxiety disorder-7 (GAD-7) scale as a screening tool. *Health Qual. Life Outcomes* **2010**, *8*, 8. [CrossRef]
51. Kroenke, K.; Spitzer, R.L.; Williams, J.B. The PHQ-9: Validity of a brief depression severity measure. *J. Gen. Intern. Med.* **2001**, *16*, 606–613. [CrossRef]
52. Barrigón, M.L.; Rico-Romano, A.M.; Ruiz-Gomez, M.; Delgado-Gomez, D.; Barahona, I.; Aroca, F.; Baca-García, E. Comparative study of pencil-and-paper and electronic formats of GHQ-12, WHO-5 and PHQ-9 questionnaires. *Rev. Psiquiatr. Salud Ment.* **2017**, *10*, 160–167. [CrossRef]
53. Bueno-Notivol, J.; Gracia-García, P.; Olaya, B.; Lasheras, I.; López-Antón, R.; Santabárbara, J. Prevalence of depression during the COVID-19 outbreak: A meta-analysis of community-based studies. *Int. J. Clin. Health Psychol.* **2021**, *21*, 100196. [CrossRef]
54. Ritchie, H.; Roser, M. *Our World in Data. Mental Health*; University of Oxford: Oxford, UK, 2021. Available online: https://ourworldindata.org/mental-health (accessed on 15 September 2021).
55. Marroquín, B.; Vine, V.; Morgan, R. Mental health during the COVID-19 pandemic: Effects of stay-at-home policies, social distancing behavior, and social resources. *Psychiatry Res.* **2020**, *293*, 113419. [CrossRef]
56. Elkin, L.; Bermejo-Martins, E.; Martinez, M.; Sarrionandia, A.; Cortes, C.; Oliveros, E.Y.; Garces, M.S.; Oron, J.V.; Fernández-Berrocal, P. Relationship between self-care activities, stress and well-being during COVID-19 lockdown: A cross-cultural mediation model. *BMJ Open* **2021**, *11*, e048469.
57. Del-Valle, M.V.; López-Morales, H.; Gelpi-Trudo, R.; Poó, F.M.; García, M.J.; Yerro-Avincetto, M.; Andrés, M.L.; Canet-Juric, L.; Urquijo, S. More than a year of pandemic: Longitudinal assessment of anxiety and depressive symptoms in the argentine general population during the COVID-19 outbreak. *Stress Health* **2022**, 1–10. [CrossRef] [PubMed]
58. Hossain, M.M.; Rahman, M.; Trisha, N.F.; Tasnim, S.; Nuzhath, T.; Hasan, N.T.; Clark, H.; Das, A.; McKyer, E.; Ahmed, H.U.; et al. Prevalence of anxiety and depression in South Asia during COVID-19: A systematic review and meta-analysis. *Heliyon* **2021**, *7*, e06677. [CrossRef] [PubMed]
59. Adams, S.H.; Schaub, J.P.; Nagata, J.M.; Park, M.J.; Brindis, C.D.; Irwin, C.E., Jr. Young Adult Anxiety or Depressive Symp-toms and Mental Health Service Utilization During the COVID-19 Pandemic. *J. Adolesc. Health* **2022**, *70*, 985–988. [CrossRef]
60. Van der Velden, P.G.; Contino, C.; Das, M.; van Loon, P.; Bosmans, M. Anxiety and depression symptoms, and lack of emo-tional support among the general population before and during the COVID-19 pandemic. A prospective national study on prevalence and risk factors. *J. Affect. Disord.* **2020**, *277*, 540–548. [CrossRef]

61. Di Fazio, N.; Morena, D.; Delogu, G.; Volonnino, G.; Manetti, F.; Padovano, M.; Scopetti, M.; Frati, P.; Fineschi, V. Mental Health Consequences of COVID-19 Pandemic Period in the European Population: An Institutional Challenge. *Int. J. Environ. Res. Public Health* **2022**, *19*, 9347. [CrossRef]
62. Fancourt, D.; Steptoe, A.; Bu, F. Trajectories of anxiety and depressive symptoms during enforced isolation due to COVID-19 in England: A longitudinal observational study. *Lancet Psychiat.* **2021**, *8*, 141–149. [CrossRef]
63. Vahratian, A.; Blumberg, S.J.; Terlizzi, E.P.; Schiller, J.S. Symptoms of Anxiety or Depressive Disorder and Use of Mental Health Care Among Adults During the COVID-19 Pandemic—United States, August 2020–February 2021. *MMWR Morb. Mortal. Wkly. Rep.* **2021**, *70*, 490–494. [CrossRef]
64. Alcover, C.M.; Rodríguez, F.; Pastor, Y.; Thomas, H.; Rey, M.; del Barrio, J.L. Group Membership and Social and Personal Identities as Psychosocial Coping Resources to Psychological Consequences of the COVID-19 Confinement. *Int. J. Environ. Res. Public Health* **2020**, *17*, 7413. [CrossRef]
65. Landi, G.; Pakenham, K.I.; Boccolini, G.; Grandi, S.; Tossani, E. Health Anxiety and Mental Health Outcome during COVID-19 Lockdown in Italy: The Mediating and Moderating Roles of Psychological Flexibility. *Front. Psychol.* **2020**, *11*, 2195. [CrossRef]
66. Lei, L.; Huang, X.; Zhang, S.; Yang, J.; Yang, L.; Xu, M. Comparison of Prevalence and Associated Factors of Anxiety and Depression among People Affected by versus People Unaffected by Quarantine during the COVID-19 Epidemic in Southwestern China. *Med. Sci. Monit.* **2020**, *26*, e924609. [CrossRef] [PubMed]
67. Pieh, C.; Budimir, S.; Delgadillo, J.; Barkham, M.; Fontaine, J.R.J.; Probst, T. Mental health during COVID-19 lockdown in the United Kingdom. *Psychosom. Med.* **2021**, *83*, 328–337. [CrossRef] [PubMed]
68. Kwong, A.; Pearson, R.M.; Adams, M.J.; Northstone, K.; Tilling, K.; Smith, D.; Fawns-Ritchie, C.; Bould, H.; Warne, N.; Zammit, S.; et al. Mental health before and during the COVID-19 pandemic in two longitudinal UK population cohorts. *BJPsych* **2021**, *218*, 334–343. [CrossRef] [PubMed]
69. Liu, C.; Liu, Y. Media exposure and anxiety during COVID-19: The mediation effect of media vicarious traumatization. *Int. J. Environ. Res. Public Health* **2020**, *17*, 4720. [CrossRef] [PubMed]

behavioral sciences

MDPI

Article

The Importance of Positive Psychological Factors among People Living with HIV: A Comparative Study

Cristina Rivera-Picón [1,*], María Hinojal Benavente-Cuesta [1], María Paz Quevedo-Aguado [1] and Pedro Manuel Rodríguez-Muñoz [2,3]

1 Faculty of Health Sciences, Nursing, Pontifical University of Salamanca, 37002 Salamanca, Spain
2 Faculty of Nursing and Physiotherapy, University of Salamanca, 37008 Salamanca, Spain
3 Departament of Nursing, Instituto Maimónides de Investigación Biomédica de Córboda, 14005 Córdona, Spain
* Correspondence: criverapi@upsa.es; Tel.: +34-923-277100 (ext. 7665)

Abstract: We aim to identify the differences in psychological well-being, resilience, and coping strategies between healthy subjects and HIV patients. The design followed in this work was empirical, not experimental, and cross-sectional with a correlational objective. The sample included a total of 399 participants (199 patients with HIV and 200 without pathology). The instruments applied for data collection were as follows: a questionnaire on socio-demographic data, the Psychological Well-being Scale, the Resilience Scale and the Coping Strategies Questionnaire. The study period was from February 2018 to January 2020. Patients with HIV had a significantly lower score than healthy subjects, in the resilience factors of perseverance and self-confidence. Subjects with HIV scored less in all dimensions of psychological well-being, with the exception of the dimension of autonomy. Finally, it was observed that HIV-positive subjects used rational coping strategies less frequently than healthy subjects, based on social support seeking and problem-solving coping. However, HIV patients scored higher in emotional coping strategies than healthy individuals.

Keywords: nursing; HIV; psychological well-being; resilience; coping strategies; adaptation

1. Introduction

Human immunodeficiency virus (HIV) infection and AIDS diagnosis are currently a global public health problem. This pathology, in addition to producing a significant burden of disease in terms of morbidity and mortality, has had an enormous impact on the demography and economy of the countries most affected [1]. Currently, estimates provided by WHO and UNAIDS in 2017 state that 36.7 million people worldwide were diagnosed with HIV at the end of 2016. In the same year, approximately 1.8 million subjects were infected [1]. In Spain, the latest data show that, until 30 June 2019, 3244 new cases of HIV were detected [2].

The history of HIV infection is broad, not only scientifically, but also sociologically, in the way that it has impacted society [3]. Thus, the diagnosis of this pathology has complex psychological and social repercussions, which apparently hinder the well-being of these patients; thus, it is necessary to develop a process of adaptation to the disease [4–6].

HIV infection is a highly complex pathology, with a multifactorial process, which must be addressed from a biopsychosocial model. The subjects living with this disease deal with numerous physiological, socio-cultural, economic and psychological stressors that constitute a potential threat to their physical and mental health [7,8].

In this way, the social stigma associated with the diagnosis of HIV is considered a significant threat to combating the disease [9]. In addition, previous studies show that stigma is associated with more severe disease symptoms such as fatigue, gastrointestinal discomfort, numbness or body changes. It is even stated that people living with pathologies with clear social stigma suffer more perceived psychological stress [10,11]. Such stress, in turn, is negatively related to health, increasing the most severe HIV symptoms, the progression of the disease and altering the CD4 count and an increased risk of mortality and development of AIDS [4].

Because the stigma of HIV is difficult to eliminate but continues to have negative implications for the health of these patients, it is essential to identify strategies to protect against the harmful effects of this stigma. Therefore, we consider it essential to carry out research in this regard, in order to determine the resilience, psychological well-being and coping strategies most used in these patients [10].

In this line, resilience is defended as a dampening variable of physical and mental health, relating to a better quality of life and adaptation to the disease [12]. Due to its importance in the health of the subjects, the influence of resilience has been studied in different chronic pathologies such as cancer, diabetes, rheumatic diseases, rheumatoid arthritis, chronic pain, multiple sclerosis, HIV, urinary incontinence, renal insufficiency and cardiovascular diseases [13–15]. The common denominator of these studies is to consider that individuals with higher levels of resilience have less depression, anxiety and somatisation, which are common conditions in patients with chronic diseases such as HIV [16–18]. In addition, resilient people are better able to cope with the processes of illness, both their own and others, coming out strengthened from the situation [19–24].

In relation to psychological well-being, we also find data on its relationship with biological indicators associated with health. It has been shown that optimal levels of psychological well-being improve the immune capacity of individuals and healthy behaviours. In addition, subjects with a better psychological state benefit from an easier and faster recovery from the disease [25]. In this way, we consider it important to know the pathologies associated with lower welfare levels.

Finally, based on the last variable studied in this project, it is highlighted that coping strategies are described as possible protective factors of health and as promoters of psychological well-being [26]. Thus, it is evident that coping is a mediating factor that allows us to adapt to the disease. Therefore, it is essential that patients develop effective coping strategies to meet the demands of different diseases.

Studies carried out with patients diagnosed with HIV show that avoidance-based coping does not protect against psychological distress, promoting levels of stress and anxiety [27]. Thus, the most active coping strategies, characterised by the mobilisation of the patient to deal with the disease, are associated with greater well-being. In addition, in a study by Milena et al. (2009) [28], which evaluated the relationship of coping strategies with anxiety and depression in 92 subjects diagnosed with HIV, showed that the use of problem-solving coping, positive reappraisal, social support seeking and religious coping were associated with lower levels of anxiety and depression.

Additionally, some studies reflect that resilience and more active coping strategies help to face the stigmatization of the disease, changing the beliefs of patients towards it and improving the psychological well-being of patients [4,29].

Thus, the positive impact on the health of HIV patients with high levels of psychological well-being and resilience, as well as the use of active coping strategies, was studied. Based on the theoretical aspects stated, which reflect the difficulties associated with the diagnosis of this disease, we consider it important to determine whether there are differences in resilience, psychological well-being and coping strategies among HIV carriers and healthy participants. This can be of great importance to nursing staff in terms of creating secondary prevention plans, focusing on the psychological aspects most frequently affected in HIV patients.

2. Materials and Methods

2.1. Aims and Design of the Study

The aim of this study was to identify the differences in psychological well-being, resilience, and coping strategies between healthy subjects and HIV patients. Thus, our intention was to determine if subjects with HIV show a different psychological pattern in relation to resilience, psychological well-being and the use of coping strategies compared to HIV-negative subjects. The study had a non-experimental cross-sectional design with a correlational objective.

2.2. Participants

The study subjects were 200 healthy subjects (HIV-negative) and 199 patients with HIV. Thus, the total sample consisted of 399 participants, with a mean age of 47.5 years (SD = 9.97).

The total sample (N = 399) was made up of subjects diagnosed with HIV (n = 199) collected at the University Assistance Complex, specifically at Salamanca University Hospital. These patients voluntarily participated in the study after attending their scheduled appointment at the nursing clinic in the infectious disease unit. Therefore, this sub-sample was obtained with an incidental sampling, and is representative since the population of HIV subjects in the Salamanca University Hospital is approximately 600 patients.

After obtaining the sample of HIV subjects, the sample of healthy patients was selected (n = 200), following a sample by quotas method according to age, sex and level of equivalent studies, with the aim of achieving homogeneous sub-samples.

As inclusion criteria, it was highlighted that the subjects had to be of legal age and participate voluntarily in the project. In the case of subjects with HIV, it was also included to have a confirmed diagnosis of said disease. On the contrary, as an inclusion criterion in healthy patients, it was necessary to have not been diagnosed with HIV. Exclusion criterion included having any illness or medical or psychological disorder that prevented the subject from completing the study or signing the informed consent.

2.3. Data Collection

The data were collected from 4 February 2018 to 30 January 2020. The information was collected through nursing consultations, through self-administered questionnaires. Those subjects who agreed to participate in the study dedicated a time that ranged between 30 and 45 min to complete all the questionnaires, detailed below:

2.3.1. Sociodemographic Data Questionnaire

Sociodemographic data were collected through an instrument made up of a series of questions of a socio-demographic nature and information related to health. The variables collected through this questionnaire were:

- Health status (subjects without pathology, HIV-positive subjects)
- Socio-demographic variables studied (age, sex, marital status and educational level)

2.3.2. Carol Ryff's Psychological Well-Being Scale (PWBS)

Carol Ryff, in 1989, developed the Scales of Psychological Well-Being (SPWB). Diaz et al. (2006) adapted it to Spanish [30].

This author proposed a multidimensional model of psychological well-being consisting of six dimensions: self-acceptance, positive relations, autonomy, environmental mastery, purpose in life and personal growth. Van Dierendonck's version consisted of a 39-item test with six answer options (from 1, totally disagree, up to 6, totally agree). The version proposed by Diaz and collaborators, used in this study, has 29 items. A total score is obtained for each dimension. Table 1 shows the psychometric properties of the Spanish version of this scale with 39 items (original) and with 29 items (version proposed by Díaz et al.).

In this research, the use of the 29-item version was chosen for two reasons: (a) its brevity, and (b) its psychometric properties, which were better in the abbreviated version.

Table 1. Psychometric properties of the Psychological Well-being scale. Spanish version.

	39 Items Version		29 Items Version	
	Number of Items	α Cronbach	Number of Items	α Cronbach
Self-acceptance	6	0.83	4	0.84
Positive relations	6	0.81	6	0.78
Autonomy	8	0.73	6	0.70
Environmental mastery	6	0.71	5	0.82
Purpose in life	7	0.83	5	0.70
Personal growth	6	0.68	4	0.71

2.3.3. Coping Strategies Questionnaire (Sandín and Chorot)

Sandín and Chorot in 2002 developed the scale of the Coping Strategies Questionnaire. This scale is based on a previous version: the Scale of Coping Strategies–Revised (EEC-R), created in 1999 by Sandín, Valiente and Chorot. The scale allows the study of seven dimensions of coping: social support seeking, overt emotional expression, religious coping, problem-solving coping, avoidance coping, negative auto-focused coping, and positive reappraisal. Two more general dimensions were performed after a second-order analysis. The first of them, emotional coping, included negative auto-focused coping and overt emotional expression. The other dimension, rational coping, included problem-solving coping, positive reappraisal and social support seeking. This questionnaire contains a scale comprising 42 items. Each item goes from 0 (never) to 4 (almost always) [31].

Table 2 shows the variance explained by each factor, as well as the associated Cronbach's α coefficient. The total variance explained by the seven factors was 55.3%. Regarding the second order structure, with the two large groups of strategies (Rational and Emotional), 49.3% of the total variance of the test will be clarified.

Table 2. Correlations between factors and Cronbach's alpha coefficients.

	Variance Explained	α Cronbach
Social Support Seeking	20.3%	0.92
overt emotional expression	11.2%	0.74
Religious coping	7.8%	0.86
Problem-solving coping	5.3%	0.85
Avoidance coping	4.7%	0.76
Negative auto-focused coping	3.2%	0.64
Overt emotional expression	2.8%	0.71

2.3.4. Resilience Scale (Wagnild and Young)

Wagnild and Young in 1993 created The Resilience Scale. In 2002, Novella adapted the scale into Spanish [32]. This questionnaire contains a scale comprising 25 items, with a response range from 1 (totally disagree) to 7 (totally agree).

The scale allows the study of five resilience factors: personal satisfaction, equanimity, feeling good alone, self-confidence, and perseverance. Regarding the psychometric properties, Table 3 shows the coefficients of each area obtained in the study by Novella (2002). The overall internal consistency measured through the Cronbach's α coefficient had a value of 0.88.

Table 3. Reliability of the Resilience Scale.

	α Cronbach
Personal satisfaction	0.78
Equanimity	0.75
Feeling good alone	0.71
Self-confidence	0.80
Perseverance	0.76
Full scale	0.87

2.4. Ethical Considerations

The study was admitted by public institutions associated with the study. Addition-ally, it received a positive report from the Ethics Committee. The participation of the subjects was voluntary, ensuring the confidentiality and anonymity of the participants, who were given an information sheet and asked to complete the informed consent form.

2.5. Statistical Analysis

Statistical analysis was performed using International Business Machines' (IBM) Statistical Package for the Social Sciences (SPSS) v25 (IBM Corp., Armonk, NY, USA).

A descriptive analysis of the socio-demographic variables was carried out in terms of sample size and percentages. The analysis of the differences between the subsamples is presented. Due to the nature of the socio-demographic variables, Pearson's χ^2 test was used, using Cramer's V to determine the effect size. The values proposed by Cohen (1988) were used to interpret the magnitude of the effect found.

To determine the differences in psychological well-being, resilience, and coping strategies between healthy subjects and HIV patients, the multivariate analysis of variance (MANOVA) was performed.

In all statistical tests, testing was significant when $p < 0.05$

3. Results

3.1. Descriptive Analysis

In total, 399 subjects participated in the study. Most of the study is made up of men ($N = 293$), and the subjects are mainly aged between 44 and 50 years ($N = 116$). The majority of the total sample is married/in a relationship ($N = 182$) and have an educational level equivalent to secondary or lower ($N = 324$) (Table 4).

According to the health status of the patients, two categories are differentiated: HIV patients ($N = 199$) and healthy subjects ($N = 200$). No significant differences were obtained with respect to sex, educational level and age ($p > 0.05$). The only significant variable was marital status (χ^2, = 49,881; $p < 0.01$). However, the effect is moderate (V = 0.354) (Table 4).

3.2. Resilience, Psychological Well-Being and Coping Strategies

Differences were observed between participant HIV-positive and healthy subjects. To determine the differences in resilience, psychological well-being and coping strategies between subjects with HIV and healthy participants, the MANOVA technique was applied. In relation to the multivariate test, in the Pillai trace it was observed that there were significant differences between groups (F(df) = 10.041 (18); $p < 0.001$). The power was high (1.000) and the size of the effect was large ($\eta_p{}^2 = 0.323$) (Table 5).

For the variables of resilience, significant differences were detected (Table 6): perseverance (F(df) = 14.699(1); $p = <0.001$) and self-confidence (F(gl) = 15.987(1); $p = <0.001$). In addition, significant differences were detected in all dimensions of psychological well-being, except in the dimension of autonomy (F(df) = 5.031(1); $p = 0.025$). The power was moderate (0.698), and the effect size was small ($\eta_p{}^2 = 0.013$). Finally, significant differences were found for the variables of coping: social support seeking (F(gl) = 32.381(1); $p = <0.001$), problem-solving coping (F(df) = 9.759(1); $p = 0.002$) and positive reappraisal. (F(df) = 51.520(1); $p = <0.001$).

Table 4. Sociodemographic variables based on health status.

	HIV		Healthy		Total		Ji	TE	*p*
	N	%	N	%	N	%			
N° participants	199	49.8%	200	50.2%	399	100%			
Sex									
Woman	48	24.1%	58	29.0%	106	26.5%	1.217	0.055	0.270
Man	151	75.9%	142	71.0%	294	73.5%			
Age									
43 years or younger	50	25.1%	59	29.5%	109	27.3%	8.509	0.146	0.037
44 to 50 years	61	30.7%	55	27.5%	116	29.1%			
From 51 to 55 years old	57	28.6%	38	19.0%	95	23.8%			
56 years or older	31	15.6%	48	24.0%	79	19.8%			
Civil status									
Married/couple	58	29.1%	124	62.0%	182	45.6%			
Single/widowed/other	117	58.8%	51	25.5%	168	42.1%	49.881	0.354	0.000
Separated/divorced	24	12.1%	25	12.5%	49	12.3%			
Level of studies									
Secondary or lower	168	84.4%	156	78.0%	324	81.2%	2.695	0.082	0.101
Superior	31	15.6%	44	22.0%	75	18.8%			

N: Number of subjects; %: percentage, χ^2 : chi − squared TE: effect size; *p*: *p*-value.

Table 5. Multivariate tests: Pillai trace.

Effect	Value	F	Hypothesis df	Error df	*p*	$\eta_p{}^2$	Observed Power
Intersection	0.985	1411.971	18	379	<0.001	0.985	1.000
Health status	0.323	10.041	18	379	<0.001	0.323	1.000

$\eta_p{}^2$: eta squared; df: degrees of freedom.

Below, using the Dunnett, the differences according to the resilience factors between the groups are shown (Table 7). As can be seen, subjects with HIV, compared to healthy subjects, show lower scores in perseverance (HIV-Healthy = −1.90, STD. ERROR = 0.497, CI = [−3.08, −0.73]) and in self-confidence (HIV-Healthy = −2.25, STD. ERROR = 0.563, CI = [−3.58, −0.92]).

HIV subjects scored significantly less than healthy subjects in all well-being variables, except in autonomy (HIV-Healthy = −1.16, STD. ERROR = 0.518, CI = [−2.38, 0.06]). For the positive relationships variable, the one with the highest effect size, HIV subjects scored slightly more than four points less than healthy subjects (HIV-Healthy = −4.21, STD. ERROR = 0.475, CI = [−5.33, −3.08]) (Table 8).

In relation to coping strategies, it was found that HIV-positive participants use social support and problem-solving coping less frequently than healthy subjects (Table 9). In addition, patients with HIV used more negative auto-focused coping, compared to healthy patients (HIV-Healthy = 2.72, STD. ERROR = 0.379, CI = [−1.82, 3.61]).

Table 6. Effects tests between subjects: health status.

Dependent Variable	F	Sig.	η_p^2	df	Observed Power
RS Personal satisfaction	4.323	0.038	0.011	1	0.545
RS Equanimity	1.971	0.301	0.003	1	0.178
RS Feeling good alone	13.389	0.110	0.006	1	0.358
RS Perseverance	14.699	<0.001	0.000	1	0.969
RS Self-confidence	15.986	<0.001	0.039	1	0.979
PWS Self-acceptance	43.336	<0.001	0.099	1	1.000
PWS Autonomy	5.031	0.025	0.013	1	0.698
PWS Purpose in life	73.559	<0.001	0.157	1	1.000
PWS Positive relations	78.408	<0.001	0.165	1	1.000
PWS Environmental mastery	29.122	<0.001	0.069	1	1.000
PWS Personal growth	36.523	<0.001	0.084	1	1.000
CS Problem-solving coping	9.759	0.002	0.024	1	0.876
CS Social support seeking	32.381	<0.001	0.076	1	1.000
CS Positive reappraisal	3.919	0.048	0.010	1	0.506
CS Negative auto-focused coping	51.520	<0.001	0.115	1	1.000
CS Overt emotional expression	2.571	0.110	0.006	1	0.359
CS Religious coping	1.199	0.274	0.003	1	0.194
CS Avoidance coping	257	0.263	0.003	1	0.201

η_p^2: eta squared; RS: resilience; PWS: psychological well-being; CS: coping strategies.

Table 7. Multiple comparisons: resilience factors.

Dependent Variable	(I) Subject Health Status	(J) Subject Health Status	Mean Difference (I-J)	Std. Error	CI 95%	
					Lower Bound	Upper Bound
RS Personal satisfaction	HIV	healthy subjects	−0.64	0.307	−1.36	0.09
RS Equanimity	HIV	healthy subjects	−0.26	0.248	−0.84	0.33
RS Feeling good alone	HIV	healthy subjects	−0.37	0.229	−0.91	0.17
RS Perseverance	HIV	healthy subjects	−1.90 *	0.497	−3.08	−0.73
RS Self-confidence	HIV	healthy subjects	−2.25 *	0.563	−3.58	−0.92

The Dunnett C test was used. * significant differences; RS: resilience; Std. error: standard error; CI: confidence interval.

Table 8. Multiple comparisons: dimensions of psychological well-being.

Dependent Variable	(I) Subject Health Status	(J) Subject Health Status	Mean Difference (I-J)	Std. Error	CI 95%	
					Lower Bound	Upper Bound
PWS Self-acceptance	HIV	Healthy subjects	−2.34 *	0.356	−3.18	−1.50
PWS Autonomy	HIV	healthy subjects	−1.16	0.518	−2.38	0.06
PWS Purpose in life	HIV	healthy subjects	−3.79 *	0.442	−4.83	−2.75
PWS Positive relations	HIV	healthy subjects	−4.21 *	0.475	−5.33	−3.08
PWS Environmental mastery	HIV	healthy subjects	−2.14 *	0.397	−3.08	−1.20
PWS Personal growth	HIV	healthy subjects	−1.94 *	0.321	−2.70	−1.18

The Dunnett C test was used. * significant differences; PWS: psychological well-being; Std. error: standard error; CI: confidence interval.

Table 9. Multiple comparisons: coping strategies.

Dependent Variable	(I) Subject Health Status	(J) Subject Health Status	Mean Difference (I-J)	Std. Error	CI 95%	
					Lower Bound	Upper Bound
CS Social support seeking	HIV	Healthy subjects	−3.73 *	0.655	−5.28	−2.18
CS Problem-solving coping	HIV	Healthy subjects	−1.61 *	0.516	−2.83	−0.39
CS Positive reappraisal	HIV	Healthy subjects	−0.89	0.452	−1.96	0.17
CS Negative auto-focused coping	HIV	Healthy subjects	2.72 *	0.379	1.82	3.61
CS Overt emotional expression	HIV	Healthy subjects	−0.62	0.385	−1.53	0.29
CS Religious coping	HIV	Healthy subjects	−0.71	0.647	−2.24	0.82
CS Avoidance coping	HIV	Healthy subjects	−0.52	0.462	−1.61	0.57

The Dunnett C test was used. * significant differences; CS: coping strategies; Std. error: standard error; CI: confidence interval.

4. Discussion

The present study showed that participants with HIV had a significantly lower score than healthy subjects in the resilience factors: perseverance and self-confidence.

This psychological variable is important because, as detailed in other investigations, there is enough published evidence that associates resilience with positive health benefits, favouring viral suppression in subjects with HIV [33] and positively impacting on their quality of life [34,35].

Other studies reflected that healthy subjects have higher levels of resilience than patients with chronic pathologies [13]. These results are in line with those obtained in our work. Similar results to those presented in our study are shown in the research by Mcgowan et al. (2018) [34], in which it was observed that the level of resilience was higher in healthy subjects than in those with a diagnosis of HIV. However, in contrast to our study, this difference was not significant. It should be noted that the presence of such research comparing the levels of resilience in HIV subjects and healthy subjects is very sparse. Therefore, we consider it necessary to develop more research in this area.

On the other hand, HIV-positive patients scored lower on all dimensions of psychological well-being compared to healthy participants, with the exception of the autonomy dimension. In a study by López et al. (2008) [36], it was suggested that patients with HIV have more psychological problems due to the stigma associated with the disease. This consideration could explain why HIV-positive participants in this study had lower levels of psychological well-being and resilience. There are not enough published projects that allow comparing the results obtained here in terms of the dimensions of psychological well-being. However, Wisk and Weitzman (2017) [37] in their study on subjects with chronic pathology and healthy subjects, observed that those individuals diagnosed with a chronic pathology had lower psychological well-being in adulthood than their healthy peers. In this way, we consider it necessary to detect which chronic pathologies are associated with lower psychological well-being. On the other hand, in a study by Chongwo et al. (2018) [38], it was evident that healthy subjects had better scores in terms of psychological well-being compared to the group of subjects with HIV. Additionally, in the study by Ramkisson et al. (2016), it was reflected that the absence of disease is associated with higher levels of psychological well-being than in subjects with HIV [39]. These findings are consistent with those of our study, where subjects diagnosed with HIV scored significantly less than healthy subjects in all dimensions of well-being, except for autonomy.

Finally, based on the coping strategies studied, it was observed that HIV subjects used strategies based on social support seeking and problem-solving coping less frequently than healthy subjects. Recalling the general classification of coping strategies, it is observed that patients with HIV use less rational strategies than participants without pathology. On the contrary, subjects with HIV used more emotional strategies, specifically in the dimension of negative self-centered coping, than healthy individuals.

These results are important because rational coping is associated with a greater ability of the patient to cope with the disease, achieving a greater adaptation to the disease and a greater degree of well-being. However, the styles of avoidance coping or emotional coping are related to negative psychological results, less adherence to treatment and worse adaptation to the disease, promoting levels of stress and anxiety [27]. Therefore, HIV-positive subjects could be using inappropriate strategies to cope with the disease. These results could be justified due to the great emotional impact of a HIV diagnosis [7]. Therefore, these patients do not feel able to actively face the consequences of the disease using strategies based on negative auto-focused coping. In addition, this greater use of emotional strategies could justify the lower levels of resilience and psychological well-being in this group of patients.

However, other projects have highlighted that problem solving, seeking social support and avoidance were the coping strategies most used by HIV patients [40,41]. These statements are contrary to the results offered in this study, which reflects the need to continue research in this area. These results do not coincide with those found in our work, in which it was observed that the strategies based on social support seeking, problem-solving coping and avoidance coping were less used by HIV-positive participants compared to healthy subjects. In addition, the social support seeking strategy was the least used by patients with HIV compared to healthy subjects. As justification for this result, different investigations show that these patients experience more fear and feelings of shame, which can prevent these patients from turning to their relatives or friends, so they use this type of coping strategy less frequently [42–44]. Heydari el al. (2020), published a study similar to ours. The aim of this study was to compare the coping styles of people living with Human immunodeficiency virus, positive and negative, in the Iranian population. In this investigation it was detected that there were no differences in coping strategies between the subgroups [45]. These results are contrary to those presented in our study. However, it could be justified by the cultural difference between the samples of both studies.

It should be noted that there is little research focused on predicting the levels of resilience, psychological well-being and coping strategies used in subjects with HIV. In this way, our results show that it is necessary to develop more research that evaluates and compares resilience in these subjects, which allows us to determine the differences in resilience depending on the pathology.

Among the limitations of this study is the presence of significant differences in the sociodemographic variable of marital status between the two studied sub-samples. However, taking into account the high percentage of single subjects in the group of subjects with HIV, justified in part by the difficulties that this group may have in maintaining relationships, makes it very difficult to obtain homogeneous subsamples in this sociodemographic variable. In addition, with regard to the analysis of differences between sub-samples, marital status was the only significant variable and the size of the effect was small. Another limitation would be access to medical care, which would make it difficult to obtain a larger sample in a shorter period of time. Finally, we also highlight as a limitation the non-inclusion of the descriptive data of all the variables analyzed, as well as the values of resilience, psychological well-being and coping of each group. However, the purpose of the work was to compare the different health states with each other. Future investigations turned out to take into account the limitations indicated above to provide more specific evidence on the results found.

5. Conclusions

By way of conclusion, patients with HIV showed a lower score than healthy subjects in the factors of resilience, perseverance and self-confidence. In addition, they scored less than healthy subjects in all dimensions of psychological well-being except in autonomy. Finally, it was observed that subjects with HIV used rational coping strategies (problem-solving coping and social support seeking) less frequently than healthy subjects, although they used more negative auto-focused coping compared to the sub-sample without pathology.

It is highlighted that high levels of resilience, psychological well-being and rational coping strategies are related to a better prognosis and health benefits in HIV subjects. However, the present study found that patients with HIV have worse levels in these psychological constructs than healthy participants.

Implications: These conclusions reflect the importance of the involvement of all health and mental health professionals who work with HIV patients, reflecting the need for a multidisciplinary team.

In addition, the development of interventions to promote resilience and active coping strategies can have a positive impact on the quality of life and well-being of people. Furthermore, it would be necessary to create public health measures that promote access to equality and reduce social stigma in HIV-positive patients.

Author Contributions: Conceptualization, C.R.-P., M.H.B.-C. and P.M.R.-M.; methodology, C.R.-P.; software, C.R.-P. and M.P.Q.-A.; validation, M.H.B.-C., M.P.Q.-A. and C.R.-P.; formal analysis, C.R.-P.; investigation, M.H.B.-C. and P.M.R.-M.; resources, P.M.R.-M.; data curation, C.R.-P. and P.M.R.-M.; writing—original draft preparation, C.R.-P.; writing—review and editing, C.R.-P. and M.P.Q.-A.; visualization, C.R.-P. and M.P.Q.-A.; supervision, M.H.B.-C. and P.M.R.-M.; project administra-tion, C.R.-P.; funding acquisition, C.R.-P., M.H.B.-C., M.P.Q.-A. and P.M.R.-M. All authors have read and agreed to the published version of the manuscript.

Funding: This research received no external funding.

Institutional Review Board Statement: The study was conducted according to the guidelines of the Declaration of Helsinki, and approved by the University Care Complex of Salamanca and by the Primary Care Management of Salamanca. It also received a favourable report from the Research with Medicines in the Health Area Ethics Committee of Salamanca, with CEIC code PI02/01/2018.

Informed Consent Statement: Informed consent was obtained from all subjects involved in the study.

Conflicts of Interest: The authors declare no conflict of interest.

References

1. Lamotte, J.A. Infection due to HIV/aids in the current world. *Medisan* **2014**, *18*, 993–1013.
2. Ministerio de Sanidad Consumo y Bienestar Social. *Vigilancia Epidemiológica del VIH y Sida en España 2018: Sistema de Información sobre Nuevos Diagnósticos de VIH y Registro Nacional de Casos de Sida;* Plan Nacional Sobre el Sida, D.G. de Salud Pública, Calidad e Innovación/Centro Nacional de Epidemiología; ISCIII: Madrid, Spain, 2019.
3. Cobos Manuel, I.; Jackson-Perry, D.; Courvoisier, C.; Bluntschli, C.; Carel, S.; Muggli, E.; Waelti Da Costa, V.; Kampouri, E.; Cavassini, M.; Darling, K. Stigmatisation et VIH: Tous concernés [Stigma and HIV: Relevant for everyone]. *Rev. Med. Suisse* **2020**, *16*, 744–748. [PubMed]
4. Earnshaw, V.A.; Bogart, L.M.; Dovidio, J.F.; Williams, D.R. Stigma and racial/ethnic HIV disparities: Moving toward resilience. *Am. Psychol.* **2015**, *1*, 60–74. [CrossRef]
5. Furlotte, C.; Schwartz, K. Mental Health Experiences of Older Adults Living with HIV: Uncertainty, Stigma, and Approaches to Resilience. *Can. J. Aging* **2017**, *36*, 125–140. [CrossRef] [PubMed]
6. Ruiz-Algueró, M.; Hernando, V.; Marcos, H.; Gutiérrez, G.; Pérez-Elías, M.J.; López-Bernaldo, J.C.; Pulido, F.; Górgolas, M.; Sanz, J.; Suarez-García, I.; et al. Self-rated health among people living with HIV in Spain in 2019: A cross-sectional study. *BMC Infect. Dis.* **2021**, *21*, 129. [CrossRef]
7. Lessa, T.; Oliveira, D.C.; Marcos, A.; Tosoli, A.M.; Formozo, G.A. Quality of life and people living with AIDS: Relationship with sociodemographic and health aspects. *Rev. Lat. Am. Enferm.* **2014**, *22*, 582–590. [CrossRef]
8. Nyongesa, M.K.; Nasambu, C.; Mapenzi, R.; Koot, H.M.; Cuijpers, P.; Newton, C.; Abubakar, A. Psychosocial and mental health challenges faced by emerging adults living with HIV and support systems aiding their positive coping: A qualitative study from the Kenyan coast. *BMC Public Health* **2022**, *22*, 76. [CrossRef] [PubMed]

9. Koerting, A.; Polo, R.; Vázquez, M.C.; Del Amo, J. The Social Pact for the Non-discrimination and Equal Treatment Associated with HIV development. *Rev. Española Salud Pública* **2019**, *93*, e201912115.
10. Earnshaw, V.A.; Lang, S.M.; Lippitt, M.; Jin, H.; Chaudoir, S.R. HIV Stigma and Physical Health Symptoms: Do Social Support, Adaptive Coping, and/or Identity Centrality Act as Resilience Resources? *AIDS Behav.* **2015**, *19*, 41–49. [CrossRef] [PubMed]
11. Yang, X.; Li, X.; Qiao, S.; Li, L.; Parker, C.; Shen, Z.; Zhou, Y. Intersectional stigma and psychosocial well-being among MSM living with HIV in Guangxi, China. *AIDS Care* **2020**, *32*, 5–13. [CrossRef]
12. Plascencia de la Torre, J.C.; Castellanos, C. Resilience assessment in mexicans diagnosed with hiv: A comparative study. *Salud Soc.* **2019**, *10*, 52–64. [CrossRef]
13. Gheshlagh, R.; Sayehmiri, K.; Ebadi, A.; Dalvandi, A.; Dalvand, S.; Nourozi, K. Resilience of Patients With Chronic Physical Diseases: A Systematic Review and Meta-Analysis. *Iran. Red Crescent Med. J.* **2016**, *18*, e38562. [CrossRef]
14. Gheshlagh, R.G.; Ebadi, A.; Dalvandi, A.; Rezaei, M.; Tabrizi, K.N. A Systematic Study of Resilience in Patients with Chronic Physical Diseases. *Nurs. Midwifery Stud.* **2017**, *6*, e36401. [CrossRef]
15. Quiceno, M.; Vinaccia, S. Resilience and sociodemographic characteristics in the chronic ill. *Psicol. Desde. Caribe.* **2012**, *29*, 87–104.
16. Fernanda, S.; Ribeiro, L.; Eugenia, M.; Borreto, M. Resilience in chronic diseases: A systematic review. *Cogent Psychol.* **2015**, *39*, 1–9. [CrossRef]
17. Min, J.; Yoon, S.; Lee, C.; Chae, J.; Lee, C.; Song, K.; Kim, T. Psychological resilience contributes to low emotional distress in cancer patients. *Support Care Cancer* **2013**, *21*, 2469–2476. [CrossRef] [PubMed]
18. Crowley, T.; Van der Merwe, A.S.; Esterhuizen, T.; Skinner, D. Resilience of adolescents living with HIV in the Cape Metropole of the Western Cape. *AIDS Care* **2021**, *2021*, 1–8. [CrossRef] [PubMed]
19. Amar, J.; Martínez, M.; Utria, L. New approach to health considering the resilience. *Salud Uninorte.* **2013**, *29*, 124–133.
20. Gonzalez, I.; Eduarda, D.S.; Paiva, L.; Rossi, L.A.; Dantas, S.; Alcalá, D. Anxiety, depression, resilience and self-esteem in individuals with cardiovascular diseases. *Rev. Lat.-Am. Enfermagem.* **2016**, *24*, 2–10. [CrossRef]
21. Quiceno, J.M.; Vinaccia, S. Resilience: A perspective from chronic disease in the adult population. *Pensam. Psicol.* **2011**, *9*, 69–82.
22. Schumacher, A.; Sauerland, C.; Silling, G.; Berdel, W.E.; Stelljes, M. Resilience in patients after allogeneic stem cell transplantation. *Support Care Cancer* **2014**, *22*, 487–493. [CrossRef] [PubMed]
23. Yang, Z.; Wang, J.; Zhang, B.; Zeng, Y.; Ma, H. Factors influencing resilience in patients with burns during rehabilitation period. *Int. J. Nurs. Sci.* **2014**, *1*, 97–101. [CrossRef]
24. Babić, R.; Babić, M.; Rastović, P.; Ćurlin, M.; Šimić, J.; Mandić, K.; Pavlović, K. Resilience in Health and Illness. *Psychiatr. Danub.* **2020**, *32*, 226–232. [PubMed]
25. Vázquez, C.; Hervás, G.; Rahona, J.J.; Gómez, D. Psychological well-being and health: Contributions from Positive Psychology. *Anu. Psicol. Clínica Salud* **2009**, *5*, 15–28.
26. Orozco-Gómez, Á.; Castiblanco-Orozco, L. Psychosocial Factors and Psychological Intervention in Chronic Non-Communicable Disease. *Rev. Colomb. Psicol.* **2015**, *24*, 203–217. [CrossRef]
27. Carrobles, J.A.; Remor, E.; Rodríguez-Alzamora, L. Coping, perceived social support and emotional distress in patients with HIV infection. *Psicothema* **2003**, *15*, 420–426.
28. Milena, G.A.; Quiceno, J.M.; Vinaccia, S.; Martínez, L.A.; Otalvaro, M.C. Copying Strategies, Anxiety and Depression in HIV/Aids Patients. *Ter. Psicológica* **2009**, *27*, 5–13.
29. Garrido-Hernansaiz, H.; Murphy, P.J.; Alonso-Tapia, J. Predictors of Resilience and Posttraumatic Growth Among People Living with HIV: A Longitudinal Study. *AIDS Behav.* **2017**, *21*, 3260–3270. [CrossRef] [PubMed]
30. Díaz, D.; Rodríguez-Carvajal, R.; Blanco, A.; Moreno-Jiménez, B.; Gallardo, I.; Valle, C.; Van Dierendock, D. Adaptation of the Ryff psychological well-being scales. *Psicothema* **2006**, *18*, 572–577. [PubMed]
31. Sandín, B.; Chorot, B. The Coping Strategies Questionnaire: Development and preliminary validation. *Rev. Piscopatoogía Piscologia Clínico* **2002**, *8*, 39–54. [CrossRef]
32. Novella, A. Incremento de la Resiliencia Luego de la Aplicación de un Programa de Psicoterapia Breve en Madres Adolescentes. Ph.D. Thesis, Universidad Nacional Mayor de San Marcos, Lima, Peru, 2002.
33. Dale, S.K.; Cohen, M.H.; Kelso, G.A.; Cruise, R.C.; Weber, K.M.; Watson, C.; Burke-Miller, J.K.; Brody, L.R. Resilience Among Women with HIV: Impact of Silencing the Self and Socioeconomic Factors. *Sex Roles* **2014**, *70*, 221–231. [CrossRef]
34. Mcgowan, J.A.; Brown, J.; Lampe, F.C.; Lipman, M.; Smith, C.; Rodger, A. Resilience and Physical and Mental Well-Being in Adults with and Without HIV. *AIDS Behav.* **2018**, *22*, 1688–1698. [CrossRef]
35. Brown, L.L.; Martin, E.G.; Knudsen, H.K.; Gotham, H.J.; Garner, B.R. Resilience-Focused HIV Care to Promote Psychological Well-Being during COVID-19 and Other Catastrophes. *Front. Public Health* **2021**, *9*, 705573. [CrossRef]
36. López, M.; Laviana, M.; Fernández, L.; López, A.; Rodríguez, A.M.; Aparicio, A. The struggle against the stigma and discrimination in mental health. A complex strategy based on available data. *Rev. Assoc. Española Neuropsiquiatría* **2008**, *28*, 43–83. [CrossRef]
37. Wisk, L.E.; Weitzman, E.R. Expectancy and Achievement Gaps in Educational Attainment and Subsequent Adverse Health Effects Among Adolescents with and without Chronic Medical Conditions. *J. Adolesc. Health* **2017**, *61*, 461–470. [CrossRef] [PubMed]
38. Chongwo, E.; Ssewanyana, D.; Nasambu, C.; Mwangala, P.N.; Mwangi, P.M.; Nyongesa, M.K.; Newton, C.R.; Abubakar, A. Validation of a Swahili version of the World Health Organization 5-item well-being index among adults living with HIV and epilepsy in rural coastal Kenya. *Glob. Health Res. Policy* **2018**, *3*, 26. [CrossRef]

39. Ramkisson, S.; Pillay, B.J.; Sartorius, B. Anxiety, depression and psychological well-being in a cohort of South African adults with Type 2 diabetes mellitus. *South Afr. J. Psychiatry* **2016**, *22*, a935. [CrossRef]
40. Grant, N.; Tarakeshwar, N.; Hansen, N.; Kochman, A.; Sikkema, K. Coping Mediates Outcome Following a Randomized Group Intervention for HIV-Positive Bereaved Individuals. *J. Clin. Psychol.* **2009**, *65*, 319–335. [CrossRef]
41. Xiao, Z.; Li, X.; Qiao, S.; Zhou, Y.; Shen, Z. Coping, social support, stigma, and gender difference among people living with HIV in Guangxi, China. *Psychol. Health Med.* **2018**, *23*, 18–29. [CrossRef] [PubMed]
42. Choi, K.H.; Gibson, D.R.; Han, L.; Guo, Y. High levels of unprotected sex with men and women among men who have sex with men: A potential bridge of HIV transmission in Beijing, China. *AIDS Educ. Prev.* **2004**, *16*, 19–30. [CrossRef]
43. Wong, W.C.W.; Zhang, J.; Wu, S.C.; Kong, T.S.K.; Ling, D.C.Y. The HIV related risks among men having sex with men in rural Yunnan, China: A qualitative study. *Sex. Transm. Infect.* **2006**, *82*, 127–130. [CrossRef] [PubMed]
44. Ye, Z.; Chen, L.; Lin, D.; Wang, S.X. The Relationship between Posttraumatic Stress Disorder Symptoms and Posttraumatic Growth among HIV-Infected Men who Have Sex with Men in Beijing, China: The Mediating Roles of Coping Strategies. *Front. Psychol.* **2018**, *9*, 1787. [CrossRef] [PubMed]
45. Heydari, M.; Karimzadeh, Y.; Faghih, M.; Heydari, Z.; Hosseini, E.; Mehraeen, M. Coping styles in HIV positives and HIV negatives. *BMC Psychol.* **2020**, *8*, 116. [CrossRef] [PubMed]

behavioral sciences

MDPI

Article

Adaptation of an Emotional Stroop Test for Screening of Suicidal Ideation in Portugal

Graça Esgalhado [1,2], Henrique Pereira [1,3,*] and Patricia Silva [1]

[1] Department of Psychology and Education, Faculty of Social and Human Sciences, University of Beira Interior, Pólo IV, Estrada do Sineiro, s/n, 6200-209 Covilhã, Portugal
[2] Institute of Cognitive Psychology, Human and Social Development (IPCDHS), 3000-115 Coimbra, Portugal
[3] Research Centre in Sports Sciences, Health Sciences and Human Development (CIDESD), 5001-801 Vila Real, Portugal
* Correspondence: hpereira@ubi.pt

Abstract: Cognitive instruments, especially those with emotional components, may be useful to address the limitations of self-report scales commonly used to assess suicidal ideation. The aim of this study was to develop an emotional Stroop test for screening suicidal ideation in Portugal. The project was developed in five phases using different samples for each phase. The first two phases were focused on the formulation of the potential words that would compose the slides. For this purpose, five biology teachers (neutral slide) and five mental health professionals (positive and negative slides) were invited to help choose the words that were most representative for each slide. The third phase validated the words defined in the previous phase. In this phase, 300 university students participated (M_{age} = 21.66; SD = 3.67; 68% female). They rated the words on a Likert scale in terms of their frequency of use, familiarity, level of understanding, and degree of image evocation. In the fourth phase, the researchers developed the complete version of the test, which consists of three slides with neutral, positive, and negative emotional stimuli, consecutively. Finally, in the fifth phase, we validated the final version of the test through a comparative study between a clinical group and a non-clinical group, each one composed by 50 participants (M_{age} = 32; SD = 9.70; 55% female). Results indicated that the clinical group demonstrated significantly higher scores for depression and suicidal ideation and lower scores for the three Stroop tasks. Words related to negative emotions were strongly correlated with suicidal ideation. Finally, the three Stroop slides explained 74.1% of the variance in suicidal ideation. These findings suggest that this test can be a viable complementary measure in the psychological assessment of suicide ideation, and intervention in the field of suicide prevention in Portugal.

Keywords: emotional Stroop test; screening; suicidal ideation; Portugal

1. Introduction

Suicide is a complex phenomenon which is classified by the World Health Organization as a serious public health concern, since 800,000 people die due to suicide every year [1]. The occurrence of suicide involves multidimensional determinants, such as biological and genetic, psychological, psychiatric, social, and environmental factors [2], with suicidal ideation being one of the main predictors of suicide attempt [3,4]. The relationship between psychological factors and suicidal ideation is complex but involves perceived burdensomeness and internal entrapment, as well as feelings of defeat, external entrapment, and thwarted belonginess [5]. Suicidal ideation is a relatively recurrent and stressful experience, given that about 10% of people have had some type of suicidal thoughts throughout the life cycle [6]. However, anticipating this type of event is not easy, as the psychological assessment of suicidal ideation involves cognitive, emotional, and behavioral measures before the occurrence of suicidal thoughts [7]. Factors such as gender (women have greater suicidal ideation than men) [8], rumination and cognitive inflexibility [9], and previous suicidal ideation and attempt experiences [10] seem to be important predictors of the occurrence of suicidal ideation.

Suicidal ideation refers to a vast set of cognitions, emotions, and behaviors associated with the thought of ending life, often associated with ideas, intentions, motivations, and plans to carry out suicide [11]. Since the assessment of suicidal ideation depends on self-report, several difficulties arise in the operationalization of this assessment, as people tend not to manifest their intentions [12] and tend to deliberately deny or hide their thoughts to avoid interventions or hospitalizations [13]. This reinforces the importance of developing viable alternatives to assess suicidal ideation, namely through the assessment of cognitive and emotional functioning.

The Stroop task [14] is a well-known cognitive task to assess the attentional processing of simultaneous information in the context of selective attention, cognitive set shifting, and inhibition of responses [15,16]. In the original version of the color-word Stroop task (CW-Stroop) [17], three slides are presented. The first slide contains words of the colors "blue", "green", "red", and "yellow" printed in black. The second slide contains rectangles printed in blue, green, red, or yellow ("color-naming" condition). The third slide shows the same words as the first slide printed in an incongruous color (for example, the word "green" printed in blue). Hence, Stroop interference allows the assessment of attentional capacity and bias.

The Emotional Stroop Test introduces changes to the CW-Stroop by replacing colored words with neutral and emotional stimuli (for example, the word "death" printed in blue compared to a neutral word of the same color) [18]. In individuals without psychopathology, the Emotional Stroop Test does not cause attentional bias. However, in individuals with psychopathology, it is common to observe some kind of attentional bias, interpreted as threatening [19]. Several studies have analyzed Stroop interference in patients with anxiety and depression disorders [20,21], post-traumatic stress [22], and suicidal behavior [8,23].

Therefore, this work aims to develop methodological procedures in order to contribute to the evaluation of the Emotional Stroop Test for the detection of suicide ideation as a measure of suicidal risk. Unlike most previous studies that focus on clinical populations [24,25], this study focuses on associating the Stroop task to assess differences in attentional functioning when compared to specific levels of suicide ideation in clinical and non-clinical populations in Portugal. We propose that individuals that report higher levels of suicide ideation will present more difficulties in attentional control, hence being at a higher risk of suicide, because they are unable to inhibit negative thoughts and direct attention toward task-relevant information. In contrast, participants with lower levels of suicide ideation will be able to control attentional functioning and are thus less likely to focus on negative thoughts. Hence, we predict that participants with more suicide ideation will show more difficulties inhibiting negative words.

2. Materials and Methods

This study took place in four phases: (1) obtaining the words for the neutral slide, (2) obtaining the words for the positive and negative slides, (3) word validation, (4) formulation of the Emotional Stroop Test, and (5) validation of the Emotional Stroop Test by comparing a clinical and a non-clinical group. For each phase, different samples were used. We explain ahead each phase with greater detail.

2.1. Phase 1—Words for the Neutral Slide

To carry out the first phase of the investigation, we used five Biology teachers from a school in the municipality of Covilhã, Portugal to become formal judges. All teachers had a university degree in biology as a minimum educational qualification. As this task had a similar structure to the classic Stroop test, the neutral slide consisted of non-activating words. We chose words belonging to the "fruits" category. For the selection of these words, the Portuguese lexicon was used, and 48 words were withdrawn from the search. An authorization was requested to apply the questionnaire to the school principal in order to allow the participation of selected judges who were present with the words and were asked to classify them as belonging or not to the fruit category. The list of the 48 words belonging to the fruit category is presented in Table 1.

Table 1. Neutral words presented to the specialists' panel.

Fruits			
Fig	Blackberry	Persimmon	Medlar
Cherry	Blueberry	Raspberry	**Apple**
Pomegranate	Currant	Nectarine	**Pear**
Date	Strawberry	Pinion	**Banana**
Grape	Olive	Peanut	Melon
Lime	Guava	Pistachio	**Watermelon**
Lemon	Lychee	Cashew	Sloe
Cider	Pineapple	Raisins	**Orange**
Tangerine	Walnut Mango	Plum	Quince
Grapefruit	Papaya	Apricot	Peach
Avocado	Coconut	Chestnut	Almond
Passion Fruit	**Kiwi**	Hazelnut	Arbutus

Note: Words belonging to the Fruit category, to integrate the neutral slide are highlighted in black.

Of these 48 words, 10 were selected to be included in the slide. The choice criterion was due to the fact that the ten words were classified by all the judges as belonging to the fruit category and taking into account the four colors to be used in the Emotional Stroop—yellow, red, blue, and green—the chosen words have the same number of syllables (in Portuguese) of the color in which they were be printed (highlighted in Table 1).

2.2. Phase 2—Words for the Positive and Negative Slides

To carry out the second phase of the investigation, an intentional sample was used, consisting of five specialists in the field of mental health. Of these five specialists, three were clinical psychologists, one was a psychiatrist, and last one was child psychiatrist. For the construction of the positive slide and negative slides—a bibliographic research was developed on words associated with the issue in question (suicide ideation) and the stage of the life cycle in which the participant was at. Seventy-four words were presented to the specialists' panel, who were then asked to classify the words on a Likert-type scale with values ranging from −2 (very negative words) to +2 (very positive words). Other words that the judges considered pertinent could be added to the initial list.

Of the initial 74 words, only 20 were selected. Ten were classified as positive and ten were classified as negative. Each ten words were chosen in accordance with an obtained common score by the five judges of above 60%—i.e., the words were validated by the five judges when their agreement was common for at least three of them. In addition to this criterion, and similar to the neutral blade, the number of syllables that the words have in Portuguese was also taken into account, such that the chosen words had the same number of syllables corresponding to the number of syllables as the color of the words in the which they were printed (Table 2).

2.3. Phase 3—Word Validation

In this phase we used a convenience sample of 300 university students who attended the University of Beira Interior in Portugal. The mean age was 21.66 (SD = 3.67), 68% were female, and 32% were male. Of this 300, 5% studied architecture, 14.7% sociology, 23.3% sports Science, 30.7% psychology, 8.7% marketing and 17.7% medicine.

After obtaining the three sets of words, a protocol consisting of five pages was elaborated. The first page contained a brief explanation of the study, as well as instructions. The second page contained sociodemographic information. The remaining pages presented a brief explanation of the task that was being asked, and three tables with words in which the participants should comment. The protocol application took place in a classroom of the university facilities after informed consent was obtained. Anonymity and confidentiality were guaranteed. This sample assessed the three sets of words stimuli—neutral, negative, and positive—on a Likert-type scale, ranging from 1 (nothing) to 4 (very) in relation to the "Frequency of Use", (if they were used in everyday life) to "Familiarity" (if they were more or less familiar), to "Level of Understanding" (if their meaning was understood), and to the "Degree of Image Evocation" (if it was easy or difficult to mental visualize the image corresponding to the word). A total of 51% of participants considered all the words frequent, familiar, understandable, and evocable.

Table 2. Positive and negative words presented to the specialists' panel.

Words					
Cry	**Life**	**Depression**	Qualities	**Loss**	**Success**
Sun	Burden	Help	**Joy**	Change	**Victory**
Wealth	Try	Ache	Conflict	Alcohol	Testament
Death	**Mourning**	Charm	**Anguish**	Beauty	Survive
Adolescence	**Wealth**	Unemployment	Affable	Development	Rejection
Crisis	**Love**	Loneliness	Aggressiveness	Praise	Parasuicide
Farewell	Appeal	Salvation	Employment	Friendship	Anxiety
Drugs	**Passing**	**Laughter**	Sexuality	**Sadness**	Confusion
Color	**Health**	Hope	End	**Recreation**	Identity
Weapon	Separation	**Disease**	Humor	Self-harm	Defects
Happiness	Transformation	Hanging	Growth	Sacrifice	Youth
Isolation	Pills	Struggle	Impulsivity	Communication	Hopelessness
				Suffering	Suicide

Note: Words belonging to the positive and negative categories to integrate the correspondent slides, are highlighted in black.

2.4. Phase 4—Formulation of the Emotional Stroop Test for Screening of Suicide Ideation

In this phase, we started to create the Stroop test for screening of suicide ideation. Like all Stroop procedures, whether classic or emotional, each slide was printed in A4 format (21 × 30 cm). Each slide contained 100 elements distributed over five columns of 20 elements. All words were randomly distributed, and the same word was not allowed to appear twice in a row in the same column, just as the same color was not allowed to appear twice in a row. The words that made up the three slides of the Emotional Stroop Test for suicide ideation are presented in Table 3.

Table 3. Neutral, positive, and negative words.

Neutral Blade	Positive Blade	Negative Blade
Tangerine	Love	Death
Banana	Joy	Farewell
Kiwi	Victory	Mourning
Watermelon	Health	Depression
Orange	Life	Passing
Apple	Laughter	Loss
Grape	Success	Sadness
Cherry	Wealth	Weapon
Lemon	Happy	Disease
Pear	Leisure	Anguish

Figures 1–3 are excerpts from the Emotional Stroop Test for screening of suicide ideation in Portuguese. The first slide printed the ten neutral words in colored ink—blue, yellow, green, and red (Figure 1).

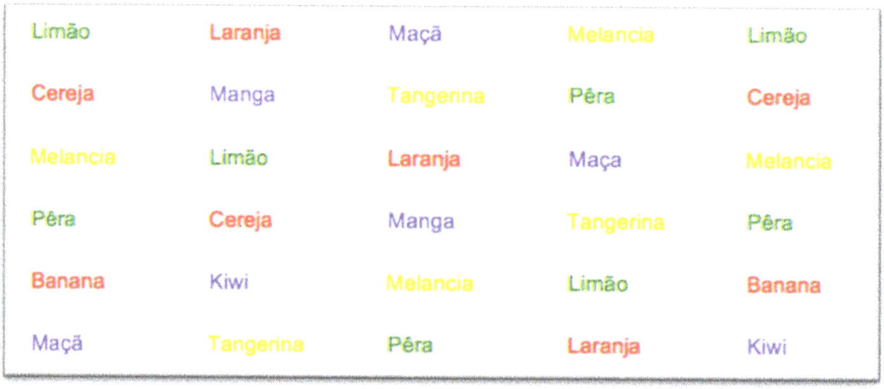

Figure 1. The ten neutral words.

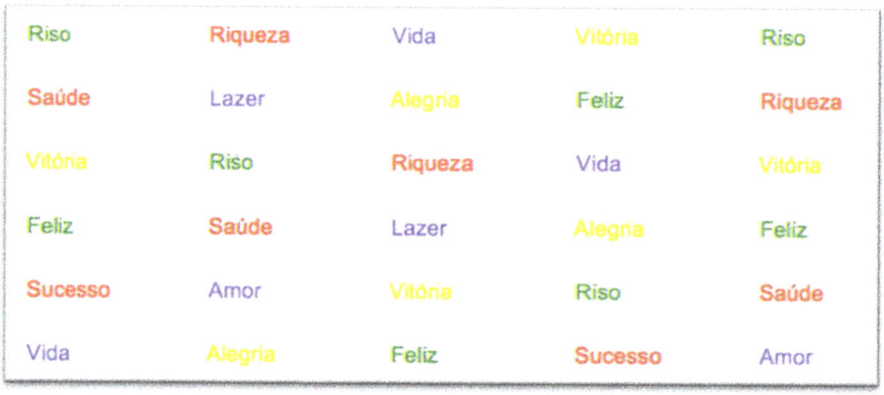

Figure 2. The ten positive words.

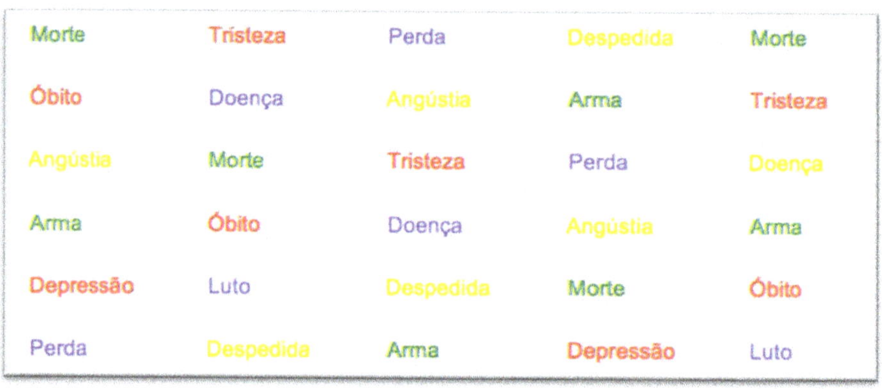

Figure 3. The ten negative words.

The second slide contained the words that were classified as positive, also printed in color. Figure 2 shows an excerpt of that slide.

The third slide contained the words that were classified as negative, also printed in color. Figure 3 shows an excerpt of that slide.

2.5. Phase 5—The Final Study: The Emotional Stroop Test for Screening of Suicide Ideation and The Suicide Ideation Questionnaire

In this final step, we used 100 participants divided into two groups: clinical ($n = 50$) and non-clinical ($n = 50$). In the clinical group, the presence of depressive symptoms was defined as an inclusion criterion, assessed through the Beck Depression Inventory [26], and the exclusion criterion was the presence of other diagnosis. In the non-clinical group, the presence of a psychopathological symptoms was used as an exclusion criterion. Participants were aged between 20 and 59 years, with an average age of 32 years (SD = 9.70). With regard to gender distribution, 55 subjects (55%) were female and 45 (45%) were male. Regarding marital status, 67% of participants were single, 30% married, and 3% divorced. A total of 27% of participants were students, 16% were unemployed, 8% were nurses, 6% were operational assistants, 5% were engineers and managers, 4% were social workers, and teachers, 3% were sociologists, 2% were psychologists, and 1% were entrepreneurs. Regarding education, 48% had a university degree, 35% had secondary diploma, and 7% had basic school diploma. Homogeneity tests were used to test similarity between the clinical and non-clinical groups for sociodemographic characteristics. The only main difference was having or not having clinical symptomatology for depression.

A sociodemographic questionnaire was used to characterize the participants on age, gender, professional status, education, and a self-assessment item to detect the presence of psychic comorbidities.

The prevalence of suicidal thoughts and cognitions was assessed using the Suicidal Ideation Questionnaire (SIQ). This instrument is a Portuguese version of the Suicide Ideation Questionnaire, originally created by Davis [27] and translated and adapted to Portuguese [28]. The SIQ allows analyzing the severity of suicidal thoughts in adolescents and adults, and assesses a hierarchy of thoughts related to suicide, which oscillate between little and very serious. It consists of 30 items on a Likert-type scale, ranging from "I never thought" to "I always thought", in a growing trend of severity. For evaluation purposes, each item is rated from 0 to 6, respectively. The total scores can range from 0 to 180. In the Portuguese version, a score of 23.04 was defined as the average for the population (SD = 25.65). A Cronbach's alpha coefficient of 0.96 was obtained in the present study, indicating excellent reliability for the SIQ.

The clinical sample was collected from the psychiatric department of a local general hospital. After obtaining a formal consent to access to patients from the ethics committee, the sociodemographic questionnaire, the Emotional Stroop Test created in this study, the Beck Depression Inventory, and the Suicidal Ideation Questionnaire were used to collect data. All ethical principles of anonymity and confidentiality were guaranteed. The non-clinical sample was collected via formal and informal community contacts using the snowball technique to collect participants' responses to the same measures.

Immediately before applying the set of instruments, a quick detection of any deficiencies in color perception (for example, achromatism, or dichromatism) was performed by presenting color squares (yellow, green, blue, and red) and asking participants to identify the respective colors. Subsequently, some indications and instructions were given in order to ensure the understanding and proper performance of the Emotional Stroop Task by naming the color in which the word was printed aloud as quickly as possible, while ignoring its meaning, in 45 s. The BDI and the SIQ were also applied. Throughout the sample collection procedure, a face-to-face approach was used. Participants needed, on average, 10 to 20 min to answer the questionnaires and requested little support in clarifying any items.

2.6. Data Analyses

Quantitative results were analyzed using IBM SPPS Statistics, Version 27.0. After data cleaning, descriptive statistics, including frequencies, means, and standard deviations were established. In order to compare differences between samples, t-student tests were conducted. Finally, correlational and linear regression analyses were also performed.

3. Results

A normal distribution was found for all variables under study after conducting the Kolmogorov–Smirnov test. Regarding depression symptoms, participants from the non-clinical group scored significantly lower than participants from the clinical group, $M_{non\text{-}clinical}$ = 3.06, SD = 2.54, and $M_{clinical}$ = 43.88, SD = 11.97, respectively [t(98) = −23.57; $p < 0.001$)]. Regarding suicide ideation, participants from the non-clinical group scored significantly lower than participants from the clinical group, $M_{non\text{-}clinical}$ = 2.22, SD = 3.12, and $M_{clinical}$ = 83.46, SD = 19.97, respectively [t(98) = −28.41; $p < 0.001$)] (Table 4).

Table 4. Depression and suicide ideation scores by non-clinical and clinical groups.

Variable	Group	n	*M* (SD)	t (df)	*p*	*Cohen's d*
Depression	Non-Clinical	50	3.06 (2.54)	−23.57 (98)	0.000 *	81.240
	Clinical	50	43.88 (11.97)			
Suicide Ideation	Non-Clinical	50	2.22 (3.12)	−28.41 (98)	0.000 *	40.820
	Clinical	50	83.46 (19.97)			

* $p < 0.001$.

For the Emotional Stroop Test for screening of suicide ideation, a comparative analysis between non-clinical and clinical groups was performed for all three types of slides with neutral, positive, and negative words, assessing the number of correct words evoked. Results shown in Table 5 indicate that significant differences were obtained for all three conditions ($p < 0.001$). Non-clinical participants scored higher for all three conditions.

Table 5. Results for neutral, positive, and negative words scores by non-clinical and clinical groups.

Variable	Group	*n*	*M* (SD)	t (df)	*p*	*Cohen's d*
Neutral words	Non-Clinical	50	60.64 (9.41)	5.92 (98)	0.000 *	−9.280
	Clinical	50	51.56 (5.84)			
Positive words	Non-Clinical	50	64.34 (7.53)	−11.61 (98)	0.000 *	−15.740
	Clinical	50	48.60 (5.93)			
Negative words	Non-Clinical	50	66.32 (7.59)	14.64 (98)	0.000 *	−20.460
	Clinical	50	45.86 (6.32)			

* $p < 0.001$.

A correlational analysis between the number of negative words on slide three (negative words) and levels of suicide ideation. A very strong, negative, and significant association was found (r = −0.840; $p < 0.001$). Table 6 describes these correlations.

Table 6. Correlation Matrix.

	1	2	3	4
1. Suicide Ideation	-			
2. Slide 1 (Neutral)	−0.558 **	-		
3. Slide 2 (Positive)	−0.773 **	0.844 **	-	
4. Slide 3 (Negative)	−0.840 **	0.801 **	0.952 **	-

** $p < 0.001$.

Finally, simple logistic regression was performed to assess the predictive value of neutral, positive, and negative words in suicide ideation. As shown in Table 7, the model was found to be significant, and indicates that the Stroop slides explain 74.1% of the variance in suicide ideation levels, with greater contribution from the negative words (slide 3).

Table 7. Simple linear regression analysis predicting the suicide ideation.

Variable	B	SE B	β
Slide 1 (Neutral)	1.515	0.461	0.318 *
Slide 2 (Positive)	0.013	0.790	0.003
Slide 3 (Negative)	−3.824	0.593	−1.098 **
R^2		0.741	
F		91.728 *	

* $p < 0.05$; ** $p < 0.001$.

4. Discussion

The present study sought to develop an Emotional Stroop Test as a suicidal risk measure for the Portuguese population. The test aims to assess differences in attentional functioning when compared to specific levels of suicide ideation. We hypothesized that people with higher levels of suicidal ideation performed worse on the Stroop task. There were then four phases of test formulation in Portuguese and one phase for the validation of the test through the application of the final questionnaire to a clinical sample (n = 50) compared to a non-clinical sample (n = 50). The clinical sample had higher scores for depression and suicidal ideation and lower scores for correct answers on the 3 slides of the Stroop task. Suicidal ideation was strongly correlated with negative words, which in turn contributed to a greater explanation of the variance in levels of suicidal ideation. All results were significant.

Our findings corroborate previous studies that demonstrated that the Emotional Stroop Test is an important tool for the assessment of suicidal ideation, as it fills gaps in commonly used self-report scales [10,29,30]. In fact, this test will be beneficial for the field of psychological assessment in Portugal, as it considers specific criteria and characteristics related to suicidal ideation that other measures are not prepared to assess. This is due to the fact that this test can measure how well a person can use their ability to control their automatic reactions to words or images, which is called the "Stroop effect" [14,18]. From the use of words with positive, negative, and neutral emotional stimuli, it is possible to assess attention bias, response inhibition, and cognitive flexibility—variables that are related to a person's emotions and affective states and have already been widely related to suicidal behavior [31–33].

In fact, the Stroop paradigm has been used to demonstrate attentional bias in different clinical populations. Studies with these populations have shown that participants have longer reaction times when exposed to stimuli associated with their dysfunctional behavior; that is, they tend to name the color of words related to their problems, or emotionally relevant stimuli, more slowly than those with neutral emotional valence. It is also verified in different investigations with the Emotional Stroop Test, that the scores obtained in the three slides by the control group are higher than those of the clinical group. We can infer that participants in the clinical group may have a psychological impairment that influences their performance, possibly with implications for a decrease in the speed of response processing, which explains why they also score less on the neutral slide than participants in the control group. However, it is in the negative slide, as would be expected, that these differences are accentuated, which corroborates the results of different versions of the Emotional Stroop Test that use the scores in the negative slide as an indicator of the interference of the meaning of the words in the execution of the requested task, the naming of the color in which they are written.

There are also operational aspects that support our tool as a useful measure for the assessment of suicidal ideation. The main one is related to the application time. This test can be used as a quick and easy way to detect suicidal tendencies (participants needed, on average, 10 to 20 min to complete the entire protocol). In addition, this type of test is especially effective for assessing these tendencies in people who would not normally present/respond to a suicide assessment [34,35], or for those who might have response biases on the self-report scales, such as people of clinical populations [10,36,37]. Hence, this is a useful and practical test in clinical settings since its application is easy and quick, providing immediate screening clues for suicidal ideation. In addition, our protocol can be administered in a variety of settings, including psychiatric hospitals, private practices, and schools, which increases the tool's reach in suicide screening.

The information obtained through this Emotional Stroop Test can be used by mental health professionals to assist in the assessment and monitoring of a person's or group's suicide risk, which would allow them to direct people with suicidal ideation to appropriate services and determine which prevention measures need to be taken. In fact, different types of treatment can be more or less effective depending on whether or not the person is conscious of the suicidal ideation and what the level of suicidal ideation is [38], which can be verified through the Emotional Stroop Test. Psychology researchers can also benefit from this tool to study suicidal ideation in different populations. With a neuropsychological dimension, this test can be useful to complement analyzes with regard to assessments, comparisons and discovery of patterns and potential risk groups. This is also the case when a differential diagnosis between impulsive behaviors associated with attention deficit with hyperactivity disorder (ADHD) and impulsive behaviors associated with depression, because the Emotional Stroop Test is sensitive to attentional biases caused by negative words related to each disorder.

In addition, we need to understand our test from a public health perspective. In Portugal, around 3 people die every day from intentional self-harm (suicide) [39]. In 2017, suicide represented a loss of about 15 potential years of life [39]. In addition, the country is the first in the European Union with more people to suffer from chronic depression, which has a direct connection with suicidal ideation [40]. According to the Lusa Agency and the National Authority for Medicines and Health Products (Infarmed), the sale of antidepressants has also increased considerably in recent years, reaching an increase of almost 100% between 2010 and 2019 [41]. For these reasons, the prevention of suicidal behavior through population screening and the implementation of intervention strategies should be identified as a public health priority [1], which demonstrates the relevance of this study in the context of public health in the country.

However, despite being an innovative work and with important contributions, this study has its limitations. The first one is related to the validation of the protocol for specific populations. Although our sample had a heterogeneous distribution, the final study was carried out with a diverse audience (different ages, academic degrees, socioeconomic status, etc.), which may have influenced our results. Future studies could benefit from the validation of this test for specific populations (adolescents, elderly people, people from minority groups, among others) and for larger and more representative samples. Validation studies are important to determine whether a psychological test can be used safely, which will contribute to the construction of knowledge on this test in Portugal.

Another limitation is related to the need to understand the colors to perform the test. In this case, those who have difficulties in identifying colors are excluded. This also applies to people with language difficulties or diminished cognitive abilities, who should not be evaluated using this test. For these people, we recommend the use of other assessment measures with a neuropsychological basis and others, which are able to complement the suicide risk assessment with more precision [37]. Finally, this test was based on computer slides and considers the importance of innovation present also in the area of psychological assessment. Future studies could verify the feasibility and relevance of using a mobile application version of this test, which would facilitate its application by professionals who do not have access to a computer at the time of the assessment [42,43].

5. Conclusions

We believe that assessing a person's attentional functioning is fundamental for suicide screening, given that individuals with suicidal ideations have greater difficulties in inhibiting their impulses than healthy individuals. In this sense, this study sought to present the development and feasibility of an Emotional Stroop Test for screening for suicidal ideation in a clinical and non-clinical sample of the Portuguese population. We describe several advantages of our study, as well as important implications for academic, clinical, and public health practice in the country. We also emphasize the importance of identifying suicidal ideation before any suicide attempt, in order to contribute to the promotion of effective actions for each case. Finally, we discuss the main limitations and future directions for research with this tool. We conclude that this Emotional Stroop Test will be beneficial for the area of psychological assessment in Portugal with a focus on cognitive functions, since the test measures selective attention, executive functions, cognitive flexibility, inhibition, and the attention biases than can appears in case of psychopathology. This test can be included in neuropsychological assessment tools that do not depend on self-harm self-report questionnaires and be an important resource to assess suicidal ideation and assist in suicide prevention in people of Portuguese language.

Author Contributions: Conceptualization, G.E.; methodology, H.P.; software, H.P.; validation, G.E., H.P. and P.S.; formal analysis, H.P.; investigation, G.E.; resources, G.E.; data curation, G.E.; writing—original draft preparation, G.E., H.P. and P.S; writing—review and editing, G.E., H.P. and P.S.; supervision, G.E.; project administration, G.E. All authors have read and agreed to the published version of the manuscript.

Funding: This research received no external funding.

Institutional Review Board Statement: The study was conducted according to the guidelines of the Declaration of Helsinki and approved by the Ethics Committee of the University of Beira Interior (Portugal).

Informed Consent Statement: Informed consent was obtained from all subjects involved in the study.

Data Availability Statement: The data presented in this study are available upon request.

Conflicts of Interest: The authors declare no conflict of interest.

References

1. World Health Organization. Suicide. Available online: https://www.who.int/news-room/fact-sheets/detail/suicide (accessed on 6 June 2022).
2. Turecki, G.; Brent, D.A.; Gunnell, D.; O'Connor, R.C.; Oquendo, M.A.; Pirkis, J.; Stanley, B.H. Suicide and suicide risk. *Nat. Rev. Dis. Primers* **2019**, *5*, 74. [CrossRef] [PubMed]
3. Baghani, E.; Fata, L.; Salehi, M.; Hasani, F. Prediction of Suicide Ideation Based on the Attentional Bias in Clinical and Non-clinical Populations. *IJPCP* **2020**, *26*, 76–101. [CrossRef]
4. King, C.A.; Jiang, Q.; Czyz, E.K.; Kerr, D.R. Suicidal ideation of psychiatrically hospitalized adolescents has one-year predictive validity for suicide attempts in girls only. *J. Abnorm. Child Psychol.* **2014**, *42*, 467–477. [CrossRef]
5. De Beurs, D.; Fried, E.I.; Wetherall, K.; Cleare, S.; O'Connor, D.B.; Ferguson, E.; O'Carroll, R.E.; O'Connor, R.C. Exploring the psychology of suicidal ideation: A theory driven network analysis. *Behav. Res. Ther.* **2019**, *120*, 103419. [CrossRef]
6. Nock, M.K.; Borges, G.; Bromet, E.J.; Cha, C.B.; Kessler, R.C.; Lee, S. Suicide and suicidal behaviors. *Epidemiol. Rev.* **2008**, *30*, 133–154. [CrossRef]
7. Franklin, J.C.; Ribeiro, J.D.; Fox, K.R.; Bentley, K.H.; Kleiman, E.M.; Huang, X.; Musacchio, K.M.; Jaroszewski, A.C.; Chang, B.P.; Nock, M.K. Risk factors for suicidal thoughts and behaviors: A meta-analysis of 50 years of research. *Psychol. Bull.* **2017**, *143*, 187–232. [CrossRef] [PubMed]
8. Chung, Y.; Jeglic, E.L. Use of the Modified Emotional Stroop Task to Detect Suicidality in College Population. *Suicide Life-Threat. Behav.* **2016**, *46*, 55–66. [CrossRef] [PubMed]
9. Miranda, R.; Valderrama, J.; Tsypes, A.; Gadol, E.; Gallagher, M. Cognitive inflexibility and suicidal ideation: Mediating role of brooding and hopelessness. *Psychiatry Res.* **2013**, *210*, 174–181. [CrossRef]
10. Cha, C.B.; Najmi, S.; Park, J.M.; Finn, C.T.; Nock, M.K. Attentional bias toward suicide-related stimuli predicts suicidal behavior. *J. Abnorm. Psychol.* **2010**, *119*, 616–622. [CrossRef]
11. Thompson, C.; Ong, E.L.C. The Association Between Suicidal Behavior, Attentional Control, and Frontal Asymmetry. *Front. Psychiatry* **2018**, *9*, 79. [CrossRef]
12. Mann, J.J.; Currier, D. A review of prospective studies of biologic predictors of suicidal behavior in mood disorders. *Arch. Suicide Res.* **2007**, *11*, 3–16. [CrossRef] [PubMed]

13. Mann, J.J.; Currier, D.; Stanley, B.; Oquendo, M.A.; Amsel, L.V.; Ellis, S.P. Can biological tests assist prediction of suicide in mood disorders? *Int. J. Neuropsychopharmacol.* **2006**, *9*, 465–474. [CrossRef] [PubMed]
14. Stroop, J.R. Studies of Interference in Serial Verbal Reactions. *J. Exp. Psychol.* **1935**, *18*, 643–662. [CrossRef]
15. MacLeod, C.M. Half a century of research on the Stroop effect: An integrative review. *Psychol. Bull.* **1991**, *109*, 163–203. [CrossRef] [PubMed]
16. Stein, M.B.; Kennedy, C.M.; Twamley, E.W. Neuropsychological Function in Female Victims of Intimate Partner Violence with and without posttraumatic stress disorder. *Biol. Psychiatry* **2002**, *52*, 1079–1088. [CrossRef]
17. Golden, C.J.; Freshwater, S.M. *Stroop Color and Word Test: A Manual for Clinical and Experimantal Uses*; Skoelting: Chicago, IL, USA, 1978.
18. Williams, J.M.; Mathews, A.; MacLeod, C. The emotional Stroop task and psychopathology. *Psychol. Bull.* **1996**, *120*, 3–24. [CrossRef]
19. El Khoury-Malhame, M.; Reynaud, E.; Soriano, A.; Michael, K.; Salgado-Pineda, P.; Zendjidjian, X.; Gellato, C.; Eric, F.; Lefebvre, M.N.; Rouby, F.; et al. Amygdala activity correlates with attentional bias in PTSD. *Neuropsychologia* **2011**, *49*, 1969–1973. [CrossRef]
20. Bar-Haim, Y.; Lamy, D.; Pergamin, L.; Bakermans-Kranenburg, M.J.; van Ijzendoorn, M.H. Threat-related attentional bias in anxious and nonanxious individuals: A meta-analytic study. *Psychol. Bull.* **2007**, *133*, 1–24. [CrossRef]
21. Epp, A.M.; Dobson, K.S.; Dozois, D.J.; Frewen, P.A. A systematic meta-analysis of the Stroop task in depression. *Clin. Psychol. Rev.* **2012**, *32*, 316–328. [CrossRef]
22. Joyal, M.; Wensing, T.; Levasseur-Moreau, J.; Leblond, J.T.; Sack, A.; Fecteau, S. Characterizing emotional Stroop interference in posttraumatic stress disorder, major depression and anxiety disorders: A systematic review and meta-analysis. *PLoS ONE* **2019**, *14*, e0214998. [CrossRef]
23. Cha, C.B.; Najmi, S.; Amir, N.; Matthews, J.D.; Deming, C.A.; Glenn, J.J.; Calixte, R.M.; Harris, J.A.; Nock, M.K. Testing the Efficacy of Attention Bias Modification for Suicidal Thoughts: Findings From Two Experiments. *Arch. Suicide Res.* **2017**, *21*, 33–51. [CrossRef] [PubMed]
24. Palmer, C.J. Suicide attempt history, self-esteem, and suicide risk in a sample of 116 depressed voluntary inpatients. *Psychol. Rep.* **2004**, *95*, 2–4. [CrossRef]
25. Klonsky, E.D.; May, A.M. Differentiating suicide attempters from suicide ideators: A critical frontier for suicidology research. *Suicide Life-Threat. Behav.* **2014**, *44*, 1–5. [CrossRef] [PubMed]
26. Campos, R.; Gonçalves, B. The Portuguese Version of the Beck Depression Inventory-II (BDI-II). *Eur. J. Psychol. Assess.* **2011**, *27*, 258–264. [CrossRef]
27. Davis, J.M. Suicidal Ideation Questionnaire. *J. Psychoeducat. Assess.* **1992**, *10*, 298–301. [CrossRef]
28. Ferreira, J.A.; Castela, M.C. Questionário da Ideação Suicida (QIS). In *Testes e Provas Psicológicas em Portugal*; Simões, M.R., Gonçalves, M.M., Almeida, L.S., Eds.; Sistemas Humanos e Organizacionais, Lda.: Braga, Portugal, 1999; Volume 2, pp. 123–130.
29. Chung, Y.; Jeglic, E.L. Detecting Suicide Risk Among College Students: A Test of the Predictive Validity of the Modified Emotional Stroop Task. *Suicide Life-Threat. Behav.* **2017**, *47*, 398–409. [CrossRef]
30. Tavakoli, P.; Jerome, E.; Boafo, A.; Campbell, K. Attentional Bias Deficits in Adolescent Suicide Attempters During an Emotional Stroop Task: An ERP Study. *Front Psychiatry* **2021**, *12*, 1695. [CrossRef]
31. Interian, A.; Myers, C.E.; Chesin, M.S.; Kline, A.; Hill, L.S.; King, A.R.; Miller, R.; Latorre, M.; Gara, M.A.; Stanley, B.H.; et al. Towards the objective assessment of suicidal states: Some neurocognitive deficits may be temporally related to suicide attempt. *Psychiatry Res.* **2020**, *287*, 112624. [CrossRef]
32. Richard-Devantoy, S.; Ding, Y.; Lepage, M.; Turecki, G.; Jollant, F. Cognitive inhibition in depression and suicidal behavior: A neuroimaging study. *Psychol. Med.* **2016**, *46*, 933–944. [CrossRef]
33. Harfmann, E.J.; Rhyner, K.T.; Ingram, R.E. Cognitive inhibition and attentional biases in the affective go/no-go performance of depressed, suicidal populations. *J. Affect. Disord.* **2019**, *1*, 228–233. [CrossRef]
34. Busch, K.A.; Fawcett, J.; Jacobs, D.G. Clinical correlates of inpatient suicide. *J. Clin. Psychiatry* **2003**, *64*, 14–19. [CrossRef] [PubMed]
35. Hom, M.A.; Stanley, I.H.; Junior-Joiner, T.E. Evaluating factors and interventions that influence help-seeking and mental health service utilization among suicidal individuals: A review of the literature. *Clin. Psychol. Rev.* **2015**, *40*, 28–39. [CrossRef] [PubMed]
36. Nock, M.K.; Park, J.M.; Finn, C.T.; Deliberto, T.L.; Dour, H.J.; Banaji, M.R. Measuring the suicidal mind: Implicit cognition predicts suicidal behavior. *Psychol. Sci.* **2010**, *21*, 511–517. [CrossRef] [PubMed]
37. Moreno, M.; Gutiérrez-Rojas, L.; Porras-Segovia, A. Implicit Cognition Tests for the Assessment of Suicide Risk: A Systematic Review. *Curr. Psychiatry Rep.* **2022**, *24*, 141–159. [CrossRef] [PubMed]
38. Rudd, M.D.; Joiner, T.; Rajab, H.M. *Treating Suicidal Behavior: An Effective, Time-limited Approach*; The Guilford Press: New York, NY, USA, 2001.
39. Instituto Nacional de Estatística. Taxa de Mortalidade por Lesões Autoprovocadas Intencionalmente (Suicídio) por 100.000 Habitantes (N.º). Available online: https://www.ine.pt/xportal/xmain?xpid=INE&xpgid=ine_indicadores&indOcorrCod=0003736&contexto=bd&selTab=tab2 (accessed on 6 June 2022).
40. Eurostat. 7.2% of People in the EU Suffer from Chronic Depression. Available online: https://ec.europa.eu/eurostat/en/web/products-eurostat-news/-/edn-20210910-1 (accessed on 6 June 2022).

41. Autoridade Nacional do Medicamento e Produtos de Saúde. Evolução da pandemia em Portugal. Available online: https://www.infarmed.pt/documents/15786/3552218/Infarmed+Not%C3%ADcias+n%C2%BA+71+julho+2020/0bd46c6f-7515-1865-f8bf-c95c3e56df60?version=1.2 (accessed on 6 June 2022).
42. Baucom, B.R.; Georgiou, P.; Bryan, C.J.; Garland, E.L.; Leifker, F.; May, A.; Wong, A.; Narayanan, S.S. The promise and the challenge of technology-facilitated methods for assessing behavioral and cognitive markers of risk for suicide among US Army National Guard Personnel. *Int. J. Environ. Res. Public Health* **2017**, *14*, 361. [CrossRef] [PubMed]
43. Meliá, R.; Francis, K.; Hickey, E.; Bogue, J.; Duggan, J.; O'Sullivan, M.; Young, K. Mobile Health Technology Interventions for Suicide Prevention: Systematic Review. *JMIR mHealth uHealth* **2020**, *8*, 1. [CrossRef]

behavioral sciences

MDPI

Article

Mediating Effect of Psychological Process Variables on the Relationship between Dysfunctional Coping and Psychopathologies: A Comparative Study on Psychopathologies during COVID-19

Nurfarah Lydia Hambali [1], Friska Ayu [2], Nicholas Tze Ping Pang [1,*], Mohd Amiruddin Mohd Kassim [1], Hafid Algristian [3], Moch. Sahri [2], Nelbon Giloi [1], Syed Sharizman Syed Abdul Rahim [1], Azizan Omar [1], Mohammad Saffree Jeffree [1] and Walton Wider [4,*]

1 Faculty of Medicine and Health Sciences, Universiti Malaysia Sabah, Kota Kinabalu 88400, Malaysia; nurfarahlydia@ums.edu.my (N.L.H.); amiruddink@ums.edu.my (M.A.M.K.); nelbon.giloi@ums.edu.my (N.G.); syedsharizman@ums.edu.my (S.S.S.A.R.); azizan.omar@ums.edu.my (A.O.); saffree@ums.edu.my (M.S.J.)
2 Faculty of Health, Universitas Nahdlatul Ulama Surabaya (UNUSA), Surabaya 60237, Indonesia; friskayuligoy@unusa.ac.id (F.A.); sahrimoses@unusa.ac.id (M.S.)
3 Faculty of Medicine, Universitas Nahdlatul Ulama Surabaya (UNUSA), Surabaya 60237, Indonesia; dr.hafid@unusa.ac.id
4 Faculty of Business and Communication, INTI International University, Nilai 71800, Malaysia
* Correspondence: nicholas@ums.edu.my (N.T.P.P.); walton.wider@newinti.edu.my (W.W.)

Abstract: The COVID-19 crisis has had repercussions on global mental wellbeing. This study aimed: (1) to identify the mediating role of psychological process variables, namely psychological mindedness, psychological mindfulness, and psychological inflexibility on the relationship between dysfunctional coping and psychopathologies in Indonesian undergraduate students subjected to national quarantine orders throughout July, 2020 and (2) to compare the level of anxiety, depression, and anxiety between Indonesian and Malaysian undergraduate students. A cross-sectional study was performed with 869 Indonesian undergraduate students from Nahdlatul Ulama University of Surabaya (UNUSA) and 515 undergraduate students from Universiti Malaysia Sabah (UMS). The BIPM, MAAS, AAQ-I, DASS-21, and Brief COPE were used to assess the research variables. The proportion who scored "moderate" and above for depression, anxiety, and stress were 20.2%, 25.0%, and 14.2%, respectively, in Malaysian samples and 22.2%, 35.0%, and 23.48% in Indonesian samples. In Study 1, psychological mindedness, psychological mindfulness, and psychological inflexibility significantly mediated the relationship between dysfunctional coping and psychopathologies. In Study 2, Indonesians demonstrated significantly higher anxiety and stress compared to Malaysian samples. Despite the contrasting COVID-19 situations in Malaysia and Indonesia, psychopathologies were more affected in Indonesia. Hence, our study suggests how crucial it is for mental health providers to consider promoting psychological mindedness, psychological mindfulness, and psychological flexibility to alleviate the corresponding psychopathologies among undergraduate students.

Keywords: COVID-19; Indonesia; Malaysia; psychological mindedness; psychological inflexibility; psychological mindfulness; psychopathologies; dysfunctional coping

1. Introduction

Coronavirus disease (COVID-19), a novel coronavirus which emerged from Wuhan, China in late 2019, was declared a pandemic on 12 March 2020 by the World Health Organization (WHO). The pandemic reached Malaysia in January 2020 from travelers in China arriving via Singapore on 25 January 2020. With the escalation of active cases in March 2020 especially after the emergence of localised clusters, the Malaysian government implemented a Movement Control Order (MCO) from 18 March 2020. The MCO comprised of restrictions on mass gathering, travelling abroad, closure of all government and private schools and universities, and closure of all government and private premises except for essential services [1,2].

Likewise, in Indonesia, Jakarta was the first to implement large-scale social restrictions, also known as *Pembatasan Sosial Berskala Besar* (PSBB) starting from 10 April 2020 [3]. The Nahdlatul Ulama University of Surabaya (UNUSA) in Surabaya, East Java province, implemented the study from home policy on 22 March 2020 before Surabaya implemented the PSBB on 26 April 2020. Many universities were forced to shift towards e-learning, which relies disproportionately on university computer lab services, poor internet connections, and excessive consumption of Internet data for video conferences. Literature suggests that college and university students were stressed about dormitory evacuation, cancellation of planned events, loss of part-time jobs, anxiety about the job market, and the potential for abuse at home [4]. Furthermore, COVID-19 negatively affected undergraduate students' mental health in terms of stress, disappointment, loneliness, financial setbacks, and relocation [5]. As asserted by Sun et al. [6], university students are considered a group of people who are vulnerable to distress and mental health disorders during COVID-19. Thus, it is pertinent to determine the risks and protective factors towards students' mental health during the pandemic.

Many factors can contribute to students' psychological distress, and analysing such underlying psychological process variables would assist in a better understanding of particular psychopathologies [7,8]. Three psychological process variables were explored in this study, namely psychological mindedness, psychological mindfulness, and psychological inflexibility. Psychological mindedness refers to the intrinsic motivation to be in touch with one's inner feelings and thoughts by monitoring and analysing them in an adaptive way [9,10]. For psychological mindfulness, there are two main elements of mindfulness in a clinical psychology perspective: the awareness of one's moment-to-moment experience nonjudgmentally and with acceptance [11]. Psychological inflexibility is a process wherein an individual depicts dysfunctional control endeavors connected with real sensations, feelings, or thoughts to try not to encounter upsetting internal or external events [12]. Studies have shown significant correlations between psychological mindedness, psychological mindfulness, psychological inflexibility, and psychopathologies. For example, psychological mindedness was found to be inversely related to symptoms of psychological distress and psychopathologies [13,14]. Meanwhile, low levels of mindfulness were found to be associated with depression, anxiety, neuroticism, dissociation, insecure attachment, negative affect, and difficulties in emotion regulation [15–18]. Likewise, extensive evidence has shown that psychological flexibility is positively associated with psychological well-being and inversely associated with a wide range of distress, including depression, anxiety, and general psychological distress [19–23].

Malaysia and Indonesia adopted fairly strict social restrictions to prevent COVID-19 transmission, resulting in large-scale quarantines and isolation. It has been known that quarantine is a risk factor for mental health issues, with longer quarantines associated with poorer psychological outcomes [24]. However, despite the measures taken to flatten the curve, there was a stark difference between the two countries. Indonesia was among the worst hit countries in the world, while Malaysia was able to handle COVID-19 relatively well. This study was hence performed to assess the effect on underlying psychological processes, namely psychological mindedness, psychological mindfulness, and psychological inflexibility, on the relationship between dysfunctional coping and psychopathologies during the COVID-19 pandemic. Moreover, it aims to determine if the difference of the COVID-19 burden in these two countries would affect the level of anxiety, depression, and stress of the respective populations.

2. Methods

2.1. Study Design and Participants

This study used a cross-sectional design by utilising survey methods to investigate the relationship between psychological mindedness, psychological mindfulness, psychological inflexibility, dysfunctional coping, and psychopathologies.

The study population from Indonesia encompassed university students in UNUSA located at Surabaya, East Java province, who were subject to the large-scale social restrictions (PSBB). As UNUSA did not have on-campus hostels, hence, respondents were not restricted within the university campus. However, they were still subjected to the implementation of PSBB in their respective provinces. The students were either staying inside Surabaya or outside of Surabaya. On the other hand, the study population from Malaysia encompassed university students in three campuses of a public university in East Malaysia (Sabah) who were subject to the nationwide Movement Control Order. All respondents were restricted to movement within the university campus only. All respondents were aged within 17–30 years old.

2.2. Ethical Considerations

The study was conducted according to the guidelines of the Declaration of Helsinki and approved by the medical ethics review committee of Universiti Malaysia Sabah (JKetika 2/20 (2), 27 April 2020).

2.3. Research Instruments

Firstly, basic sociodemographic characteristics were assessed in both groups. Secondly, in the Indonesian students, five scales were used: the DASS-21 measuring depression, anxiety, and stress (psychopathologies); the Balanced Index of Psychological Mindedness (BIPM) for psychological mindedness; the Acceptance and Action Questionnaire-II (AAQ-II) for psychological inflexibility; Coping Orientation to Problems Experienced Inventory (Brief COPE) Inventory for dysfunctional coping; and the Mindfulness Attention and Awareness Scale (MAAS) for psychological mindfulness. The DASS-21 has been validated both in the Malay and Indonesian language. The BIPM, AAQ-II, and MAAS are only available in Malay language validations. However, Malay and Indonesian languages are mutually intelligible; hence, the lead researchers from Indonesia made minor adjustments to all three Malay scales in order to ensure full intelligibility. Due to time pressures in the dynamic urgency of COVID-19, there was insufficient time to perform a full validation. For the Malaysian students, data were extracted from a separate project in a similar cohort of university students where only DASS-21 scores were measured.

2.3.1. The Depression, Anxiety and Stress Scale—21 Items (DASS-21)

The DASS-21 questionnaire is a set of scale consisting of 21 items measuring the emotional states of depression, anxiety, and stress [25]. Respondents were requested to complete the DASS-21 based on the presence of a symptom over the previous week. They rated each item on a four-point scale ranging from 1 (*did not apply to me at all over the last week*) to 4 (*applied to me very much or most of the time over the past week*), with higher scores indicating greater severity. The Malay version of DASS-21 has reasonable internal consistency with Cronbach's alpha values ranges from 0.74 to 0.84 [26].

2.3.2. Balanced Index of Psychological Mindedness (BIPM)

The BIPM is a self-report psychological instrument that measures psychological mindedness and was developed by [27]. It comprises of 14 items and 2 factors: Interest and Insight. *Interest* refers to attending to one's internal feelings, and *Insight* refers to understanding these feelings [28,29]. Each item is rated on a five-point Likert scale ranging from 1 (not true) to 5 (very much true). The Interest and Insight subscales of the BIPM showed good internal consistency (Cronbach's alphas = 0.85 and 0.76, respectively), test-retest reliability ($r = 0.63$ and 0.71, respectively), and construct validity (e.g., $r > 0.40$ with related constructs). The Malay version of the BIPM was preliminarily validated and has a Cronbach's alpha for total scores of 0.79, as well as for the "Interest" (0.76) and "Insight" (0.75) subscales, which are acceptable [30,31].

2.3.3. Acceptance and Action Questionnaire-II (AAQ-II)

The AAQ-II is an instrument to assess experiential avoidance and psychological inflexibility [32]. Experiential avoidance is defined as the attempt of the individual to ignore unpleasant thought, feelings, and physical sensations that leads to measures against one's values, causing continuing harm. Meanwhile, psychological inflexibility refers to rigid psychological reaction against one's value in order to avoid distress, uncomfortable feelings, and thought and tend to ignore the present moment [33]. AAQ-II is a unidimensional scale with 7 items and is rated based on 7-point scale. AAQ-II has good internal consistency (Cronbach's alpha = 0.88) and good test retest reliability over 3 and 12 months at 0.81 and 0.79, respectively [32]. Higher AAQ-II scores reflected significant psychological inflexibility and were also found to be associated with greater levels of depressive symptoms, anxiety and stress, thought suppression, and psychological distress.

2.3.4. Mindful Attention Awareness Scale (MAAS)

The MAAS measures the level of awareness and attention to the present-moment experience [16]. It consists of 15 items, and participants respond to each item using a six-point scale ranging from 1 (*almost always*) to 6 (*almost never*). Higher scores indicate higher levels of psychological mindfulness [34]. The Malay version of MAAS showed an acceptable internal consistency with Cronbach's alpha of 0.851 [35].

2.3.5. Coping Orientation to Problems Experienced Inventory (Brief COPE) Inventory

The Brief COPE is a self-report instrument containing 28 items that enquire regarding the frequency of various coping methods [36]. Individuals use a 4-point scale to respond regarding the frequency of specific coping methods, from 1 (*I usually don't do this at all*) to 4 (*I usually do this a lot*). The scale yields scores on three factors: problem-oriented coping styles, emotion-oriented coping styles, and dysfunctional coping styles. For the entire Malay scale, the internal consistencies ranged from 0.51 to 0.99. The test–retest Intraclass Correlation Coefficient (ICC) ranged from < 0.00 to 0.98 [37]. For the purpose of this study, we only used the dysfunctional coping style.

2.4. Data Analysis

In Study 1, we applied partial least squares–structural equation modeling (PLS-SEM) to assess measurement models and structural models for the Indonesian sample. We utilized PLS-SEM because of the inborn appropriateness of this methodology for exploratory investigations [38]. In addition, the comparison of anxiety, depression, and stress among Indonesian and Malaysian samples was performed using SPSS Version 27.

2.5. Reliability and Validity

For the Indonesian sample, a total of 869 samples were used to evaluate the measurement and structural models. At first, the reliability and validity of the reflective constructs (psychological mindedness, psychological mindfulness, psychological inflexibility, dysfunctional coping, and psychopathologies) were assessed. In order to confirm reliability, the composite reliability (CR) should be higher than 0.7, whereas for convergent validity to be established, the average variance extracted (AVE) should be higher than 0.5 [38]. Twenty-five indicators were removed due to weak outer loadings. Table 1 presents a summary for all reflective constructs, demonstrating that reliability and convergent validity had been verified. Next, to ascertain the discriminant validity, we used the Fornell–Larcker criterion [39]. According to Table 2, the Fornell–Larcker results demonstrated that the square root of the AVE for each construct (bold) was higher than its correlation with other constructs; discriminant validity was therefore established.

Table 1. Results of measurement model.

Construct	Items	Loadings	CR	AVE	Mean	SD
Psychopathologies	A4	0.655	0.920	0.511	1.93	0.65
	A5	0.713				
	A7	0.650				
	D3	0.755				
	D4	0.790				
	D5	0.674				
	D6	0.690				
	S4	0.748				
	S5	0.797				
	S6	0.690				
	S7	0.684				
Dysfunctional Coping	DC4	0.796	0.805	0.582	1.97	0.64
	DC5	0.658				
	DC7	0.824				
Psychological Mindfulness	MAAS1	0.701	0.904	0.513	3.84	1.03
	MAAS10	0.705				
	MAAS14	0.74				
	MAAS2	0.718				
	MAAS3	0.772				
	MAAS4	0.709				
	MAAS5	0.617				
	MAAS8	0.733				
	MAAS9	0.739				
Psychological Mindedness	INSIGHT1	0.769	0.899	0.504	2.39	0.88
	INSIGHT2	0.587				
	INSIGHT3	0.724				
	INSIGHT4	0.812				
	INSIGHT5	0.799				
	INSIGHT6	0.716				
	INTEREST1	0.522				
	INTEREST3	0.546				
	INTEREST5	0.834				
Psychological Inflexibility	AAQ1	0.768	0.911	0.594	3.35	1.39
	AAQ2	0.835				
	AAQ3	0.851				
	AAQ4	0.773				
	AAQ5	0.733				
	AAQ6	0.695				
	AAQ7	0.729				

Table 2. Discriminant validity: Fornell–Larcker.

No	Variables	1	2	3	4	5
1	Dysfunctional Coping	**0.763**				
2	Inflexibility	0.498	**0.771**			
3	Mindedness	0.440	0.621	**0.710**		
4	Mindfulness	−0.302	−0.364	−0.436	**0.716**	
5	Psychopathologies	0.436	0.574	0.673	−0.428	**0.715**

Note. Square root of the AVE for each construct (bold) was higher than its correlation with other constructs; discriminant validity was therefore established.

3. Results

3.1. Descriptive Statistics

Table 3 shows the respondent profiles who participated in this study. Out of 869 Indonesian respondents, 736 (84.7%) were females. The mean age for Indonesian respondents was 20.5 years old. Out of 515 Malaysian respondents, 357 (69.3%) were females. The mean age for the Malaysian respondents was 22.2 years old. Furthermore, the descriptive analyses of DASS-21 revealed that the majority of Indonesian respondents had a normal level of depression (61.0%), whereas the majority of Malaysian respondents had mild levels of depression (38.1%). In terms of anxiety, the majority of Indonesian respondents had a normal level (46.3%), whereas the majority of Malaysian respondents had a mild level (41.7%). Last but not least, for stress, the majority of Indonesian respondents had a normal level (64.6%), whereas the majority of Malaysian respondents had moderate level (40.4%).

Table 3. Descriptive analysis of respondents.

		Indonesian (N = 869)			Malaysian (N = 515)		
		Mean	**Frequency**	**Percent**	**Mean**	**Frequency**	**Percent**
Age		20.5			22.2		
Gender	Male		133	15.3		158	30.7
	Female		736	84.7		357	69.3
Depression	Normal		530	61.0		156	30.3
	Mild		146	16.8		196	38.1
	Moderate		98	11.3		142	27.6
	Severe		72	8.3		18	3.5
	Extra Severe		23	2.6		3	0.6
Anxiety	Normal		402	46.3		171	33.2
	Mild		163	18.8		215	41.7
	Moderate		141	16.2		118	22.9
	Severe		73	8.4		11	2.1
	Extra Severe		90	10.4		0	0.0
Stress	Normal		561	64.6		126	24.5
	Mild		104	12.0		158	30.7
	Moderate		141	16.2		208	40.4
	Severe		48	5.5		20	3.9
	Extra Severe		15	1.7		3	0.6

3.2. Study 1

Table 1 shows the mean scores and standard deviations (SD) for research variables for Study 1. The mean score for psychopathologies was 1.93 (SD = 0.65); 1.97 for dysfunctional coping (SD = 0.64); 3.84 for psychological mindfulness (SD = 1.03); 2.39 for psychological mindedness (SD = 0.88); and 3.35 for psychological inflexibility (SD = 1.39).

Table 4 also shows that all inner VIF values were below 5, therefore indicating that there was no issue of collinearity among the predictor constructs in the structural model [40]. To assess the direct effect and indirect effect, we assessed the structural model by computing the path coefficient (β), t-values, p-values, and R^2 using a 5000-sampling bootstrapping technique [40]. According to Table 4 and Figure 1, all direct effects were significant. With regard to the ΔR^2 value, the findings showed that the ΔR^2 value ranged from 0.091 to 0.515, which was acceptable [40] and accounted for 9.1% to 51.5% of the exploratory variance.

To assess the mediator in this study, the product of the coefficient approach using the bootstrapping resampling method was applied [41]. Our study showed that psychological mindedness, psychological mindfulness, and psychological inflexibility significantly mediate the relationship between dysfunctional coping and psychopathologies (refer Table 4).

Table 4. Results of direct and indirect effect.

Relationship	β	t	p	ΔR^2	VIF	Supported
Dysfunctional Coping → Psychological Inflexibility	0.498	16.987	0.00	0.248	1.000	Yes
Dysfunctional Coping → Psychological Mindedness	0.440	13.948	0.00	0.193	1.000	Yes
Dysfunctional Coping → Psychological Mindfulness	−0.302	8.253	0.00	0.091	1.000	Yes
Dysfunctional Coping → Psychopathologies	0.100	3.492	0.00	0.515	1.395	Yes
Psychological Inflexibility → Psychopathologies	0.197	7.598	0.00		1.658	Yes
Psychological Mindedness → Psychopathologies	0.450	14.512	0.00		1.776	Yes
Psychological Mindfulness → Psychopathologies	−0.129	4.966	0.00		1.257	Yes
Dysfunctional Coping → Psychological Inflexibility → Psychopathologies	0.117	6.658	0.00			Yes
Dysfunctional Coping → Psychological Mindfulness → Psychopathologies	0.042	4.068	0.00			Yes
Dysfunctional Coping → Psychological Mindedness → Psychopathologies	0.206	9.634	0.00			Yes

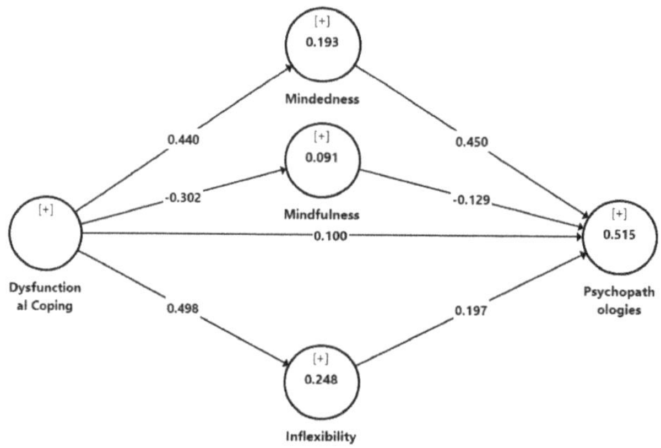

Figure 1. Results of structural model.

3.3. Study 2

In Study 2, the information was obtained from secondary data source, namely a separate but similar project performed by a similar research group. Combining the Indonesian study with the Malaysian data, there was a total of 1382 respondents consisting of 291 males (21.0%) and 1091 females (78.8%). Both studies utilized students from undergraduate age groups. As per Table 5, there was a significant difference in anxiety and stress between both countries. Specifically, Indonesian participants (M = 1.78, SD = 0.55) compared to the Malaysian participants (M = 1.64, SD = 0.52) demonstrated significantly higher anxiety: t(1380) = 3.342, p = 0.001. In addition, Indonesian participants (M = 1.93, SD = 0.63) compared to the Malaysian participants (M = 1.82, SD = 0.59) demonstrated significantly higher stress: t(1380) = 4.509, p = 0.000. There were no differences in depressive symptoms between both countries.

Table 5. Mean scores for anxiety, depression, and stress for Indonesia and Malaysia.

Variables	Indonesia		Malaysia	
	Mean	SD	Mean	SD
Anxiety	1.78 **	0.55	1.64 **	0.52
Depression	1.67	0.59	1.72	0.60
Stress	1.93 **	0.63	1.82 **	0.59

Note: ** $p < 0.01$.

4. Discussion and Conclusions

The COVID-19 pandemic has resulted in major impacts on many sectors such as economy, health, and education. With multiple nations imposing stay-at-home orders and lockdowns, mental wellbeing is paramount as there is a restriction of freedom alongside changes in routine. Many previous studies show the long term effects on people who were subjected to quarantine even months after the quarantine was over. This study aspires to understand the underlying psychological processes that cause people to either have a dysfunctional coping style or psychopathology symptoms, with the clinical implication of contributing to prospective interventions to mitigate emotional distress in individuals impacted by this pandemic.

The Indonesian data demonstrates that 22.2% of respondents scored "moderate" and above (severe and extremely severe) for depression, 35.0% scored "moderate" and above for anxiety, and 23.48% scored "moderate" and above for stress. This is also consistent with a previous study conducted in China in assessing the impact of COVID-19 on anxiety in Chinese university students [42]. Dysfunctional coping styles were significantly related to psychopathologies, which is consistent with previous studies [30,43]. The three psychological process variables, namely psychological mindedness, psychological mindfulness, and psychological inflexibility, completely mediated the relationship between dysfunctional coping mechanisms and psychopathologies. Specifically, dysfunctional coping is shown to have a negative effect on psychological mindfulness, which in turn had a negative impact upon the psychopathologies of participants. Since mindfulness is an emotion-regulating tool [11], our findings indicate that psychological mindfulness can be an indicator of the degree to which a person feels aware and accepting his or her experiences without bias judgments and thus serves as a buffer on psychopathologies. Additionally, dysfunctional coping was shown to have a positive effect on psychological inflexibility and psychological mindedness, which in turn have a positive effect on psychopathologies, probably because psychological inflexibility represents the opposite emotional states: disconnected with real sensations, feelings, or thoughts. Therefore, individuals in turn develop greater psychopathologies. However, an unexpected finding was that dysfunctional coping had a positive effect on psychological mindedness, which in turn has a positive effect on psychopathologies. Nevertheless, Hansell et al. [44] reported that psychological mindedness was positively correlated with psychopathologies. Due to the fact that highly psychologically minded individuals are more attuned than others to inner contradictions and dilemma, therefore, individuals are more likely to feel guilty and insecure [45]. In this sense, highly psychologically minded individuals are highly in introspective but also miserable. Essentially, the findings of this study suggest that the benefits of psychological mindedness during the COVID-19 pandemic are inextricably linked to its costs: greater psychopathologies.

This is a crucial finding as it suggests that if specific interventions that target psychological mindedness, psychological mindfulness, and psychological flexibility are performed, which are crucial components of Acceptance and Commitment Therapy (ACT), and we increase the levels of both constructs, clinically, it is implied that dysfunctional coping mechanisms will then no longer lead to psychopathologies, as the effect of the improved mediators reduces that relationship to non-significance. This concurs well with ACT theoretical models that suggest that instead of attempting to eliminate psychopathologies, which are unrealistic targets, the focus of therapy should be to learn to live with the distress better using psychological mindedness and mindfulness skills and to be more psychologically flexible so that one can live a more meaningful and value-driven life despite the pain. This is especially prescient in COVID-19, where the trigger is unseen, potentially carried by asymptomatic carriers, untreatable, and not vaccinated at the point of the study being performed. Hence, as the source of the distress clearly cannot be ameliorated, is worsening in certain countries, and is unlikely to go away anytime soon due to the lack of treatment and vaccine, this study supports wholeheartedly the assertion that it is better and more efficacious to be kind to oneself and to have more skills in the armamentarium to be more psychologically flexible in order to ride through and weather the COVID-19 storm.

The alarming COVID-19 situation in Indonesia had certainly caused significant psychological distress, as evidenced by higher anxiety and stress levels among the Indonesian respondents compared to Malaysian respondents. This corroborates with findings of other studies that proposed that there is a linear relationship between the number of cases and psychological distress suffered, especially those in high-risk areas [46,47]. Although this may reflect a normal physiological reaction, however, with the number of positive cases and total deaths steadily increasing, authorities should consider large-scale mental health intervention to address and alleviate the trepidation suffered by the Indonesians and Malaysians.

Stress is the most prominent psychopathologies among the students, looking into the findings. More intervention on alleviating stress symptoms among students should be refined, and this study corroborates overwhelming evidence that show that psychological mindedness, psychological mindfulness, and psychological flexibility are efficacious in dealing with psychopathology symptoms. These three psychological processes can aid in responding to the unpredictable and untenable stress of COVID-19, with awareness of physical and emotional reactions in the present moment, rather than simply acting instinctively without an awareness of motives. This allows more adaptive reactions to difficult situations, of which the dynamic and flexible COVID-19 situation is most certainly one. By practicing psychological mindfulness, individuals can learn to maintain a relaxed mind and concentrate on the present moment [48]. Hence, this study's important clinical implication is that psychosocial interventions and also needs assessments should be inclined towards risk groups; i.e., females and those in Indonesia, and should be grounded in mindedness, mindfulness, and flexibility-oriented psychological approaches.

Limitation and Implication

There are a few limitations of this study. Firstly, it is a cross sectional study, and hence causal inferences cannot be made. Secondly, due to the dearth of available Indonesian language questionnaires for psychological process variables, validated Malay questionnaires were used and adapted with Indonesian variations to accommodate for UNUSA respondents. Due to the urgency and dynamic requirements of the COVID-19 pandemic, there was insufficient time to perform a formal validation study on the adapted Indonesian questionnaires. As the Malay and Indonesian language are largely mutually intelligible, the face validity of the Malay versions was confirmed with Indonesian researchers in this study; but for future research purposes, the validation of all three psychological process variables into Bahasa Indonesia are in progress by the same teams. Thirdly, the survey was performed through online methods due to social distancing and lockdowns; hence there may be higher levels of social desirability.

Nevertheless, quarantine orders implemented by both countries most certainly will create difficulties in implementing psychological interventions. However, creative approaches have been encouraged and implemented. Online counselling has evolved in COVID-19 to be more approachable, private, secure, and more easily accessed. Mindfulness training especially has started to evolve into video- or audio-guided home practice daily with specialised trainers in small groups. For psychological flexibility, online Acceptance and Commitment Therapy (ACT) programs, with their focus on discrete skill building, can supplant face-to-face approaches. It is a constructive method to shape behavior with a target to enhance the quality of life, with an aim to support clients to adopt life goal-directed behaviors to manage anxiety [48].

In conclusion, this study has provided an insight on the importance of various psychological process students' psychopathologies during the COVID-19 pandemic. In light of this, factors such as psychological mindedness, psychological mindfulness, and psychological flexibility are important. The high level of stress and anxiety among the Indonesian sample compared to the Malaysian sample in this study showed that most Indonesian students are uniquely susceptible to mental health difficulties during COVID-19. Hence, this study aspires to develop a more refined and polished intervention especially for students in Malaysian and Indonesian public universities who are subjected to the quarantine order as implemented by both government authorities.

Author Contributions: Conceptualization, N.L.H., F.A. and N.T.P.P.; methodology, N.T.P.P. and W.W.; software, N.T.P.P. and W.W.; formal analysis, N.T.P.P. and W.W.; investigation, N.L.H. and F.A.; resources, N.L.H., F.A., N.T.P.P., M.A.M.K., H.A., M.S.; data curation, N.L.H., F.A. and N.T.P.P.; writing—original draft preparation, N.L.H., F.A. and N.T.P.P.; writing—review and editing, N.L.H., F.A., N.T.P.P., M.A.M.K., H.A., M.S., N.G., S.S.S.A.R., A.O., M.S.J. and W.W.; visualization, N.L.H.; supervision, N.T.P.P.; project administration, N.L.H. and F.A. All authors have read and agreed to the published version of the manuscript.

Funding: This research received no external funding.

Institutional Review Board Statement: The study was conducted according to the guidelines of the Declaration of Helsinki and approved by the medical ethics review committee of Universiti Malaysia Sabah [JKetika 2/20 (2), 27 April 2020].

Informed Consent Statement: Informed consent was obtained from all patients involved in the study.

Data Availability Statement: Data can be available upon reasonable request.

Conflicts of Interest: The authors declare no conflict of interest.

References

1. Muhamad, A.B.; Pang, N.T.P.; Salvaraji, L.; Rahim, S.S.S.A.; Jeffree, M.S.; Omar, A. Retrospective Analysis of Psychological Factors in COVID-19 Outbreak Among Isolated and Quarantined Agricultural Students in a Borneo University. *Front. Psychiatry* **2021**, *12*, 483. [CrossRef] [PubMed]
2. Salvaraji, L.; Rahim, S.S.S.A.; Jeffree, M.S.; Omar, A.; Pang, N.T.P.; Ahmedy, F.; Hayati, F.; Yeap, B.T.; Giloi, N.; Saupin, S. The importance of high index of suspicion and immediate containment of suspected COVID-19 cases in institute of higher education Sabah, Malaysia Borneo. *Malays. J. Public Health Med.* **2020**, *20*, 74–83. [CrossRef]
3. Sutrisno, B. Indonesia to Evaluate Partial Lockdown as Companies, Factories Continue Business as Usual. Available online: https://www.thejakartapost.com/news/2020/04/20/indonesia-to-evaluate-partial-lockdown-as-companies-factories-continue-business-as-usual.html (accessed on 21 April 2020).
4. Lee, J. Mental health effects of school closures during COVID-19. *Lancet* **2020**, *395*, 912–920. [CrossRef]
5. Brown, S.; Kafka, A.C. Has Worsened the Student Mental-Health Crisis. Can Resilience Training Fix It? Available online: https://www.chronicle.com/article/covid-19-has-worsened-the-student-mental-health-crisis-can-resilience-training-fix-it/ (accessed on 11 May 2022).
6. Sun, S.; Goldberg, S.B.; Lin, D.; Qiao, S.; Operario, D. Psychiatric symptoms, risk, and protective factors among university students in quarantine during the COVID-19 pandemic in China. *Glob. Health* **2021**, *17*, 1–14.
7. Pang, N.T.P.; James, S.; Giloi, N.; Rahim, S.S.S.A.; Omar, A.; Jeffree, M.S.; Hayati, F.; Lim, M.C.; Kassim, M.A.M.; Ng, J.R. Relationships between psychopathology, psychological process variables, and sociodemographic variables and comparison of quarantined and non-quarantined groups of Malaysian University students in the COVID-19 pandemic. *Int. J. Environ. Res. Public Health* **2021**, *18*, 9656. [CrossRef] [PubMed]
8. Pang, N.T.P.; Nold Imon, G.; Johoniki, E.; Mohd Kassim, M.A.; Omar, A.; Syed Abdul Rahim, S.S.; Hayati, F.; Jeffree, M.S.; Ng, J.R. Fear of COVID-19 and COVID-19 stress and association with sociodemographic and psychological process factors in cases under surveillance in a frontline worker population in Borneo. *Int. J. Environ. Res. Public Health* **2021**, *18*, 7210. [CrossRef]
9. Denollet, J.; Nyklicek, I. Psychological mindedness: A forgotten emotion-focused coping style? In *Emotional Expression and Health: Advances in Theory, Assessment and Clinical Applications*; Brunner-Routledge: Hove, UK, 2004; pp. 185–203.
10. Koep, L.L.; Biggs, M.L.; Rhodes, J.R.; Elkins, G.R. Psychological mindedness, attitudes toward hypnosis, and expectancy as correlates of hypnotizability. *Int. J. Clin. Exp. Hypn.* **2020**, *68*, 68–79. [CrossRef]
11. Keng, S.-L.; Smoski, M.J.; Robins, C.J. Effects of mindfulness on psychological health: A review of empirical studies. *Clin. Psychol. Rev.* **2011**, *31*, 1041–1056. [CrossRef]
12. Arslan, G.; Yıldırım, M.; Tanhan, A.; Buluş, M.; Allen, K.-A. Coronavirus stress, optimism-pessimism, psychological inflexibility, and psychological health: Psychometric properties of the Coronavirus Stress Measure. *Int. J. Ment. Health Addict.* **2021**, *19*, 2423–2439. [CrossRef]
13. Nyklíček, I.; Majoor, D.; Schalken, P.A. Psychological mindedness and symptom reduction after psychotherapy in a heterogeneous psychiatric sample. *Compr. Psychiatry* **2010**, *51*, 492–496. [CrossRef]
14. Nyklíček, I.; Poot, J.C.; van Opstal, J. Psychological mindedness in relation to personality and coping in a sample of young adult psychiatric patients. *J. Clin. Psychol.* **2010**, *66*, 34–45. [CrossRef] [PubMed]
15. Baer, R.A.; Smith, G.T.; Hopkins, J.; Krietemeyer, J.; Toney, L. Using self-report assessment methods to explore facets of mindfulness. *Assessment* **2006**, *13*, 27–45. [CrossRef] [PubMed]
16. Brown, K.; Ryan, R. The benefits of being present: Mindfulness and its role in psychological well-being. *J. Personal. Soc. Psychol.* **2003**, *84*, 822–848. [CrossRef] [PubMed]
17. Pepping, C.A.; O'Donovan, A.; Davis, P.J. The differential relationship between mindfulness and attachment in experienced and inexperienced meditators. *Mindfulness* **2014**, *5*, 392–399. [CrossRef]
18. Pepping, C.A.; Duvenage, M.; Cronin, T.J.; Lyons, A. Adolescent mindfulness and psychopathology: The role of emotion regulation. *Personal. Individ. Differ.* **2016**, *99*, 302–307. [CrossRef]
19. Masuda, A.; Anderson, P.L.; Wendell, J.W.; Chou, Y.-Y.; Price, M.; Feinstein, A.B. Psychological flexibility mediates the relations between self-concealment and negative psychological outcomes. *Personal. Individ. Differ.* **2011**, *50*, 243–247. [CrossRef]
20. Masuda, A.; Tully, E.C. The role of mindfulness and psychological flexibility in somatization, depression, anxiety, and general psychological distress in a nonclinical college sample. *J. Evid.-Based Complementary Altern. Med.* **2012**, *17*, 66–71. [CrossRef]
21. Tull, M.T.; Gratz, K.L.; Salters, K.; Roemer, L. The role of experiential avoidance in posttraumatic stress symptoms and symptoms of depression, anxiety, and somatization. *J. Nerv. Ment. Dis.* **2004**, *192*, 754–761. [CrossRef]
22. Bond, F.; Bunce, D. Mediators of change in emotion-focused and problem-focused worksite stress management interventions. *J. Occup. Health Psychol.* **2000**, *5*, 156–163. [CrossRef]
23. Kashdan, T.B.; Barrios, V.; Forsyth, J.P.; Steger, M.F. Experiential avoidance as a generalized psychological vulnerability: Comparisons with coping and emotion regulation strategies. *Behav. Res. Ther.* **2006**, *44*, 1301–1320. [CrossRef]

24. Brooks, S.K.; Webster, R.K.; Smith, L.E.; Woodland, L.; Wessely, S.; Greenberg, N.; Rubin, G.J. The psychological impact of quarantine and how to reduce it: Rapid review of the evidence. *Lancet* **2020**, *395*, 912–920. [CrossRef]
25. Lovibond, S.H.; Lovibond, P.F. *Manual for the Depression Anxiety Stress Scales*; Psychology Foundation of Australia: Sydney, Australia, 1996.
26. Musa, R.; Fadzil, M.A.; Zain, Z. Translation, validation and psychometric properties of Bahasa Malaysia version of the Depression Anxiety and Stress Scales (DASS). *ASEAN J. Psychiatry* **2007**, *8*, 82–89.
27. Nyklícek, I.; Denollet, J. Development and evaluation of the Balanced Index of Psychological Mindedness (BIPM). *Psychol. Assess.* **2009**, *21*, 32–44. [CrossRef] [PubMed]
28. Giromini, L.; Brusadelli, E.; Di Noto, B.; Grasso, R.; Lang, M. Measuring psychological mindedness: Validity, reliability, and relationship with psychopathology of an Italian version of the Balanced Index of Psychological Mindedness. *Psychoanal. Psychother.* **2015**, *29*, 70–87. [CrossRef]
29. Takagishi, Y. Factor structure, validity, and reliability of the Japanese version of the Balanced Index of Psychological Mindedness (BIPM). *Jpn. Psychol. Res.* **2020**, *62*, 56–64. [CrossRef]
30. Ping Pang, N.T.; Masiran, R.; Tan, K.A.; Kassim, A. Psychological mindedness as a mediator in the relationship between dysfunctional coping styles and depressive symptoms in caregivers of children with autism spectrum disorder. *Perspect. Psychiatr. Care* **2020**, *56*, 649–656. [CrossRef]
31. MK, M.A.; TP, N.P.; Wendy, D.; LT, M.W.; Yeoh, Y.X. Validation of Bahasa Malaysia version of psychological mindedness in a university population. *IIUM Med. J. Malays.* **2021**, *20*. [CrossRef]
32. Shari, N.I.; Zainal, N.Z.; Guan, N.C.; Ahmad Sabki, Z.; Yahaya, N.A. Psychometric properties of the acceptance and action questionnaire (AAQ II) Malay version in cancer patients. *PLoS ONE* **2019**, *14*, e0212788. [CrossRef]
33. Bond, F.W.; Hayes, S.C.; Baer, R.A.; Carpenter, K.M.; Guenole, N.; Orcutt, H.K.; Waltz, T.; Zettle, R.D. Preliminary psychometric properties of the Acceptance and Action Questionnaire–II: A revised measure of psychological inflexibility and experiential avoidance. *Behav. Ther.* **2011**, *42*, 676–688. [CrossRef]
34. Carlson, L.E.; Brown, K.W. Validation of the Mindful Attention Awareness Scale in a cancer population. *J. Psychosom. Res.* **2005**, *58*, 29–33. [CrossRef]
35. Zainal, N.; Nor-Aziyan, Y.; Subramaniam, P. Psychometric properties of the Malay-translated Mindfulness, Attention and Awareness Scale (MAAS) in a group of nursing students in Malaysia. *Malays. J. Psychiatry* **2015**, *24*, 33–41.
36. Carver, C.S. You want to measure coping but your protocol'too long: Consider the brief cope. *Int. J. Behav. Med.* **1997**, *4*, 92–100. [CrossRef] [PubMed]
37. Yusoff, N.; Low, W.Y.; Yip, C.H. Reliability and validity of the Brief COPE Scale (English version) among women with breast cancer undergoing treatment of adjuvant chemotherapy: A Malaysian study. *Med. J. Malays.* **2010**, *65*, 41–44.
38. Ali, F.; Rasoolimanesh, S.M.; Sarstedt, M.; Ringle, C.M.; Ryu, K.S. An Assessment of the Use of Partial Least Squares Structural Equation Modeling (PLS-SEM) in Hospitality Research. *Int. J. Contemp. Hosp. Manag.* **2018**, *30*, 514–538. [CrossRef]
39. Voorhees, C.M.; Brady, M.K.; Calantone, R.; Ramirez, E. Discriminant validity testing in marketing: An analysis, causes for concern, and proposed remedies. *J. Acad. Mark. Sci.* **2016**, *44*, 119–134. [CrossRef]
40. Hair Jr, J.F.; Sarstedt, M.; Ringle, C.M.; Gudergan, S.P. *Advanced Issues in Partial Least Squares Structural Equation Modeling*; SAGE Publications: Thousand Oaks, CA, USA, 2017.
41. Nitzl, C.; Roldán Salgueiro, J.L.; Cepeda-Carrión, G. Mediation analysis in partial least squares path modeling: Helping researchers discuss more sophisticated models. *Ind. Manag. Data Syst.* **2016**, *116*, 1849–1864. [CrossRef]
42. Qiu, J.; Shen, B.; Zhao, M.; Wang, Z.; Xie, B.; Xu, Y. A nationwide survey of psychological distress among Chinese people in the COVID-19 epidemic: Implications and policy recommendations. *Gen. Psychiatry* **2020**, *33*, e100213. [CrossRef]
43. Kulip, J.; Jeffree, M.S.; Pang, N.T.P.; Nasirruddin, N.; Wider, W. Relationships between Coping Styles, Emotional Distress, and Fear of COVID-19 among Workers in the Oil and Gas Industry in Malaysia during the COVID-19 Pandemic. *Sustainability* **2022**, *14*, 5398. [CrossRef]
44. Hansell, S.; Mechanic, D.; Brondolo, E. Introspectiveness and adolescent development. *J. Youth Adolesc.* **1986**, *15*, 115–132. [CrossRef]
45. Farber, B.A. Psychological-mindedness: Can there be too much of a good thing? *Psychother. Theory Res. Pract. Train.* **1989**, *26*, 210. [CrossRef]
46. Holingue, C.; Badillo-Goicoechea, E.; Riehm, K.E.; Veldhuis, C.B.; Thrul, J.; Johnson, R.M.; Fallin, M.D.; Kreuter, F.; Stuart, E.A.; Kalb, L.G. Mental distress during the COVID-19 pandemic among US adults without a pre-existing mental health condition: Findings from American trend panel survey. *Prev. Med.* **2020**, *139*, 106231. [CrossRef] [PubMed]
47. Holingue, C.; Kalb, L.G.; Riehm, K.E.; Bennett, D.; Kapteyn, A.; Veldhuis, C.B.; Johnson, R.M.; Fallin, M.D.; Kreuter, F.; Stuart, E.A. Mental distress in the United States at the beginning of the COVID-19 pandemic. *Am. J. Public Health* **2020**, *110*, 1628–1634. [CrossRef] [PubMed]
48. Eifert, G.H.; Forsyth, J.P.; Arch, J.; Espejo, E.; Keller, M.; Langer, D. Acceptance and commitment therapy for anxiety disorders: Three case studies exemplifying a unified treatment protocol. *Cogn. Behav. Pract.* **2009**, *16*, 368–385. [CrossRef]

behavioral sciences

MDPI

Article

Causal Analysis and Prevention Measures for Extreme Heavy Rainstorms in Zhengzhou to Protect Human Health

Qingwei Xu [1,*], Liu Han [1] and Kaili Xu [2]

1 College of Information and Management Science, Henan Agricultural University, Zhengzhou 450046, China; 343572775@163.com
2 School of Resources and Civil Engineering, Northeastern University, Shenyang 110819, China; xukaili@mail.neu.edu.cn
* Correspondence: xuqingwei@henau.edu.cn

Abstract: This study focused on the extreme heavy rainstorm that occurred in Zhengzhou in July 2021; approximately 380 people were killed or missing as a result of this storm. To investigate the evolution behaviors of this rainstorm and take corresponding prevention measures, several methods and models were adopted, including cloud modeling, preliminary hazard analysis (PHA), fault tree analysis (FTA), bow-tie modeling, and chaos theory. The main reasons for this rainstorm can be divided into the following three aspects: force majeure, such as terrain and extreme weather conditions, issues with city construction, and insufficient emergency rescue. The secondary disasters caused by this rainstorm mainly include urban water logging, river flooding, and mountain torrents and landslides. The main causes of the subway line-5 accident that occurred can be described as follows: the location of the stabling yard was low, the relevant rules and regulations of the subway were not ideal, insufficient attention was given to the early warning information, and the emergency response mechanism was not ideal. Rainstorms result from the cross-coupling of faults in humans, objects, the environment, and management subsystems, and the evolution process shows an obvious butterfly effect. To prevent disasters caused by rainstorms, the following suggestions should be adopted: vigorously improve the risk awareness and emergency response capabilities of leading cadres, improve the overall level of urban disaster prevention and mitigation, reinforce the existing reservoirs in the city, strengthen the construction of sponge cities, and improve the capacity of urban disaster emergency rescue.

Keywords: rainstorm; cloud model; PHA; FTA; bow-tie model; chaos theory

1. Introduction

From 17–23 July 2021, Henan Province in China suffered a rare heavy rainstorm and severe flooding. On 20 July 2021, many deaths, missing persons, and property losses occurred in Zhengzhou city. From 4 p.m. to 5 p.m. on 20 July 2021, the 1 h precipitation in Zhengzhou reached 201.9 mm according to the China Meteorological Administration (CMA) [1]. These disasters caused a total of 14.786 million people in 150 counties (cities and districts) in Henan Province to be affected, and 398 people were killed or missing, including 380 people in Zhengzhou city, accounting for 95.5% of the total casualties in the province; the direct economic loss was 120.06 billion *yuan*, of which 40.9 billion *yuan* was in Zhengzhou, accounting for 34.1% of the direct economic loss in the province [2]. A rainstorm is a weather phenomenon that produces strong rainfall over a short period, and many countries are plagued by rainstorms worldwide [3–5]. Risk assessment of accidents caused by rainstorms is of great significance to improve the environment and protect lives.

Within a certain period, the greater the rainfall is, the more serious the consequences are. Determining the grade of precipitation plays an important role in taking targeted prevention measures. Geng et al. [6] investigated the flood risk in Quzhou city, China, based on fuzzy comprehensive evaluation. Falck et al. [7] adopted a stochastic error model to generate an ensemble of rainfall fields. The fuzzy comprehensive evaluation method can solve problems with uncertainty and fuzziness, but it cannot solve randomness problems. The stochastic model is suitable for problems with uncertainty and randomness, but it is difficult to deal with the problem of fuzziness. The cloud model can realize the uncertainty transformation between qualitative concepts and quantitative data, and this uncertainty transformation has fuzziness and randomness [8,9]. Since rainfall is affected spatiotemporally and has uncertainty, fuzziness, and randomness, this study adopted the qualitative and quantitative assessment functions of the cloud model to determine the grade of the Zhengzhou rainstorm. The cloud model has been widely used in the field of safety assessment, including in chemical plants [8] and casting workshops [9]. The cloud model used to evaluate the grade of the Zhengzhou rainstorm has a certain theoretical basis and can obtain reliable results.

To simplify the forecasting procedures, some scholars have adopted pure mathematical models to forecast rainfall in recent years. To predict disasters, Pontoh et al. [10] constructed a model of rainfall forecasting using a nonlinear autoregressive exogenous neural network. To determine long-term hydrological system trends, Lin et al. [11] proposed a hybrid grey model for forecasting annual maximum daily rainfall. Zhao et al. [12] proposed an hourly rainfall forecast model based on a supervised learning algorithm to predict rainfall with high accuracy and high time resolution. For mathematical prediction models, grey system theory focuses mainly on issues, such as partial information unknowns [13]. The GM(1,1) model is one of the most important models in the grey model group. There have been research reports on the use of grey system theory in the prediction of rainfall, and the prediction results were consistent with the actual situation [11]. It is an approximate model and effective if the data series shows a behavior of exponent distribution. Therefore, the GM(1,1) model was adopted to predict the rainfall in Zhengzhou. However, the formation of rainstorms requires certain conditions, such as the supply of water vapor, the vertical upward movement of the air, and the duration of rainfall. The intensity of rainstorms can be predicted by the numerical simulation of these factors. However, the duration of rainfall is affected spatiotemporally, and the movement of the air is quite complex and affected by terrain, underlying surfaces, and human activities. It is difficult to predict rainfall without knowledge of these basic data. The main purpose of researching rainfall forecasting in Zhengzhou was to show that the rainstorm is affected by multiple factors, and the reasons for the rainstorm are analyzed in detail later.

Rainstorms are severe weather phenomena, and a series of accidents can occur because of a rainstorm. Brazdil et al. [14] reported that rain led to 205 fatalities in the Czech Republic from 2000 to 2019, and the results showed that nearly half of the fatalities (49.8%) occurred in the summer months. Tobin et al. [15] estimated the relative risk of crashes during rain using a matched-pair analysis in Kansas for 1995–2014. Yoon et al. [16] collected data of traffic accidents during rainy conditions from 2007 to 2017 in Seoul, South Korea. Rainstorms can lead to a series of secondary disasters, such as flash floods, landslides, mudslides, house collapses, and traffic and communication interruptions, which can bring serious harm to the national economy and people's lives and property. Previous studies have mainly focused on the accidents caused by rainstorms [14–16], but they have failed to conduct a deep analysis of the causes, consequences, and prevention measures of these accidents. Preliminary hazard analysis (PHA) [17,18], fault tree analysis (FTA) [19,20], and bow-tie models [21,22] are widely used to identify the causes, consequences, and prevention measures for fatal accidents, and the results have shown that these methods can obtain accurate accident data and reduce the risk of accidents. Therefore, PHA [17,18], FTA [19,20], and the bow-tie model [21,22] were adopted to analyze rainstorms and secondary disasters.

The evolution mechanism of rainstorms plays an important role in preventing rainstorm disasters. Luini [23] investigated the evolution of rain fields based on the spatiotemporal dimensions. You et al. [24] analyzed the evolution, energetics, and trend of heavy rain-producing terrestrial low-pressure systems over the East Asian summer monsoon region. Lawal et al. [25] reported the temporal evolution of atmospheric parameter profiling on rain height over two geo-climatic regions in Nigeria. The evolution of rainstorms is affected not only by natural factors but also by human factors. With the development of the social economy and science and technology, the influence of human factors on the evolution of rainstorms is increasing. In addition, the evolution process of rainstorms is affected not only by deterministic factors but also by random factors, showing certain randomness. Previous studies have mainly focused on the influence of natural factors on the evolution of rainstorms [23–25], but there is a lack of focus on the influence of human and management factors on the evolution of rainstorms. Fortunately, chaos theory [26,27] has been adapted to explore the comprehensive influence of humans, objects, the environment, and management on the evolution process of accidents. For example, Xu et al. [27] investigated the cross-coupling function of employee, object, environment, and management subsystems on hydraulic support failure. In this study, chaos theory [26,27] was adopted to investigate the influence of humans, objects, environments, and management factors on the evolution process of rainstorms. Chaos theory has been theoretically and practically researched for accidents. In this study, chaos theory was used to investigate the evolution process of rainstorms, with the hope to expand the application scope of chaos theory.

This study proposed a composite risk assessment method for rainstorms. According to the rainfall data in Zhengzhou and the national standard *grade of precipitation* (GB/T 28592-2012) [28], the precipitation grade of Zhengzhou on 20 July 2021 was determined using a cloud model [8,9]. To explore the predictability of extreme weather from the evaluation results of the cloud model, the GM(1,1) model [13] was adopted to predict the rainfall in Zhengzhou in July 2021, and the validity and influencing factors of the prediction results were analyzed. The PHA [17,18] was adopted to analyze the causes of rainstorms in Zhengzhou, as well as secondary disasters caused by rainstorms. For flood disasters caused by rainstorms, FTA [19,20] was used to investigate the basic reasons. For the Zhengzhou subway line-5 accident that occurred due to the flood disaster, the bow-tie model [21,22] was adopted to analyze the causes in detail. Chaos theory [26,27] was used to investigate the cross-coupling effect of human, object, environment, and management factors on rainstorms. Finally, suggestions were given to prevent rainstorms and secondary disasters.

2. Methods

2.1. About the Rainstorm

From 17–23 July 2021, Zhengzhou experienced a rare heavy rainstorm and severe flooding. On 20 July 2021, Zhengzhou suffered heavy casualties and property losses. Zhengzhou lost 380 people due to the disaster, accounting for 95.5% of Henan Province; the direct economic loss was 40.9 billion *yuan*, accounting for 34.1% of Henan Province [2]. This round of rainfall is equivalent to nearly 4 billion cubic meters of water, which is the most extensive and strongest rainstorm process in Zhengzhou since meteorological observation records have been available [2]. From 4 p.m. to 5 p.m. on 20 July 2021, the 1 h precipitation in Zhengzhou reached 201.9 mm [1]. Three major rivers, including Jialu River, Shuangji River, and Ying River in Zhengzhou city, all experienced large floods that exceeded the guaranteed water level, and the process floods all exceeded the historical maximum. This rainstorm far exceeded Zhengzhou's existing drainage capacity and planned drainage standards. There are 38 drainage zones in the main urban area of Zhengzhou, and only 1 reached the planned drainage standards [2].

On 20 July, the 04502 train of subway line-5 was flooded and forced to stop due to a power outage while traveling from Haitansi Station to Shakoulu Station. After evacuation and rescue, 953 passengers were safely evacuated, and 14 passengers died [2]. This event is one of the most severe urban water logging events caused by an extremely heavy rainstorm.

The factors that led to the extreme heavy rainstorm disaster in Zhengzhou mainly include the following aspects: the subtropical high was abnormally northerly, and the summer monsoon was stronger than usual; the typhoons that formed in the same period converged to transport the water vapor from the sea, which was superimposed with the convective system above; the uplift due to Funiu Mountain and Taihang Mountain; and the terrain of Zhengzhou is high in the southwest and low in the northeast, which is a transitional zone from hilly mountains to plains.

To prevent disasters caused by rainstorms, the following suggestions should be adopted: vigorously improve the risk awareness and emergency response capabilities of leading cadres; improve the overall level of urban disaster prevention and mitigation; reinforce the existing reservoirs in the city; strengthen the construction of sponge cities; and improve the capacity of urban disaster emergency rescue. These suggestions are analyzed in detail later in this paper.

2.2. Framework and Theoretical Models

The framework of the rainstorm risk assessment method proposed in this study is shown in Figure 1.

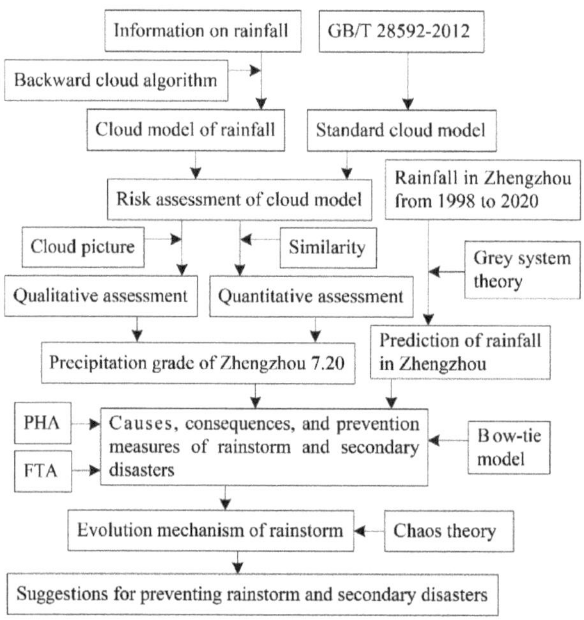

Figure 1. The framework of the risk assessment method proposed in this study.

Figure 1 shows the flow of this study, as well as the methods and data adopted. To obtain the precipitation grade in Zhengzhou on 20 July 2021, it was necessary to first determine the cloud model of the Zhengzhou rainstorm and the standard cloud model. The cloud model [8,9] of the Zhengzhou rainstorm could be achieved according to the information on rainfall and the backward cloud algorithm. The standard cloud model could be obtained by the national precipitation standard. The qualitative assessment result of the precipitation grade could be achieved by mapping the cloud model of the Zhengzhou rainstorm and the standard cloud models into a cloud picture. The quantitative assessment result of the precipitation grade could be obtained by calculating the similarity between the cloud model of the Zhengzhou rainstorm and the standard cloud model. The precipitation grade of Zhengzhou could be achieved according to the qualitative and quantitative assessment results. The Zhengzhou rainstorm that occurred in July 2021 was an extremely heavy rainstorm. Although the error test of the GM(1,1) model [13] met the accuracy requirements, the rainfall in Zhengzhou could not be accurately predicted, indicating that the rainfall in Zhengzhou in July 2021 was greatly affected by external factors. According to the FTA [19,20], the external factors of this rainstorm can be divided into the following three aspects: force majeure, such as terrain and extreme weather conditions, issues with city construction, and insufficient emergency rescue. The main causes of the subway line-5 accident can be described as follows based on the bow-tie model [21,22]: the location of the stabling yard was low, the relevant rules and regulations of the subway were not ideal, insufficient attention was given to the early warning information, and the emergency response mechanism was not ideal. Using chaos theory [26,27], we comprehensively investigated the influence of human, object, environmental, and management factors on rainstorms and analyzed the sensitivity of the evolution process to initial conditions. Finally, suggestions were given to prevent rainstorms and secondary disasters, which are analyzed in detail later in this paper.

2.2.1. Cloud Model

The cloud model describes the features of a concept by three numerical characteristics (*Ex*, *En*, and *He*) [9]. The expectation *Ex* is the center value of the qualitative concept, which is the most representative cloud drop. The entropy *En* indicates the fuzziness and randomness of the qualitative concept. The hyper entropy *He* is the fuzziness and randomness of the entropy *En*, which reflects the thickness of the cloud.

En is the uncertainty degree of the qualitative concept, which represents the cloud drops that are accepted by the qualitative concept in the domain. The larger the *En* is, the larger the range covered by the cloud model is [9]. Cloud drops that contribute to the qualitative concept in the universe domain of discourse mainly fall in the interval $[Ex - 3En, Ex + 3En]$, and the contribution rate of these cloud drops in this interval is approximately 99.74% [29]. Cloud drops other than $[Ex - 3En, Ex + 3En]$ have a negligible contribution to the qualitative concept.

(1) Forward cloud algorithm

Random variables are the basic tool for studying random phenomena, and the distribution function is an important probability characteristic of random variables that can describe the statistical behaviors of random variables [30]. Normal distribution exists widely in natural phenomena, social phenomena, scientific research, and production activities, and many random variables in real life obey or approximately obey a normal distribution. For example, random measurement errors, temperature or rainfall in a certain area all obey a normal distribution. According to the central limit theorem [31], if a given random variable is dominated by a large number of tiny, independent random factors, the individual effects of each factor are relatively uniform and no one factor has a clear advantage, andthe random variable approximately obeys a normal distribution. The normal distribution is the limiting distribution of many important probability distributions [32]. Therefore, the use of a normal probability distribution to evaluate rainfall has a certain theoretical basis.

Input. The numerical characteristics (*Ex*, *En*, and *He*) of the qualitative concept and the number of cloud drops n.

Output. The location in the domain and the membership degree $u(x)$ of each cloud drop.

① Generate a random number En' that is normally distributed and has a mean En and a standard deviation *He*; that is, $X \sim N(Ex, En'^2)$ [29]. The normal probability distribution function of the random number En' can be described as follows [32]:

$$f_{En'}(x) = \frac{1}{\sqrt{2\pi}He} e^{-\frac{(x-En)^2}{2He^2}} \quad (1)$$

② Generate a random number X that is normally distributed and has a mean Ex and standard deviation En'; that is, $X \sim N(Ex, En'^2)$ [29]. The normal probability distribution function of the random number X can be described as follows [32]:

$$f_X(x) = \frac{1}{\sqrt{2\pi}En'} e^{-\frac{(x-Ex)^2}{2En'^2}} \quad (2)$$

③ The membership degree $u(X)$ can be calculated as follows [33]:

$$\mu(x) = e^{\frac{-(x-Ex)^2}{2(En')^2}} \tag{3}$$

④ Repeat steps 1–3 until n cloud drops are generated.

(2) Backward cloud algorithm

Input. Cloud drops x_i (i = 1,2, … n).
Output. Numerical characteristics (*Ex*, *En*, and *He*) of the cloud drops.
The numerical characteristics (*Ex*, *En*, and *He*) can be calculated as follows [33].

$$Ex = \frac{1}{n}\sum_{i=1}^{n} x_i \tag{4}$$

$$En = \sqrt{\frac{\pi}{2}} \times \frac{1}{n}\sum_{i=1}^{n} |x_i - Ex| \tag{5}$$

$$He = \sqrt{\left|\frac{1}{n-1}\sum_{i=1}^{n}(x_i - Ex)^2 - En^2\right|} \tag{6}$$

(3) Standard cloud model

For an indicator with bilateral constraints, the numerical characteristics of the standard cloud model can be calculated as follows [9].

$$Ex = \frac{C_{\max} + C_{\min}}{2} \tag{7}$$

$$En = \frac{C_{\max} - C_{\min}}{6} \tag{8}$$

$$He = k \times En \tag{9}$$

where $C_{\max}$ and $C_{\min}$ are the upper and lower bounds of an indicator, respectively, and k is a constant that changes according to the randomness and fuzziness of different indicators. Usually, k is no more than one-third, and we set $k = 0.1$ in this study [9].

(4) Similarity

The similarity between the cloud model and the standard cloud model can be characterized as follows [33].

$$\lambda_j = e^{-\frac{(Ex-Ex_j)^2}{2(En_j)^2}} \tag{10}$$

where Ex is the expectation of the assessment indicator, Ex_j is the entropy of the jth standard cloud model, and En_j is the hyperentropy of the jth standard cloud model.

The level of the standard cloud model corresponding to the maximum similarity λ_j is the quantitative evaluation result according to the maximum membership principle.

2.2.2. GM(1,1) Model

Let $X^{(0)} = (x^{(0)}(1), x^{(0)}(2), \ldots, x^{(0)}(n))$ be the original data series and $X^{(1)} = (x^{(1)}(1), x^{(1)}(2), \ldots, x^{(1)}(n))$ be the first-order accumulating data series, where $x^{(1)}(k)$ can be calculated as follows based on the first-order accumulating generation operator (1-AGO) [34].

$$x^{(1)}(k) = \sum_{i=1}^{k} x^{(0)}(i), k = 1, 2, \cdots, n \tag{11}$$

where $x^{(0)}(k)$ indicates the original data, and $x^{(1)}(k)$ indicates the 1-AGO data.

Assume the matrix $X^{(1)}$ accords with the exponential change law, and the whitenization equation of the GM(1,1) model is shown as follows [34].

$$\frac{dx^{(1)}}{dt} + ax^{(1)} = b \tag{12}$$

where t indicates the time; a indicates the developing coefficient; and b indicates the grey input.

Let $\hat{x}^{(1)}(1) = x^{(0)}(1)$ be the initial condition. Solve Equation (12), and the predictive formula of $X^{(1)}$ can be obtained, as shown in Equation (13) [35].

$$\hat{x}^{(1)}(k+1) = \left[x^{(0)}(1) - \frac{b}{a}\right]e^{-ak} + \frac{b}{a}, \quad k = 0,1,2,\cdots \tag{13}$$

where $\hat{x}^{(1)}(k+1)$ indicates the predictive value of 1-AGO.

The predictive formula $X^{(0)}$ of the original data series is shown in Equation (14) and is calculated as $x^{(1)}(k+1) - x^{(1)}(k)$.

$$\hat{x}^{(0)}(k+1) = (1-e^{a})\left[x^{(0)}(1) - \frac{b}{a}\right]e^{-ak}, \quad k = 1,2,3,\cdots \tag{14}$$

where $\hat{x}^{(0)}(k+1)$ indicates the predictive value of the original data series.

The developing coefficient a and grey input b are based on the least square estimation of the GM(1,1) model, as shown in Equation (15) [35].

$$\hat{a} = \left(B^{T}B\right)^{-1}B^{T}Y = (a,b)^{T} \tag{15}$$

where the matrices B and Y are described as follows.

$$B = \begin{pmatrix} -Z^{(1)}(2) & 1 \\ -Z^{(1)}(3) & 1 \\ \cdots & \cdots \\ -Z^{(1)}(n) & 1 \end{pmatrix}, \quad Y = \begin{pmatrix} x^{(0)}(2) \\ x^{(0)}(3) \\ \cdots \\ x^{(0)}(n) \end{pmatrix}$$

The background value $Z^{(1)}$ is the mean series of $X^{(1)}$, as calculated by the following equation [35]:

$$Z^{(1)}(k+1) = \frac{1}{2}\left[X^{(1)}(k+1) + X^{(1)}(k)\right], \quad k = 1,2,\cdots,n-1 \tag{16}$$

where $Z^{(1)}(k+1)$ indicates the background value.

As time t increases, the predicted result exhibits an infinite value. To avoid this situation, we added the following content to the text.

As the prediction time increases, the error of the prediction result of the GM(1,1) model also increases. The GM(1,1) model has better prediction results for recent data (such as prediction of the next issue), and the prediction results for long-term data have a larger error. When the forecast time is very large, the forecast result may appear to be an infinite value, which is seriously inconsistent with the actual situation because as the system develops, the role of old data (such as $x^{(0)}(1)$) in characterizing the evolution of the system gradually decreases. In this case, we need to add new information (such as $x^{(0)}(n+1)$) in time, remove some old information (such as $x^{(0)}(1)$), and rebuild the model to reflect the behavioral characteristics of the system; therefore, the prediction results are consistent with the actual values.

2.2.3. Bow-Tie Model

The bow-tie model consists of a fault tree on the left and an event tree on the right [21,22], as shown in Figure 2. In the bow-tie model, both the fault tree and event tree are simplified. There is no obvious logical relationship among the causes of the fault tree, and the results of the event tree also show only one state.

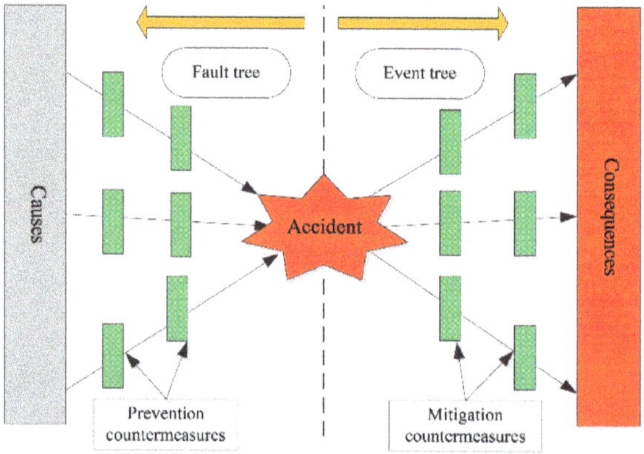

Figure 2. Flow chart of the bow-tie model.

Figure 2 indicates the frame of the bow-tie model. For the causes and consequences of the accident, the bow-tie model can take corresponding countermeasures to ensure the safety of the system.

3. Results

3.1. Precipitation Grade of the Zhengzhou Rainstorm

According to the CMA [1], the precipitation grade can be divided based on the 24 h precipitation, as shown in Table 1.

Table 1. Information about precipitation.

Grade	Precipitation (mm)	Standard Cloud Model	Similarity
Drizzle	(0, 0.1)	(0.05, 0.017, 0.0017)	0
Light rain	[0.1, 9.9]	(5, 1.63, 0.16)	0
Moderate rain	[10, 24.9]	(17.45, 2.48, 0.25)	0
Heavy rain	[25, 49.9]	(37.45, 4.15, 0.42)	0
Rainstorm	[50, 99.9]	(74.95, 8.32, 0.83)	0
Heavy rainstorm	[100, 249.9]	(174.95, 24.98, 2.5)	0
Extremely heavy rainstorm	≥250	(1000, 250, 25)	0.3713

As shown in Table 1, the grade of precipitation can be divided into seven levels in China. The corresponding standard cloud model can be calculated according to the precipitation of each grade. However, the precipitation index is required to be a bilateral constraint; that is, the precipitation grade should include both upper and lower bounds. For extremely heavy rainstorms, only the lower bound is specified in the standard, and the upper bound is missed. In reality, the upper bound of an extreme heavy rainstorm is not infinite. According to the World Meteorological Organization [36], the largest 24 h precipitation record is 1748.5 mm in China. Therefore, the bilateral constraints of 24 h precipitation in extreme heavy rainstorms are extreme heavy rainstorms (EHRSs) [250, 1750].

According to the bilateral constraints of the precipitation grade, the standard cloud model corresponding to the precipitation grade could be obtained, as shown in Table 1.

According to the CMA [1], from 6 a.m. on 20 July to 6 a.m. on 21 July 2021, the 24 h precipitation in Houzhai, Erqi District, Zhengzhou city, reached 672 mm; from 8 a.m. on

20 July to 8 a.m. on 21 July 2021, the 24 h precipitation in Zhengzhou city reached 624.1 mm. According to the backward cloud algorithm, the cloud model for the Zhengzhou rainstorm is (648.05, 30.01, 15.71).

The cloud model of the Zhengzhou rainstorm and the standard cloud models are shown on a cloud map, and the qualitative assessment of the precipitation grade could be achieved, as shown in Figure 3.

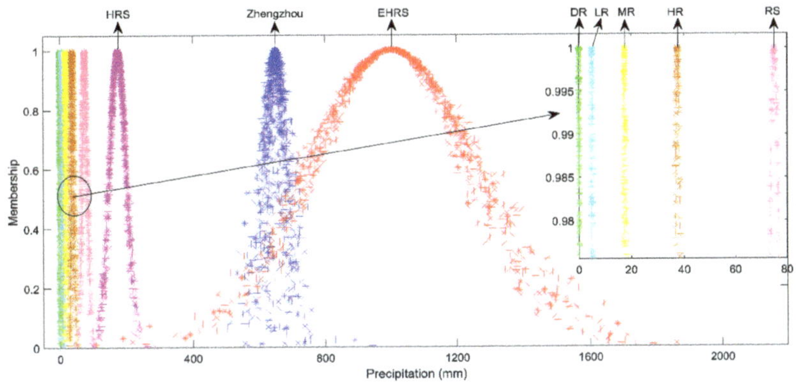

Figure 3. Qualitative assessment of the precipitation grade.

Figure 3 shows the cloud map of the precipitation grade. DR is drizzle; LR is light rain; MR is moderate rain; HR is heavy rain; RS is rainstorm; and HRS is heavy rainstorm.

As shown in Figure 3, the cloud map of the Zhengzhou rainstorm mainly falls between the HRS and EHRS cloud maps. To accurately determine the precipitation grade of the Zhengzhou rainstorm, it was also necessary to calculate the similarity between the cloud model of the Zhengzhou rainstorm and the standard cloud model, as shown in Table 1. According to the maximal membership principle, the Zhengzhou rainstorm belongs to the grade of extremely heavy rainstorm.

The qualitative assessment result of the Zhengzhou rainstorm lies between HRS and EHRS. The quantitative assessment result of the Zhengzhou rainstorm belongs to EHRS. Therefore, the Zhengzhou rainstorm was an extremely heavy rainstorm.

3.2. *Prediction of Rainfall in Zhengzhou*

The annual and July rainfall in Zhengzhou could be obtained according to the National Bureau of Statistics [37], as shown in Figure 4.

Figure 4 shows the rainfall in Zhengzhou from 1998 to 2020. The rainfall in Zhengzhou varies greatly. The maximum annual rainfall in Zhengzhou was 1010.6 mm in 2003, the average rainfall is 654.77 mm, and the minimal rainfall was 353.2 mm in 2013. The maximal rainfall in July was 309.7 mm in 2008, the average rainfall is 147.83 mm, and the minimal rainfall was 45.1 mm in 2013. July had the largest percentage of rainfall at 47.05% in 2008 and the lowest at 9.12% in 2014.

The original rainfall data in Zhengzhou are $X^{(0)}$. The parameters a = 0.0033 and b = 675.4202 could be achieved based on grey system theory [38]. Then, the prediction formula of rainfall could be calculated as follows.

$$\hat{x}^{(1)}(k+1) = -203,890.9879e^{-0.0033t} + 204,672.7879$$

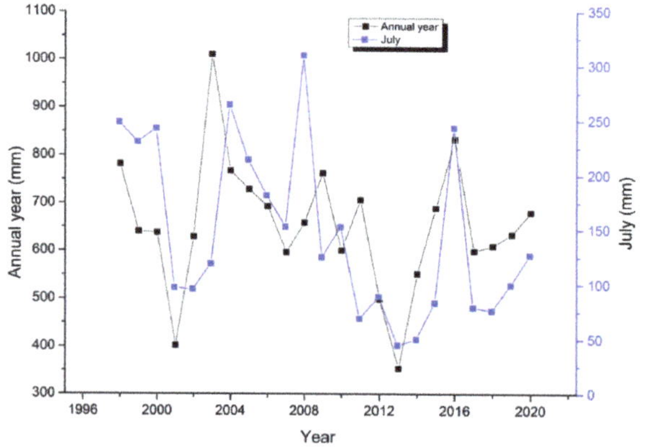

Figure 4. Rainfall in Zhengzhou.

In the case of the GM(1,1) model established using the original rainfall data, the maximal relative error of the simulation results was 81.6%, and the average relative error of the simulation results was 15.76%. The error test failed, indicating that the GM(1,1) model established by the original rainfall data cannot be used for prediction. The main reason is the large difference between the maximum and minimum rainfall in Zhengzhou. The maximum rainfall is approximately three times the minimum rainfall. To lessen this difference, the original rainfall data needed to be processed. The first-order average weakening buffer operator [39] was introduced in this case, as shown below.

$$x(k)d = \frac{1}{n-k+1}[x(k) + x(k+1) + \cdots + x(n)], \quad k = 1,2,\cdots,n \tag{17}$$

The new GM(1,1) model was established with $x(k)d$ as the basic data, and the parameters a = −0.0004 and b = 639.2562 could be achieved. The new prediction formula of rainfall could be calculated as follows.

$$\overset{*(1)}{x}(k+1) = 1,598,922.3e^{0.0004t} - 1,598,140.5$$

The maximum relative error of the simulation results was 5.06%, and the average relative error of the simulation results was 2.65%. The error test met the accuracy requirements, indicating that the new GM(1,1) model established based on $x(k)d$ can be used for prediction. The results showed that the predicted value of Zhengzhou's rainfall in 2021 was 645.3 mm. The variation range of rainfall in July in the proportion of the annual year was [9.12%, 47.05%]. The predicted interval of Zhengzhou's rainfall in July 2021 was [58.85 mm, 303.61 mm]. During the extremely heavy rainstorm in Zhengzhou on 20 July 2021,the rainfall in one day was basically equal to the annual rainfall, indicating that the rainfall cannot be predicted by conventional models. The main reason is that this rainfall was greatly affected by external factors, such as geographical location, atmospheric circulation, and typhoons, which are analyzed in detail later in this paper.

3.3. Preliminary Hazard Analysis (PHA) of Hazards Caused by Rainstorms

PHA is a qualitative method that analyzes the risk factors in the system [17,18]. Before the activities of the system, the PHA conducts a macroscopic analysis of the hazard categories, occurrence conditions, and possible accident consequences of the system. PHA of hazards caused by the rainstorm was carried out, as shown in Table 2.

Table 2. PHA of hazards caused by rainstorms.

Hazards	Causes	Results	Prevention Measures
Rainstorm	Abundant moisture. Vertical movement of moisture.	Ponding. Obstructed travel. Device is soaked in water and damaged. Some crop failure or total crop failure.	Artificial rain reduction [1]. Try not to go out. Find a safe shelter from disasters. Close doors and windows.
Flood	Rainstorm or continuous rain. Low terrain.	Dam failure. Landslide. Mud-rock flow.	Review the safety conditions of flood protection structures/infrastructures to extreme weather events. Move to a high place nearby. Turn off the gas valve and power switch.
House collapse	Flood erosion. Dilapidated house or low terrain house.	Casualties. Property loss.	Improve the quality of housing construction. Pay attention to abnormal noise in the house.
Tunnel ponding	Rainstorm or continuous rain. Tunnel drainage system is not smooth.	Casualties. Vehicle damage.	Improve tunnel drainage capacity. Drivers or pedestrians should avoid tunnels during rainy weather.
Indoor electric shock	Ponding or leaking house. Power is not cut off.	Casualties.	Cut off the power. Ground metal shell of electrical equipment. Use well-insulated household electrical equipment. Use a quality insulated ground wire.
Outdoor electric shock	Ponding or raining. Leakage of road lighting wires.	Casualties.	Do not take shelter from the rain under transformers or overhead lines. Do not touch trees near power lines. Do not go near utility poles.
Road collapse	Ground seepage. Soil is collapsible.	Casualties. Property loss.	Strengthen urban geological survey. Strengthen the construction supervision of road projects to ensure that the road quality meets the standard requirements. Strengthen the daily maintenance of roads. Strengthen the inspection of underground pipelines.
Fall into a manhole in the pavement	Too much water on the road. Did not choose the correct route.	Casualties.	Move ahead to avoid the manhole area. Pay attention to surroundings and walk close to buildings.
Fall down	Wet and slippery road. Did not choose the correct route.	Casualties.	Move ahead to avoid wet and slippery roads. Walk slowly with the help of a stick.
Plague	Drinking water pollution. Food contamination.	Casualties.	All food must be cooked at a high temperature before eaten. Do not eat spoiled food. Pay attention to environmental hygiene and do not litter. Avoid soaking hands and feet in water for a long time.

The disaster in Zhengzhou was a particularly major natural disaster caused by extremely heavy rainstorms. Secondary disasters mainly included urban water logging, river floods, mountain torrents, and landslides.

Artificial rain reduction attempts to change the moisture condition of natural clouds, thereby reducing the efficiency of precipitation, to make the moisture in the clouds form precipitation in advance, or to delay the precipitation process and redistribute the precipitation spatially. At present, the influence of artificial rain reduction is relatively limited. Ideal results can be achieved for small-scale, weak-intensity precipitation weather processes. However, in the case of heavy precipitation weather processes, artificial rain reduction can not achieve ideal results.

After heavy rains and floods, the water supply system was destroyed, and the water source was contaminated by harmful substances from human and animal excrement and carcasses. People who drink contaminated water may likely experience intestinal infections. Food soaked in floodwater is prone to mold and spoilage. Eating moldy and spoiled food can lead to food poisoning and intestinal infections. To prevent the occurrence of the plague, the public should pay attention to food hygiene and promptly dispose of the food that becomes soaked in a flood. Do not eat food that has been soaked in floodwater, and eat well-heated food. Avoid unwashed fruits and vegetables.

The series of accidents caused by the Zhengzhou extremely heavy rainstorm had causalities. The analysis of the causes and consequences of PHA accidents was relatively rough. Then, FTA [19,20] was used to deeply analyze the flood disaster caused by EHRSs and explore the logical relationships among the causes of flood disasters.

3.4. Fault Tree Analysis (FTA) of Flood Disasters

The Zhengzhou extremely heavy rainstorm also caused a flood disaster. The Changzhuang Reservoir in Zhongyuan District, Zhengzhoucity, was in danger of flooding, and the flood discharge began at 10:30 a.m. on 20 July 2021. The water line of the Guojiazui Reservoir in Erqi District, Zhengzhou city, rose rapidly. On 21 July 2021, the downstream dam of Guojiazui Reservoir collapsed over a large area. After continuous rescue work, the danger due to the flooding of the Guojiazui Reservoir was relieved.

FTA [19,20] was conducted on the flood disaster caused by the Zhengzhou extremely heavy rainstorm, and the causes of the flood disaster were discovered, as shown in Figure 5.

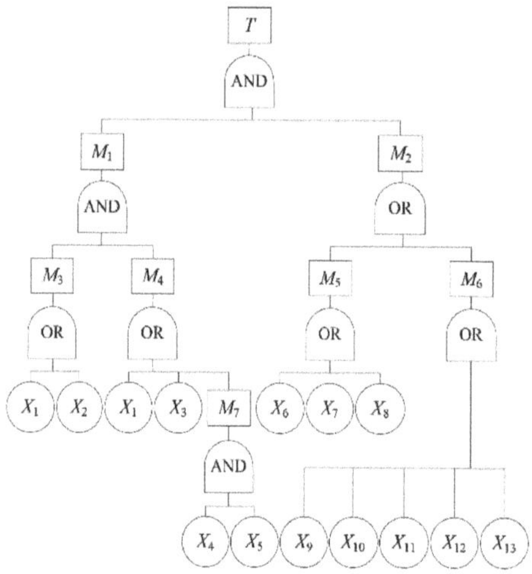

Figure 5. FTA of the flood disaster.

Figure 5 shows the FTA of the flood disaster, as well as the causes of the flood disaster. In Figure 5, T indicates the top event, that is, flood disaster; M_1 indicates the extremely heavy rainstorm; M_2 indicates insufficient countermeasures; M_3 indicates abundant moisture; M_4 indicates vertical movement of moisture; M_5 indicates insufficient urban construction; M_6 indicates insufficient emergency capacity; M_7 indicates the terrain of

Zhengzhou; X_1 indicates the subtropical anticyclone; X_2 indicates Typhoon In-fa; X_3 indicates continental plateau; X_4 indicates Taihang Mountains; X_5 indicates Funiu Mountains; X_6 indicates insufficient embankment project for the reservoir; X_7 indicates that the tunnel design was unreasonable; X_8 indicates that the drainage system design was unreasonable; X_9 indicates that the precipitation forecast was not accurate; X_{10} indicates that the early warning information did not receive enough focus; X_{11} indicates the lack of special emergency plans; X_{12} indicates that the emergency plan for flood control and rescue of the reservoir was not fully implemented;and X_{13} indicates that the public did not know what to do.

The structural equation of the flood disaster is shown below.

$$T = M_1 \times M_2$$

According to the Boolean algorithm [40], there were 24 minimal cut sets for flood disasters, indicating that there were 24 ways to cause flood disasters. The minimal cut sets can be found in the Supplementary Materials. Through the analysis of the minimal cut set, we could find the combination of basic events leading to flood disasters.

According to the Boolean algorithm [40], there were four minimal path sets for flood disasters, indicating that there were four ways to prevent flood disasters. The minimal path sets can be found in the Supplementary Materials. The optimal plan to prevent flood disasters could be selected based on the minimal path sets.

Zhengzhou was on the verge of a subtropical anticyclone in July 2021. On 18 July 2021, Typhoon In-fa was generated and approached China. Affected by the periphery of Typhoon In-fa and the subtropical anticyclone, a large amount of moisture was transported from the sea to mainland China, providing a continuous and abundant source of moisture for this rainfall in Zhengzhou. Zhengzhou is also affected by the subtropical anticyclone in the western Pacific and continental plateau, which leads to low-pressure weather in Zhengzhou. Low-pressure weather is conducive to the vertical upward movement of the atmosphere and produces rainfall. In addition, Zhengzhou is located in the pincer area in Taihang Mountains and Funiu Mountains, which has an uplift and convergence effect on the transportation of moisture, making the vertical upward movement of moisture more intense, and as a result, the rainfall increasingly strengthens.

According to the FTA of the flood disaster, the main reasons can be divided into the following three aspects: force majeure, such as terrain and extreme weather conditions, issues with city planning, and insufficient emergency rescue. For the first issue, there is nothing we can do. For the second issue, city construction is difficult to improve over a short period. To prevent disasters due to rainstorms and floods, we must pay more attention to the construction of emergency rescues.

3.5. *Bow-Tie Analysis of the Zhengzhou Subway Line-5 Accident*

The causes, consequences, and prevention measures for the subway line-5 accident are shown in Figure 6.

Figure 6 shows the causes and consequences of the subway accident, as well as the corresponding prevention measures.

The Wulongkou stabling yard of the Zhengzhou subway line-5 is on lower terrain than its surroundings. The Zhengzhou Subway Group moved the Wulongkou stabling yard eastward by 30 m, and the ground position sank by 1.973 m. This position did not meet the subway design specifications, but the Zhengzhou Subway Group did not submit it for approval as needed. In addition, the drainage function of the open ditch near the Wulongkou stabling yard was seriously damaged. Moreover, the quality of the water-retaining wall of the stabling yard is poor. The Zhengzhou extremely heavy rainstorm caused a large amount of rainwater to flood into the Wulongkou stabling yard. An increasing amount of rainwater gathered in the stabling yard, broke down the water-retaining wall, and flowed into the mainline of subway line-5. This was the direct reason for the subway line-5 accident. For this issue, the following measures can be adopted: reselect the location of the stabling yard and strengthen the water-retaining wall and increase its height.

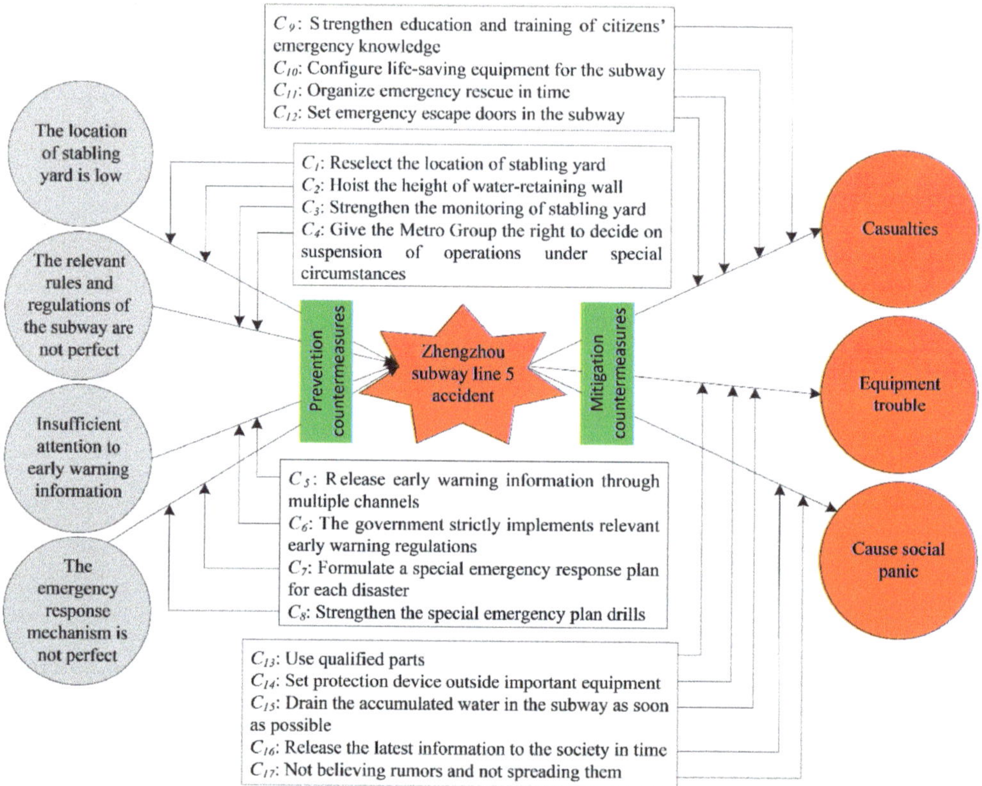

Figure 6. Bow-tie analysis of the Zhengzhou subway line-5 accident.

Another important reason for the subway line-5 accident was the inadequate rules and regulations of the subway. The water-retaining wall is the last line of defense to prevent rainwater from flowing into the mainline of the subway. According to the Code for Design of Metro [41], there is no clear specification of whether monitoring equipment or special personnel are required for the water-retaining wall. For this issue, take the following measures: improve relevant standards, set up monitoring equipment for important facilities, or arrange for special personnel to be on duty.

From 9:59 p.m. on July 19 to 4:01 p.m. on 20 July 2021, the Zhengzhou Meteorological Service [42] issued five red warnings for rainstorms. According to the CMA [1], the defense guidelines of the rainstorm red warning should be adopted as follows: the government and relevant departments need to perform well during emergency rescues and for rainstorm prevention based on their duties; stop gatherings and classes, and close businesses, except for special industries; and diligence is needed in the prevention of disasters and in undertaking rescues during disasters, such as mountain torrents, landslides, and mudslides. Although five red warning signals for rainstorms were issued, the defense guidelines have not been implemented well. On 20 July 2021, people went to work as usual, and the government did not take appropriate emergency measures. At 5 p.m. on 20 July 2021, the extreme heavy rainstorm superimposed on the peak off-work time, which contributed to the Zhengzhou subway line-5 accident. To prevent similar subway accidents, we must strictly implement the defense guidelines for rainstorm warning signals.

Although the meteorological department issued rainstorm red warnings many times, the Zhengzhou Subway Group failed to strengthen inspections as required by the relevant plans, and the investigation of flooding hazard factors was not in place. By 6:04 p.m. on 20 July 2021, the Zhengzhou Subway Group issued an order to stop the line network, but the subway lost power and was forced to stop at this time. The Zhengzhou Subway Group did not implement a major danger reporting system and did not initiate an emergency response during the incident.

The Zhengzhou Subway Group failed to command and dispatch. At approximately 5 p.m. on 20 July 2021, the water logging broke down the water-retaining wall and rushed into the subway tunnel. A failure alarm occurred, and the subway was stopped at Haitansi Station. However, the command room was released again at 5:46 p.m. on 20 July 2021, without determining the reason or understanding the danger. After 5:47 p.m. on 20 July 2021, the water flooded over the tracks, and the chief dispatcher instructed the train to move back. After approximately 30 m, the train lost power and was forced to stop [2]. As a result, the elevation of the location of the train was approximately 75 cm lower than before moving backward, which increased the water depth in the train and aggravated the danger to the trapped passengers.

If the Subway Group can suspend line-5 in the early stage of a danger, this type of accident will not occur. In fact, on the afternoon of 20 July 2021, rainwater had already begun to pour into the mainline of the subway. However, in this case, the Subway Group did not stop the subway. The suspension of the subway needs to be reported to the appropriate department of transportation, as it can be implemented after approval, and there is a certain hysteretic time. Therefore, to prevent subway accidents, we must give the Subway Group the right to suspend operations under special circumstances.

In the case of a subway accident, if the correct mitigation measures can be taken, the consequences of the accident can be greatly reduced. A major issue exposed by the Zhengzhou subway line-5 accident is that citizens do not know what to do or how to take action in the face of sudden disasters. In the future, we should focus on popularizing emergency escape skills for all kinds of sudden disasters to protect citizens' lives.

3.6. Chaos Characteristics of an Extremely Heavy Rainstorm

The original meaning of chaos refers to the scene before the universe opened, and the basic meaning mainly refers to a state of confusion and disorder. In scientific research, chaos refers to the random behavior that occurs in a deterministic nonlinear system without any additional random factors, and the deterministic nonlinear system exhibits unpredictable, random-like motions that are sensitive to initial conditions [43]. Chaos theory mainly addresses the evolution of the system from order to chaos and how to control chaos [44]. Chaos theory emphasizes the complexity of the natural world and human society that is not fully understood by humans, and it advocates interdisciplinary research to explore nonlinear objective processes. Chaos theory is a science that investigates system processes and system evolution. Chaos theory explains the random outcomes that a system can produce, which can obtain definite aperiodic outcomes using simple models [45]. Rainstorms are affected by multiple factors, and the influencing factors change dynamically, which makes the occurrence of rainstorms random. The randomness of the rainstorm evolution process provides the possibility to use chaos theory to investigate the rainstorm evolution process. Chaos features mainly include sensitivity, inherent randomness, and fractals [46]. In this study, chaos theory was introduced into the analysis of the evolution process of rainstorms, and the sensitivity of the evolution process of rainstorms is discussed.

According to the accident causation model of system theory, the occurrence of accidents is the result of the comprehensive effects of human, object, environment, and management subsystems [47]. Similarly, extremely heavy rainstorms are also affected by the cross-coupling of human, object, environmental, and management subsystems. The evolution process has an obvious butterfly effect, as shown in Figure 7.

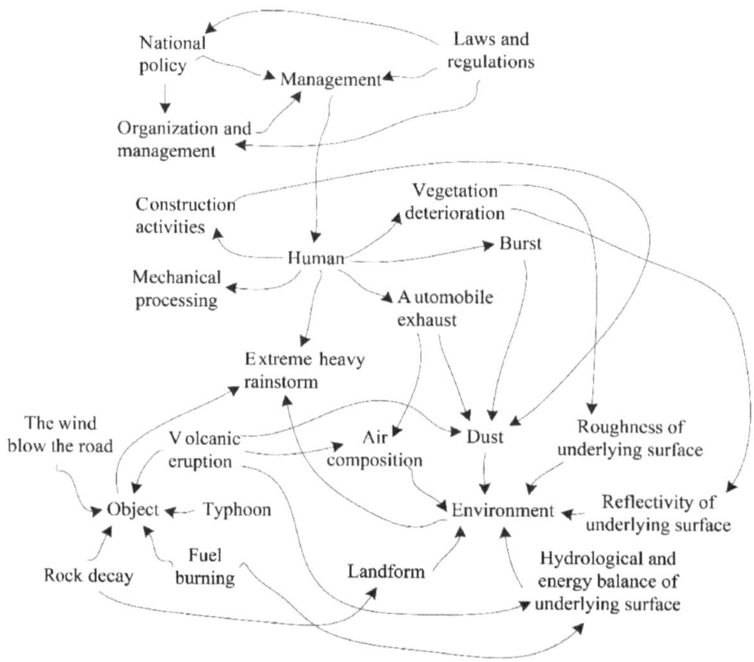

Figure 7. The butterfly effect in the evolution process of an extremely heavy rainstorm.

Figure 7 shows the influence of human, object, environment, and management subsystems on the evolution process of extremely heavy rainstorms. Factors located at the beginning of the arrow have an effect on the end factors. For example, once a volcano erupts, it changes the composition of the air. The management factors do not directly affect the rainstorm process. In fact, management factors indirectly affect the evolution of rainstorms mainly by restricting human behaviors and reducing damage to the environment. The dust generated by human activities and natural conditions can be used as condensation nuclei in the process of rainfall, creating favorable conditions for the formation of rainfall and increasing the possibility of precipitation. The impact of human activities on rainfall can be summarized as follows: changing the roughness and reflectivity of the underlying surface; generating dust and change the composition of the atmosphere; and generating energy and affecting airflow movement.

The direct impact of global warming on rainfall is changing the amount of moisture in the atmosphere. The rise in temperature means the atmosphere contains more moisture. The impact of global warming on rainfall is not unidirectional but bidirectional. Global warming has made humid areas more humid and dry areas drier, showing a phenomenon of polarization.

The indirect effects of human activities on rainfall mainly include construction activities, vegetation deterioration, bursts, automobile exhaust, and mechanical processing. In addition, human activities can also directly generate rainfall, such as artificial rainfall. Artificial rainfall is based on the principle of natural rainfall, artificially supplementing certain necessary conditions for the formation of rainfall, causing cloud droplets to condense or increase raindrops and make raindrops fall to the ground. According to the physical characteristics of different clouds, artificial rainfall involves selecting an appropriate time and using airplanes or rockets to spread catalysts, such as dry ice, silver iodide, and salt powder, into clouds to make the clouds produce rain or increase the amount of precipitation already occurring [1,48]. Artificial rainfall needs to meet the following operating conditions [1]: the cloud system develops to a certain thickness, such as more than two kilometers; the cloud lacks ice crystals and has abundant super-cooled water; and there is sufficient water vapor outside the cloud body to continuously replenish the cloud body through auxiliary uplift. Generally, artificial rainfall is relatively small, natural rainfall may be large, and artificial rainfall can only incite rainfall under certain conditions.

In the evolution of rainstorms, management factors are the basic causes, human factors are indirect causes, and environmental factors are the direct causes. The object factors can increase or decrease the grade of a rainstorm.

According to chaos theory, a rainstorm is the result of cross-coupling and infinite amplification of the faults in human, object, environment, and management subsystems, and the evolution process shows an obvious butterfly effect (Figure 7). For a nonlinear system, the small errors of a certain factor are not always small [44]. Under appropriate conditions, the small errors can evolve and develop infinitely; this can lead to consequences, such as the system being difficult to estimate. According to chaos theory [45], the small input error of the system can cause a large drift in output under certain conditions for the nonlinear system. In the actual production process, since the system is inevitably be disturbed by external factors, the small error at the initial moment can be amplified over time and lead to unpredictable consequences, such as rainstorms.

4. Discussion

Rainfall is affected spatiotemporally, and the evolution process has strong uncertainty, fuzziness, and randomness. Atmospheric motion is a very complicated process and is affected by the terrain, distribution of land and sea, and conditions of the underlying surface. Moreover, human activities also have a certain impact on atmospheric motion, resulting in a certain degree of uncertainty with rainstorms (Figure 7). The fuzzy comprehensive evaluation method can solve problems with uncertainty and fuzziness [6], but it can do nothing about randomness problems. The stochastic model is suitable for problems with uncertainty and randomness [7], but it is difficult to deal with the problem of fuzziness. In this study, the cloud model [8,9] was introduced to address the uncertainty, fuzziness, and randomness in the evolution process of the rainstorm, and the assessment result was in line with the national standard GB/T 28592-2012 [28].

Generally, accurate prediction of the grade and duration of rainfall is the most economical way to reduce the losses due to rainstorms. Rainstorm forecasting is mainly based on observational data and numerical forecasts. Forecasters use their knowledge and experience to make judgments and corrections of the forecast results. A rainstorm is the result of the time and spatial scales. Without a comprehensive analysis of various conditions and data, it is difficult to obtain accurate forecast results within a certain spatiotemporal range. Although the accuracy of the GM(1,1) model met the requirements, it was still unable to accurately predict the rainfall in Zhengzhou. The accuracy of rainstorm forecasts is not high world wide and is approximately 25% in the United States [1]. Rainstorm forecasts cannot be completely dependent on numerical forecasts, and subjective initiatives of forecasts must be fully applied.

Previous studies have mainly focused on accidents caused by rainstorms [3–5], but they have failed to deeply analyze the causes, consequences, and prevention measures of these accidents. In this study, PHA [17,18], FTA [19,20], and the bow-tie model [21,22] were adopted to comprehensively analyze rainstorms and secondary disasters. Secondary disasters mainly include urban water logging, river floods, and mountain torrents and landslides. The factors that led to the extremely heavy rainstorm disaster in Zhengzhou mainly include the following aspects: the subtropical high was abnormally northerly, and the summer monsoon was stronger than usual; a typhoon formed in the same period and converged to transport the water vapor from the sea, which was superimposed with the convective system above; the uplift due to Funiu Mountain and Taihang Mountain; and the terrain of Zhengzhou is high in the southwest and low in the northeast, which is a transitional zone from mountains to plains.

If the public paid enough attention to the warning information of EHRSs, the Zhengzhou subway line-5 accident may not have occurred. During the same period, Shaanxi Province, Luonan County, was also affected by a rainstorm, and the 24 h rainfall in Lixikou village, Maping town, was 239.3 mm from 2 p.m. 22 July to 2 p.m. 23 July 2021. A total of 77,961 people in Luonan County were affected by this rainstorm, but no one was injured [1]. The Shangluo city government of Shaanxi Province issued a commendatory report to the Luonan Meteorological Administration and awarded one hundred thousand *yuan*. The report pointed out that the Luonan Meteorological Administration accurately issued rainstorm warning information five times during the process of preventing and responding to the heavy rainstorm disaster from 22–23 July 2021. Time was gained for the advanced deployment of flood prevention and rescue work, rapid evacuation, and proper resettlement of people in dangerous areas, which effectively guaranteed the safety of people's lives and property.

The evolution of rainstorms in different countries and regions has different characteristics. Siswanto et al. [49] conducted a statistical analysis of the maximum 1h rainfall at the observation station in Jakarta, Indonesia, during 1866–1950 and 1959–2010, and the results showed that there was no significant difference in the five-year moving average of the maximum 1h rainfall during these two periods. The 1 h and 24 h rainstorms with different rainfall reappearance periods during 1956–1980 and 1981–2005 in three districts of Washington State in the United States showed different degrees of growth [50]. The 10 min maximum rainfall in Japan from 1951 to 2010 showed a significant upward trend [51]. The annual maximum rainfall of 1 h in Hong Kong and Shanghai also showed a significant upward trend [52,53]. Global warming has led to frequent extreme weather. The 1 h rainfall of the Zhengzhou extreme heavy rainstorm is a new record for China's maximum 1 h rainfall.

The process of urbanization makes extremely heavy rainstorms increasingly frequent [54–56]. Zhengzhou had a population of 6.659 million and an urbanization rate of 55.1% in 2020. At the end of 2019, the population and urbanization rate were 10.352 million and 74.6% in Zhengzhou, respectively [57]. The main issues in the process of urbanization are employment, housing, transportation, and other problems related to human survival. Due to the large investment, long construction period, and slow construction efficiency, embankment projects are often ignored by urban decision makers. In the process of urbanization, there is a phenomenon in which above ground and underground development do not match. The impact of urbanization on rainstorms and floods includes the following aspects: the impervious area of the city increases; the natural vegetation is destroyed; the space for rivers and lakes is limited; and underground parking lots, flyovers, tunnels, and subways are subject to the formation of floods.

To simplify the discussion, the parameter k in Equation (3) was set to 0.1. Future studies should focus on the influence of this parameter on the assessment result of precipitation grade. Due to the lack of sufficient basic data on EHRSs, this study did not explore the rainstorm fractal. To fully understand the characteristics of rainstorms, more rainstorm data should be collected in the future to investigate the fractals of rainstorms.

5. Suggestions

Vigorously improve the risk awareness and emergency response capabilities of leading cadres. Coordinate the two major issues of development and safety, and enhance risk awareness and bottom-line thinking. Increase the ability and level of disaster prevention, mitigation, and relief to effectively respond to various disaster risks and challenges, and consider the safety of people's lives first. Establish the major disaster investigation and evaluation system, investigate all accidents causing major casualties, and summarize the experience and lessons in a timely manner.

Enhance the overall level of urban disaster prevention and mitigation. Integrate the extreme weather response and natural disaster prevention into urban development and construction. Enhance the flood control and water logging drainage standards and disaster-resistant fortification standards for hospitals, subways, and other public service facilities so that urban disaster prevention and mitigation capabilities are compatible with economic and social development. Carry out in-depth emergency management system reform and operation evaluation. Conduct a comprehensive evaluation and revision of emergency plans, and strengthen the integrated management of early warning and response.

The existing reservoirs in the city should be reinforced. The reservoir not only plays an important role in flood prevention and disaster reduction but also benefits irrigation, water supply, hydroelectric power, aquaculture, and tourism. All aspects of the impact of the reservoir must be considered in the reinforcement to achieve comprehensive benefits from a one-time reinforcement. If the government wanted to build a new reservoir, it involves terrain, climate, capital investment, and other factors, and may cause damage to the original ecosystem; it needs to be repeatedly demonstrated. The discussion in this study did not involve a newly built reservoir. Reinforcement of the reservoir has also indirectly improved the flood prevention grade of the reservoir.

To optimize the urban drainage system, the concept of a sponge city came into being in China. The concept of a sponge city can be described as follows: more focus is placed on the recycling of rainwater, sewage treatment, and the improvement of the ecological environment in the design of rainwater discharge; the pressure of urban rainstorms on the drainage system is reduced; the risk of flooding in the city is reduced; and the ability of the city to respond to environmental changes and resist natural disasters is enhanced [58]. Zhengzhou began construction of a sponge city in 2017. The sponge city construction in Zhengzhou has required the investment of 19.63 billion *yuan*, but only 32% of the investment is related to the construction of the sponge city, and nearly 56% is used for the landscape and greening. Although the Zhengzhou extreme heavy rainstorm has caused the construction of the sponge city to be questioned, the role of the sponge city can not be denied. The Zhengzhou extreme heavy rainstorm broke the rainfall record in China. The drainage system of any city in the world may be powerless in the face of such a large amount of rainfall in a short period.

Enhance the capacity of urban disaster emergency rescue. Improve the disaster prediction accuracy, release the disaster warning information through multiple channels, and evacuate the disaster-affected areas in time. For different types of disasters, formulate specific emergency rescue plans and implement prompt rescues when dangerous situations occur. Disseminate the knowledge of disasters to residents, and enhance their awareness of risk prevention. Residents should familiarize themselves with the disaster risk in the jurisdiction, as well as master escape skills and understand the setting and use of surrounding shelters and disaster prevention and mitigation facilities. Enhance the broad risk awareness, self-rescue, and mutual rescue capabilities for the whole society. Finally, carry out publicity and education on disaster prevention, mitigation, and relief for the whole society, as well as explanations of typical cases in simple terms and enhancement of the vigilance of the public to prevent risks.

6. Conclusions

A composite risk assessment model for rainstorms was constructed in this study. The main conclusions are described below.

The disaster in Zhengzhou was a particularly major natural disaster caused by EHRSs. Secondary disasters mainly included urban water logging, river floods, and mountain torrents and landslides. The factors that led to the extremely heavy rainstorm disaster in Zhengzhou mainly include the following aspects: the subtropical high was abnormally northerly, and the summer monsoon was stronger than usual; a typhoon formed in the same periodand converged to transport water vapor from the sea, which was superimposed with the convective system above; uplift due to Funiu Mountain and Taihang Mountain; and the terrain of Zhengzhou is high in the southwest and low in the northeast, which is a transitional zone from mountains to plains. We must pay more attention to the sensitivity of the evolution process of rainstorms. The process of urbanization makes extremely heavy rainstorms increasingly more frequent. Therefore, we must propose countermeasures to rainstorms and secondary disasters along with urbanization, such as reinforcing the existing reservoirs, strengthening the construction of the sponge city, and improving the capacity of urban disaster emergency rescue. Future studies should focus on rainstorm fractals.

Supplementary Materials: The following supporting information can be downloaded at: https://www.mdpi.com/article/10.3390/bs12060176/s1, The minimal cut and path sets of flood disasters have been uploaded in the electronic supplementary materials.

Author Contributions: Data curation, Q.X.; methodology, K.X. and L.H.; writing—original draft, Q.X.; writing—review & editing, Q.X. All authors have read and agreed to the published version of the manuscript.

Funding: This study was supported by the Federation Research Project of Henan Social Science (SKL-2021-2531).

Institutional Review Board Statement: Not applicable.

Informed Consent Statement: Not applicable.

Data Availability Statement: All relevant data are within the paper.

Acknowledgments: The authors thank the anonymous reviewers for their valuable comments and suggestions.

Conflicts of Interest: The authors have no conflict of interest to declare.

References

1. China Meteorological Administration. 2021. Available online: http://www.cma.gov.cn/ (accessed on 10 August 2021).
2. The Central People's Government of the People's Republic of China. 2022. Available online: http://www.gov.cn/xinwen/2022-01/21/content_5669723.htm (accessed on 18 February 2022).
3. Ding, Y.; Wang, P.; Liu, X.; Zhang, X.; Hong, L.; Cao, Z. Risk assessment of highway structures in natural disaster for the property insurance. *Nat. Hazards* **2020**, *104*, 2663–2685. [CrossRef]
4. Greco, R.; Comegna, L.; Damiano, E.; Marino, P.; Olivares, L.; Santonastaso, G.F. Recurrent rainfall-induced landslides on the slopes with pyroclastic cover of Partenio Mountains (Campania, Italy): Comparison of 1999 and 2019 events. *Eng. Geol.* **2021**, *288*, 106160. [CrossRef]
5. Kean, J.W.; Staley, D.M. Forecasting the Frequency and Magnitude of Postfire Debris Flows Across Southern California. *Earths Future* **2021**, *9*, e2020EF001735. [CrossRef]
6. Geng, Y.F.; Zheng, X.; Wang, Z.L.; Wang, Z.W. Flood risk assessment in Quzhou City (China) using a coupled hydrodynamic model and fuzzy comprehensive evaluation (FCE). *Nat. Hazards* **2020**, *100*, 133–149. [CrossRef]
7. Falck, A.S.; Tomasella, J.; Diniz, F.L.R.; Maggioni, V. Applying a precipitation error model to numerical weather predictions for probabilistic flood forecasts. *J. Hydrol.* **2021**, *598*, 126374. [CrossRef]
8. Song, Q.; Jiang, P.; Zheng, S. The application of cloud model combined with nonlinear fuzzy analytic hierarchy process for the safety assessment of chemical plant production process. *Process Saf. Environ. Prot.* **2021**, *145*, 12–22. [CrossRef]
9. Xu, Q.; Xu, K.; Zhou, F. Safety assessment of casting workshop by cloud model and cause and effect-LOPA to protect employee health. *Int. J. Environ. Res. Public Health* **2020**, *17*, 2555. [CrossRef]
10. Pontoh, R.S.; Toharudin, T.; Ruchjana, B.N.; Sijabat, N.; Puspita, M.D. Bandung Rainfall Forecast and Its Relationship with Nino 3.4 Using Nonlinear Autoregressive Exogenous Neural Network. *Atmosphere* **2022**, *13*, 302. [CrossRef]
11. Lin, Y.-J.; Lee, P.-C.; Ma, K.-C.; Chiu, C.-C. A Hybrid Grey Model to Forecast the Annual Maximum Daily Rainfall. *KSCE J. Civ. Eng.* **2019**, *23*, 4933–4948. [CrossRef]
12. Zhao, Q.; Liu, Y.; Yao, W.; Yao, Y. Hourly Rainfall Forecast Model Using Supervised Learning Algorithm. *IEEE Trans. Geosci. Remote Sens.* **2022**, *60*, 4100509. [CrossRef]
13. Yao, H.; Zhang, Q.; Niu, G.; Liu, H.; Yang, Y. Applying the GM(1,1) model to simulate and predict the ecological footprint values of Suzhou city, China. *Environ. Dev. Sustain.* **2021**, *23*, 11297–11309. [CrossRef]
14. Brazdil, R.; Chroma, K.; Dolak, L.; Rehor, J.; Reznickova, L.; Zahradnicek, P.; Dobrovolny, P. Fatalities associated with the severe weather conditions in the Czech Republic, 2000–2019. *Nat. Hazards Earth Syst. Sci.* **2021**, *21*, 1355–1382. [CrossRef]
15. Tobin, D.M.; Kumjian, M.R.; Black, A.W. Effects of precipitation type on crash relative risk estimates in Kansas. *Accid. Anal. Prev.* **2021**, *151*, 105946. [CrossRef]
16. Yoon, S.S.; Ji, U.; Bae, I. Influence of Radar and Gauge Rainfall Data Sources on the Analysis of Spatial Distribution of Traffic Accidents and Rainfall Events. *Appl. Sci.* **2020**, *10*, 7327. [CrossRef]
17. Mateu, J.M.; Fernandez, P.M.; Franco, R.I. Setting safety foundations in the Hyperloop: A first approach to preliminary hazard analysis and safety assurance system. *Saf. Sci.* **2021**, *142*, 105366. [CrossRef]

18. Yan, F.; Xu, K. Methodology and case study of quantitative preliminary hazard analysis based on cloud model. *J. Loss Prev. Proc. Ind.* **2019**, *60*, 116–124. [CrossRef]
19. Jung, S.J.; Yoo, J.; Lee, Y.J. A Software Fault Tree Analysis Technique for Formal Requirement Specifications of Nuclear Reactor Protection Systems. *Reliab. Eng. Syst. Saf.* **2020**, *203*, 107064. [CrossRef]
20. Shu, X.; Guo, Y.; Yang, H.; Zou, H. Reliability study of motor controller in electric vehicle by the approach of fault tree analysis. *Eng. Fail. Anal.* **2021**, *121*, 105165. [CrossRef]
21. Brown, K.R.; Van Berkel, P.; Khan, F.I.; Amyotte, P.R. Application of bow tie analysis and inherently safer design to the novel coronavirus hazard. *Process Saf. Environ. Prot.* **2021**, *152*, 701–718. [CrossRef] [PubMed]
22. Xu, Q.; Xu, K.; Li, L.; Xu, X.; Yao, X. Energy release and countermeasures for sand casting explosion accidents. *Hum. Ecol. Risk Assess.* **2020**, *26*, 2078–2090. [CrossRef]
23. Luini, L. Modeling the Space-Time Evolution of Rain Fields. *IEEE Antennas Propag. Mag.* **2021**, *63*, 12–20. [CrossRef]
24. You, Y.; Ting, M.; Camargo, S.J. Heavy Rain-Producing Terrestrial Low Pressure Systems over the East Asian Summer Monsoon Region: Evolution, Energetics, and Trend. *J. Clim.* **2021**, *34*, 4539–4552. [CrossRef]
25. Lawal, Y.B.; Falodun, S.E.; Ojo, J.S. Temporal evolution of atmospheric parameter-profiling on rain height over two geoclimatic regions in Nigeria. *J. Atmos. Sol.-Terr. Phys.* **2020**, *211*, 105482. [CrossRef]
26. Anter, A.M.; Gupta, D.; Castillo, O. A novel parameter estimation in dynamic model via fuzzy swarm intelligence and chaos theory for faults in wastewater treatment plant. *Soft Comput.* **2020**, *24*, 111–129. [CrossRef]
27. Pourasad, Y.; Ranjbarzadeh, R.; Mardani, A. A New Algorithm for Digital Image Encryption Based on Chaos Theory. *Entropy* **2021**, *23*, 341. [CrossRef]
28. *GB/T 28592-2012*; Grade of Precipitation. Standards Press of China: Beijing, China, 2012.
29. Yang, X.; Zeng, L.; Feng, L.; Wang, S. Cloud hierarchical analysis. *J. Inf. Comput. Sci.* **2010**, *7*, 2468–2477.
30. Pawlas, P.; Szynal, D. On a model of ordering random variables—The (i,k)-th record values. *Commun. Stat. Theory Methods* **2022**, *51*, 895–908. [CrossRef]
31. Belovas, I. Central Limit Theorems for Combinatorial Numbers Associated with Laguerre Polynomials. *Mathematics* **2022**, *10*, 865. [CrossRef]
32. Pei, Z.; Lu, H.; Jin, Q.; Zhang, L. Target-based distributionally robust optimization for single machine scheduling. *Eur. J. Oper. Res.* **2022**, *299*, 420–431. [CrossRef]
33. Xu, Q.; Xu, K. Quality evaluation of Chinese red wine based on cloud model. *J. Food Biochem.* **2019**, *43*, e12787. [CrossRef]
34. Xu, G.; Lu, T.; Chen, X.; Liu, Y. The convergence level and influencing factors of China's digital economy and real economy based on grey model and PLS-SEM. *J. Intell. Fuzzy Syst.* **2022**, *42*, 1575–1605. [CrossRef]
35. Xu, Q.; Xu, K. Statistical Analysis and Prediction of Fatal Accidents in the Metallurgical Industry in China. *Int. J. Environ. Res. Public Health* **2020**, *17*, 3790. [CrossRef]
36. World Meteorological Organization. 2021. Available online: https://public.wmo.int/en (accessed on 11 August 2021).
37. National Bureau of Statistics. 2021. Available online: http://www.stats.gov.cn/ (accessed on 15 November 2021).
38. Comert, G.; Begashaw, N.; Huynh, N. Improved grey system models for predicting traffic parameters. *Expert Syst. Appl.* **2021**, *177*, 114972. [CrossRef]
39. Zeng, B.; Zhou, M.; Liu, X.; Zhang, Z. Application of a new grey prediction model and grey average weakening buffer operator to forecast China's shale gas output. *Energy Rep.* **2020**, *6*, 1608–1618. [CrossRef]
40. Yazdi, M.; Korhan, O.; Daneshvar, S. Application of fuzzy fault tree analysis based on modified fuzzy AHP and fuzzy TOPSIS for fire and explosion in the process industry. *Int. J. Occup. Saf. Ergon.* **2020**, *26*, 319–335. [CrossRef]
41. *GB50157-2013*; Code for Design of Metro. Architecture & Building Press: Beijing, China, 2013.
42. Zhengzhou Meteorological Service. 2021. Available online: http://zzqx.zhengzhou.gov.cn/ (accessed on 10 August 2021).
43. Azmoodeh, E.; Eichelsbacher, P.; Thale, C. Optimal Variance-Gamma approximation on the second Wiener chaos. *J. Funct. Anal.* **2022**, *282*, 109450. [CrossRef]
44. Xu, Q.; Xu, K. Importance-Based Key Basic Event Identification and Evolution Mechanism Investigation of Hydraulic Support Failure to Protect Employee Health. *Sensors* **2021**, *21*, 7240. [CrossRef]
45. Xu, Q.; Xu, K. Safety assessment of sand casting explosion accidents through on-site testing and numerical simulation of the temperature variation in sand molds to protect employee health. *Process Saf. Environ. Prot.* **2022**, *159*, 452–463. [CrossRef]
46. Jing, W.; Zhen, M.; Guan, H.; Luo, W.; Liu, X. A prediction model for building energy consumption in a shoppingmall based on Chaos theory. *Energy Rep.* **2022**, *8*, 5305–5312. [CrossRef]
47. Zhu, C.; Tang, S.; Li, Z.; Fang, X. Dynamic study of critical factors of explosion accident in laboratory based on FTA. *Saf. Sci.* **2020**, *130*, 104877. [CrossRef]
48. Wang, L.; Li, R.; Zhang, S.; Li, R.; Bai, W.; Xiao, H. Function of a Deep-Buried Isolated Trench and Its Effect on Cracking Failure Characteristics of a Slope under Artificial Rainfall. *Water* **2022**, *14*, 1123. [CrossRef]
49. Siswanto, S.; van Oldenborgh, G.J.; van der Schrier, G.; Jilderda, R.; van den Hurk, B. Temperature, extreme precipitation, and diurnal rainfall changes in the urbanized Jakarta city during the past 130 years. *Int. J. Climatol.* **2016**, *36*, 3207–3225. [CrossRef]
50. Rosenberg, E.A.; Keys, P.W.; Booth, D.B.; Hartley, D.; Burkey, J.; Steinemann, A.C.; Lettenmaier, D.P. Precipitation extremes and the impacts of climate change on stormwater infrastructure in WashingtonState. *Clim. Chang.* **2010**, *102*, 319–349. [CrossRef]

51. Fujibe, F. Clausius-Clapeyron-like relationship in multidecadal changes of extreme short-term precipitation and temperature in Japan. *Atmos. Sci. Lett.* **2013**, *14*, 127–132. [CrossRef]
52. Lenderink, G.; Mok, H.Y.; Lee, T.C.; van Oldenborgh, G.J. Scaling and trends of hourly precipitation extremes in two different climate zones—Hong Kong and the Netherlands. *Hydrol. Earth Syst. Sci.* **2011**, *15*, 3033–3041. [CrossRef]
53. Liang, P.; Ding, Y. The Long-term Variation of Extreme Heavy Precipitation and Its Link to Urbanization Effects in Shanghai during 1916–2014. *Adv. Atmos. Sci.* **2017**, *34*, 321–334. [CrossRef]
54. Bai, X.; Shi, P.; Liu, Y. Realizing China's urban dream. *Nature* **2014**, *509*, 158–160. [CrossRef]
55. Singh, J.; Vittal, H.; Karmakar, S.; Ghosh, S.; Niyogi, D. Urbanization causes nonstationarity in Indian Summer Monsoon Rainfall extremes. *Geophys. Res. Lett.* **2016**, *43*, 11269–11277. [CrossRef]
56. Yang, P.; Ren, G.; Yan, P. Evidence for a Strong Association of Short-Duration Intense Rainfall with Urbanization in the Beijing Urban Area. *J. Clim.* **2017**, *30*, 5851–5870. [CrossRef]
57. Zhengzhou Bureau of Statistics. 2020. Available online: http://tjj.zhengzhou.gov.cn/ (accessed on 11 August 2021).
58. Guan, X.; Wang, J.; Xiao, F. Sponge city strategy and application of pavement materials in sponge city. *J. Clean. Prod.* **2021**, *303*, 127022. [CrossRef]

behavioral sciences

MDPI

Article

The Relationship between Personality Traits and COVID-19 Anxiety: A Mediating Model

V. Vineeth Kumar * and Geetika Tankha

Department of Psychology, Manipal University Jaipur, Jaipur 303007, India; geetika.tankha@jaipur.manipal.edu
* Correspondence: vineeth.kumar@jaipur.manipal.edu

Abstract: The COVID-19 pandemic has created a lot of fear and anxiety globally. The current study attempted to investigate the association among the big five personality traits and the two factors of COVID-19 pandemic anxiety (fear and somatic concern). Further, sleep quality as a mediator between personality traits and pandemic anxiety was also assessed. The study involved a cross-sectional sample of 296 adult Indians who were administered the 10-item short version of BFI along with the COVID-19 Pandemic Anxiety Scale and Sleep Quality Scale. Path analysis was used to test the theoretical model that we proposed. The overall model has explained 6% and 36% of the variance, respectively, for the factors of fear and somatic concern of COVID-19 pandemic anxiety. The path analysis model indicated that only the trait of neuroticism showed a significant direct and indirect effect on pandemic anxiety in the sample. Those scoring high on neuroticism indicated high levels of fear as well as somatic concern. Neuroticism also showed partial mediation through sleep quality on the factor of somatic concern. Agreeableness was the only other personality trait that indicated a significantly negative relationship with the factor of somatic concern. These relationships were independent of age, gender, and occupational status. These findings provide a preliminary insight into the slightly different relationship which has emerged between personality and COVID-19 pandemic anxiety in comparison to general anxiety.

Keywords: PAS-10; fear; somatic concern; COVID-19; personality traits; neuroticism

1. Introduction

The COVID-19 pandemic has threatened the lives of human beings and has impacted every aspect of human life. The pandemic has affected those infected by the virus and those who were not. The life-threatening nature of the virus combined with an uncertain environment has created anxiety among the masses. It has altered the way people work, travel, communicate, and live their everyday lives. Any disruption of this kind can have an adverse psychological impact on individuals. Being anxious is part of human nature. However, when the anxiety level goes high and becomes chronic, it may adversely impact an individual's well-being. Most of the time, for individuals suffering from general anxiety, the cause is unknown. One of the differentiating factors between general anxiety and pandemic anxiety is that the cause of worry points to the pandemic (e.g., COVID-19) for human uneasiness and worry.

It seems COVID-19 pandemic anxiety stems from two components, i.e., fear and somatic concern [1]. First, continuous information overload related to the virus spreads triggered fear in individuals. People feared that if the virus infected them, it could lead to a painful death. It led them to be wary of going out to public places or meeting people. They started isolating themselves. Lockdowns and restrictions to move around added more fear to the tense environment. The need to continuously check and monitor any symptoms related to the pandemic created pressure and disrupted the daily functioning of individuals. The insecurity due to the lack of control over the situation and subsequent overindulgence in performing safety behaviors have also enhanced fear. Second, any slight perceived physiological symptoms like palpitations, shortness of breath and giddiness, or changes in eating and sleep patterns made people hyper-vigilant and concerned that they may have the coronavirus. Thus, the anxiety-driven apprehensions made people dysfunctional at psychological and social levels. With the spread of coronavirus across the world, this phenomenon of COVID-19 anxiety became more evident. Studies have demonstrated that the COVID-19 pandemic has had a severe negative bearing on mental health [2] and the psychological well-being of people across the world [3].

Since the onset of the current COVID-19 pandemic, it has been observed that the number of COVID-19 cases across nations keeps fluctuating. The virus is mutating, and the medical fraternity finds it quite challenging to make any concrete prediction regarding the end of the current pandemic. As the pandemic has been ravaging the planet for the last two years and with no end in sight, people can develop a sort of pandemic fatigue. This fatigue can prevent people from taking and maintaining precautionary measures against COVID-19. The probability of the current pandemic becoming an endemic also seems a possibility. The mental health challenges among the masses during the current pandemic can be pretty severe. Thus, identifying behavior that can help alleviate the mental health burden on individuals is quite significant. A highly anxious individual often finds it challenging to analyze, face, and successfully navigate challenging problems or situations. Somehow, the current COVID-19 pandemic has become a challenge for everyone. Identifying psychological variables that can help mitigate the mental health burdens of individuals can be beneficial in this scenario. An individual's personality plays an essential role in facilitating or obstructing how they perceive and respond to day-to-day events in unique or critical times. Personality traits can be markers for understanding the individual differences found in the way people show concern, readiness, and adaptability to environmental tragedies and exigencies. Similarly, improving sleep quality may help reduce anxiety due to the pandemic. Understanding the relationship between the variables can enable researchers and mental health professionals to develop intervention programs to help individuals manage COVID-19 pandemic anxiety.

1.1. Literature Review

1.1.1. Big Five Personality Traits and COVID-19 Anxiety

To a great extent, personality traits guide and shape an individual's responses to life events through their thoughts, emotions, and behavioral actions [4,5]. For example, individuals high on agreeableness and extraversion traits experience positive emotions. They also positively evaluate their daily activities [6]. In a study on students, openness to experience has been associated with coronavirus anxiety. However, there was a negative relation between conscientiousness with pandemic-related stress [7]. Thus, openness emerged as a risk factor, and conscientiousness was a protective personality factor. Another study reported a significant negative association for four of the big five traits, except neuroticism, which is positively associated with COVID-19 anxiety [8].

Research studies have substantiated that those individuals who are high on the personality trait of neuroticism could have a significantly increased risk perception of a pandemic [9,10]. Additionally, studies have indicated that neurotics have shown weaker mental well-being even in regular times, whereas extraverts have demonstrated stronger mental health [11–13]. It is a general belief that individuals who score highly on the trait of neuroticism report more negative rather than positive emotions. As a result, they are more susceptible to adverse outcomes when faced with traumatic experiences. These individuals are more anxious and insecure [14], predisposed to psychological distress [15], and more impulsive in their behavior in comparison to individuals who score low on neuroticism [16]. Studies have also indicated that individuals with high neuroticism scores experience higher generalized anxiety, depression [17], and negative affect [18,19]. They also experience more significant discomfort due to the work/study restrictions and a lower level of subjective well-being [20].

A recent study reported that neuroticism was positively and significantly related to high anxiety during the Covid-19 outbreak [21]. Further studies indicated that neuroticism and extroversion personality traits are strongly associated with mental health [11–13,15,22]. In general, the expectation is that an extravert will have better adjustment levels and a lower degree of anxiety. However, extraverts who desire higher levels of social and physical activity and interpersonal interaction could find the enforced isolation and restrictions of free movement during the current pandemic particularly difficult compared to introverts. Researchers have reported that the strict measures associated with the pandemic, like social isolation and social distancing, would be more natural for introverts than outgoing and social extraverts [23,24].

On the other hand, the expectation is that people with a high level of neuroticism might generally be less disturbed with being forced to stay at home rather than going out to face the everyday hassles of life. Nevertheless, increased uncertainty about being infected by the virus could offset this effect. Thus, it indicates that personality traits predispose an individual's intensity and experience of anxiety.

1.1.2. Big Five Personality Traits and Sleep Quality

Sleep is a common element of life and an essential quality health and well-being component. Conversely, poor sleep and disruptive sleeping patterns can lead to physical and psychological problems [25–28]. Past research has indicated that the personality trait of neuroticism is inversely related to good sleep quality [29–35]. On the other hand, the relation between conscientiousness and sleep is mixed. Some studies show a positive association with better quality sleep [31–33,35,36], while others indicate no association [29,30].

Similarly, high extraversion and low neuroticism are closely associated with better sleep [37]. Thus, the best predictor of sleep quality has been neuroticism. However, when all the predictors were put together in a single model, only agreeableness became a significant predictor of sleep quality [30]. Furthermore, sleep duration is also one of the critical indicators of good sleep quality. For example, individuals scoring high on traits of neuroticism and openness were short sleepers [38]. Thus, the past research indicates that neuroticism is outrightly inversely related to sleep quality, whereas the other four traits have a mixed or no association with sleep quality. However, these studies were done before the COVID-19 pandemic, and the studies done post-COVID-19 have focused on the clinical population [39] or frontline workers [40].

1.1.3. Sleep Quality and COVID-19 Anxiety

The research studies suggest that good sleep quality and anxiety are inversely related [41–44]. A study found that students who had poor sleep the previous night reported higher anxiety levels [45]. Research has also indicated that poor sleep quality can change anxiety symptoms [46,47]. In another study on university students, perceived anxiety was negatively associated with sleep quality [48]. They also confirmed that sleep education and sleep improvement-based intervention programs could help improve students' mental health and reduce stress and anxiety levels. A meta-analysis involving randomized controlled trials revealed that improving sleep quality had, on average, a medium-sized effect on mental health.

Furthermore, research indicates that sleep quality reduces depression, anxiety, and stress [49]. Nevertheless, a few studies have also indicated a bi-directional relationship between sleep quality and anxiety [50,51]. However, these relationships have not been explored in the context of COVID-19 anxiety. In addition, there is a paucity of research investigating the possible mediating role of sleep quality in the relationship between personality traits and COVID-19 anxiety in adults. Similarly, most contemporary researchers have focused on assessing the COVID-19 pandemic anxiety using instruments of general anxiety, e.g., Depression Anxiety and Stress-21 [52], Self-rating Anxiety Scale [53], and Generalized Anxiety Disorder 7-item [54]. However, as pandemics are rare and each pandemic is unique in nature, symptoms, duration, and impact, each pandemic has to be dealt with differently. Therefore, understanding whether the big five personality traits predict COVID-19 anxiety and exploring the role of sleep quality in mediating the relationship could assist mental health professionals in developing individually tailored guidance and interventions for managing COVID-19 anxiety.

1.2. The Present Study

The present study explores the relationship of big five personality traits with the two factors of COVID-19 pandemic anxiety, namely, fear and somatic concern. Quality sleep is often associated with reduced anxiety and enhanced psychological well-being. Thus, we also intend to study the role of sleep quality as a mediator between personality traits and the COVID-19 anxiety factors, i.e., fear and somatic concern, in the general adult population. The study aims to explore the extent to which the big five traits predict fear and somatic concern directly and indirectly through sleep quality. It was hypothesized that all five personality traits would predict fear and somatic concern directly and indirectly mediated through sleep quality. Therefore, a hypothetical model was proposed and tested. The model (Figure 1) included age, gender, and occupational status control variables.

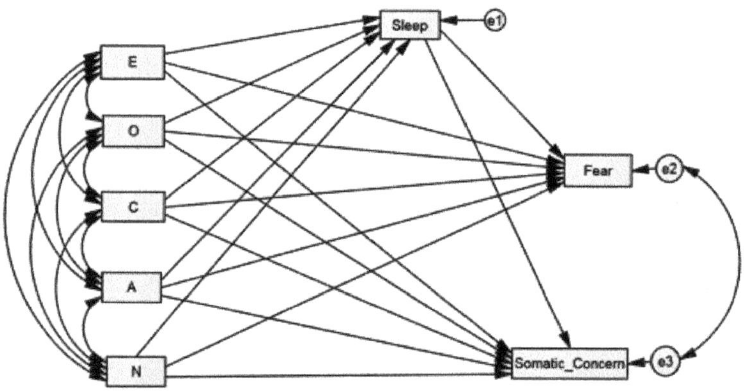

Figure 1. Conceptual model showing the relationship between the big five personality traits (E = Extraversion, O: Openness, C: Conscientiousness, A: Agreeableness, N: Neuroticism) and COVID-19 anxiety components (Fear and Somatic Concern) mediated through sleep quality.

2. Methodology

2.1. Study Design, Data Collection, and Procedures

A cross-sectional study design was followed for the research study. Data was collected using non-probability, convenience sampling methodology. Participation in the study was voluntary, and the participants were informed about the nature of the study. Furthermore, they were informed that they consented to participate in the study by filling the survey as per the Declaration of Helsinki (59th WMA General Assembly, 2009). No personally sensitive information was taken from the participants. The inclusion criteria in the study were that the participants should be of a minimum of 18 years of age, have completed a minimum of 12 years of schooling, and should be residing in India. A total of 308 participants completed the Google form consisting of the battery of questionnaires circulated through emails, WhatsApp, and Facebook during the period between 25 July 2021 to 20 September 2021. After the initial data screening, 12 incomplete forms were excluded. Excluding these 12 left a total sample of 296.

2.2. Measures for the Study

2.2.1. Sociodemographic Information

Participants were asked to state their age, gender, occupation (employed or not), and highest educational qualification. The analysis included age, gender, and occupational status as control variables. The age of the participants ranged between 18 to 77 years, and the mean age was 32.57 years (SD = 14.92 years). Table 1 illustrates the sociodemographic profile of the sample.

Table 1. Sociodemographic profile of the sample.

S. No.	Socio-Demographic Variable		*N*	Percentage
1.	Gender	Females	183	61.80
		Males	113	38.20
2.	Marital Status	Married	149	50.34
		Unmarried	138	46.62
		Others	9	3.04
3.	Education	Higher secondary	74	25.00
		Undergraduate	7	2.360
		Graduate	103	34.80
		Postgraduate	100	33.78
		PhD	12	4.05
4.	Occupational Status	Not employed	168	56.76
		Employed	129	43.24

2.2.2. Big Five Inventory-10(BFI-10)

BFI-10 [55] is a short measure of personality traits. It has two items related to each of the five traits, i.e., Openness, Extraversion, Conscientiousness, Neuroticism, Agreeableness. The responses are on a 5-point rating scale, and a higher score indicates a high trait level. The authors have reported that the scale has good validity and reliability across the different samples. However, no Cronbach alpha was calculated as only two items per factor are present in the scale (e.g., Soto and John [56]).

2.2.3. COVID-19 Pandemic Anxiety Scale (COVID-19 PAS)

COVID-19 PAS [57] is a 10-item short scale to assess the anxiety related to COVID-19 pandemic. A confirmatory factor analysis that tested the factor structure of COVID-19 PAS suggested a two-factor model with six items in factor one (fear) and four items in factor two (somatic concerns). The fear factor assessed the fear of going to markets, meeting strangers, listening to news updates, possible painful death due to the virus, and fear of lockdowns. The somatic concern factor assessed the perceived bodily concerns linked with COVID-19 (see Supplementary Figure S2). The higher scores on the scale indicated a high degree of COVID-19 anxiety. In addition, the scale's Cronbach alpha (α = 0. 80) indicated good reliability for the scale. The Cronbach alpha for fear and somatic concern components was 0.78 and 0.82, respectively.

2.2.4. Sleep Quality Scale (SQS)

SQS [58] was a single-item measure of sleep quality with strong reliability and validity. Sleep quality had to be rated from 0 to 10, with a higher rating indicating good sleep quality.

3. Results

3.1. Data Analysis

Statistical analyses have been conducted using SPSS version 21 and AMOS version 28. First, to determine the presence of common method bias, Herman's single factor test was assessed. Next, t-test and bivariate correlations were computed using SPSS version 21. Cohen's criteria were used to analyze and interpret the effect size of correlation coefficients [59]. Next, using AMOS 28, the multivariate normality of the data was assessed using Mardia's coefficient [60,61]. The kurtosis coefficient of −2.982 with a critical ratio of 1.471 indicated multivariate normality. However, the skewness and kurtosis for individual study variables indicated univariate non-normality (Supplementary Materials, Table S2). Thus, path analysis using Maximum Likelihood (ML) estimation with bootstrapping (1000 resamples) was performed to generate accurate estimations of the regression coefficients with accompanying confidence intervals (bias-corrected at the 95% confidence level) and *p*-values [62,63]. Effects with $p < 0.05$ were considered statistically significant. Path analysis allows the assessment of the direct impact of independent variables on dependent variables and allows the studying of other relations like indirect and spurious. Further, it also enables comparison of the strength of relationships and identification of the mediators. Thus, path analysis was conducted to assess the effect of personality traits on COVID-19 pandemic anxiety factors, i.e., fear and somatic concern. Also, a mediational analysis was performed to examine the mediating role of sleep quality (mediator variable) between the big five personality traits (independent, exogenous variables) and fear (F) and somatic concerns (SC) (dependent, endogenous variables). In addition, age, gender, and occupational status were added to the model as control variables. To assess whether the drawn-out model from the bootstrapped sample provides model fit, χ^2 and the Bollen–Stine bootstrap p [64] were assessed. Further, as per Hu and Bentler's criteria, SRMR, RMSEA, and CFI were also assessed for model fit [65,66]. An excellent model fit is indicated by SRMR ≤ 0.08, RMSEA ≤ 0.06, and CFI ≥ 0.95.

3.2. Testing for Common Method Bias

Exploratory factor analysis of all the observed study variables using principal axis factoring indicated that the total variance explained by a single factor was 17.528%. This was significantly lower than the threshold of 50% (See Supplementary Table S1). Thus, it indicated no serious common method bias with the data.

3.3. Descriptive Analysis

Table 2 presents the means, standard deviations, and independent t-test results for the variables under study. Independent t-test results revealed significantly higher scores for women on neuroticism, fear, and somatic concerns. However, men had scored significantly higher on quality of sleep. However, because assessing gender differences was not an aim of this study and the number of participants was unsatisfactory to test the hypothesized model separately in men and women, all following analyses were conducted in the total sample [66]. Table 3 presents the bivariate correlation between all the study variables. All the correlations were below 0.50, indicating no strong relation between independent variables as per Cohen's criteria [59].

Table 2. Means (M), standard deviations (SD), and independent sample t-tests on all measures.

Variable	Total (N = 296)		Females (*n* = 183)		Males (*n* = 113)		t	*p*
	M	SD	M	SD	M	SD		
Extraversion	6.35	2.23	6.17	2.41	6.65	1.88	−1.77	0.078
Conscientiousness	7.16	1.73	7.02	1.65	7.39	1.82	−1.79	0.075
Neuroticism	5.95	2.13	6.44	2.17	5.15	1.81	5.30	0.000
Openness	6.79	1.56	6.79	1.63	6.79	1.43	0.00	0.997
Agreeableness	7.76	1.71	7.80	1.71	7.70	1.70	0.51	0.611
Sleep	6.80	2.34	6.43	2.45	7.42	2.01	−3.60	0.000
Fear	5.90	3.62	6.33	3.58	5.20	3.59	2.62	0.009
Somatic Concern	2.35	2.54	2.99	2.79	1.32	1.61	5.80	0.000

Table 3. Correlations for the study variables.

Variables	1	2	3	4	5	6	7	8
Extraversion (1)	1							
Conscientiousness (2)	0.243 **	1						
Neuroticism (3)	−0.252 **	−0.327 **	1					
Openness (4)	−0.002	−0.067	0.009	1				
Agreeableness (5)	0.186 **	0.053	−0.163 **	0.045	1			

Table 3. *Cont.*

Variables	1	2	3	4	5	6	7	8
Sleep (6)	0.146 *	0.146 *	−0.295 **	0.052	0.083	1		
Fear (7)	−0.046	−0.074	0.171 **	−0.021	−0.116 *	−0.091	1	
Somatic Concern (8)	−0.244 **	−0.268 **	0.401 **	−0.076	−0.208 **	−0.470 **	0.318 **	1

Note: ** $p < 0.01$; * $p < 0.01$.

3.4. Path Analysis: Direct and Indirect Associations

The current investigation aimed to extend our understanding of vulnerability and protective factors to COVID-19 related anxiety. Thus, we tested a model. It was hypothesized that the personality traits of extraversion, openness to experience, conscientiousness, agreeableness, and neuroticism would directly affect the factors of COVID-19 anxiety, i.e., fear and somatic concern. Similarly, that sleep quality will mediate the relationship between personality traits and the factors of COVID-19 anxiety. The sociodemographic variables of gender, age, and occupational status were added to the models as control variables. Based on the hypothesis, a path model was developed. The resulting model (M1) was fully saturated (i.e., degree of freedom is zero) with 77 parameters. Fully saturated models always produce a perfect fit to the data. Therefore, model fit indices were neither examined nor reported. The model explained 7% of fear and 39% of somatic concern variance. In model 1, certain paths were not statistically significant, e.g., the direct relationship of extraversion on fear and somatic concern; the direct effect of openness on fear and somatic concern; the direct effect of agreeableness on fear; and the direct effect of neuroticism on fear (Table 4). Also, there was no significant effect of extraversion, openness, conscientiousness, and agreeableness on sleep. Similarly, sleep had no significant effect on fear (see Supplementary Figure S1). Thus, these non-significant paths were omitted one by one, and the model was recalculated. Age, gender, and occupational status remained in the model as control variables. The resulting (Figure 2) alternate model (M2) indicated that neuroticism had a significant direct effect on the factors of COVID-19 anxiety, i.e., fear (0.143, 95% CI (0.017, 0.247), $p = 0.02$). and somatic concern (0.213, 95% CI (0.099, 0.324), p = 0.003). Neuroticism had significant effect on quality of sleep (0.255, 95% CI (−0.364, −0.142), $p = 0.003$). Similarly, agreeableness had significant direct effect on somatic concern (−0.137, 95% CI (−0.235, −0.058), $p = 0.002$). Regarding mediation analysis, bootstrap indirect mediation analysis revealed a partial mediation by sleep quality in the relationship between neuroticism and somatic concerns (0.089, 95% CI (0.05, 0.14), $p = 0.002$). The resulting model indicated a non-significant chi-square test ($\chi 2 = 4.547$, $p = 0.208$, Bollenstine $p = 0.226$). The analysis of the indices indicates a good model fit (CMIN/DF = 1.516, RMSEA = 0.042 (95% CI, 0.000, 0.114), CFI = 0.995, TLI = 0.952, SRMR = 0.0209) as per the existing accepted criteria [64,65]. All the paths were statistically significant, and the model accounted for 6% of fear and 36% of somatic concerns. The mediator, sleep quality, also directly predicted decreased somatic concern (−0.351), indicating that somatic concerns decreased as sleep quality improved (Figure 2). However, there was no significant effect of sleep quality on fear (see Supplementary Tables S3–S10).

Table 4. Standardized effects and corresponding 95% bias-corrected bootstrap CIS for model 1.

Model Pathways	Direct (95% CI)				Indirect via Sleep (95% CI)				Total Effects (95% CI)			
	β	Lower	Upper	*p*	β	Lower	Upper	*p*	β	Lower	Upper	*p*
E → F	0.013	−0.096	0.136	0.747	−0.001	−0.022	0.007	0.496	0.012	−0.102	0.130	0.791
O → F	−0.022	−0.157	0.088	0.627	−0.001	−0.018	0.006	0.451	−0.023	−0.163	0.088	0.608
C → F	−0.014	−0.130	0.117	0.845	−0.001	−0.016	0.007	0.561	−0.016	−0.130	0.109	0.813
A → F	−0.109	−0.213	0.011	0.071	−0.001	−0.017	0.005	0.546	−0.110	−0.215	0.010	0.065
N → F	0.115	−0.010	0.232	0.081	0.005	−0.028	0.036	0.723	0.121	−0.003	0.236	0.055
E → SC	−0.086	−0.181	0.021	0.095	−0.020	−0.072	0.019	0.299	−0.106	−0.209	0.009	0.068
O → SC	−0.068	−0.172	0.023	0.130	−0.019	−0.060	0.020	0.340	0.086	−0.194	0.011	0.083
C → SC	−0.109	−0.214	0.007	0.062	−0.017	−0.064	0.027	0.390	−0.126	−0.234	−0.011	0.029
A → SC	−0.142	−0.245	−0.050	0.004	−0.012	−0.049	0.024	0.541	−0.154	−0.262	−0.051	003
N → SC	0.167	0.057	0.289	0.007	0.075	−0.038	0.124	0.002	0.243	0.131	0.361	0.001

Note: E: Extraversion, O: Openness, C: Conscientiousness, A: Agreeableness, N: Neuroticism; F: Fear, SC: Somatic Concern.

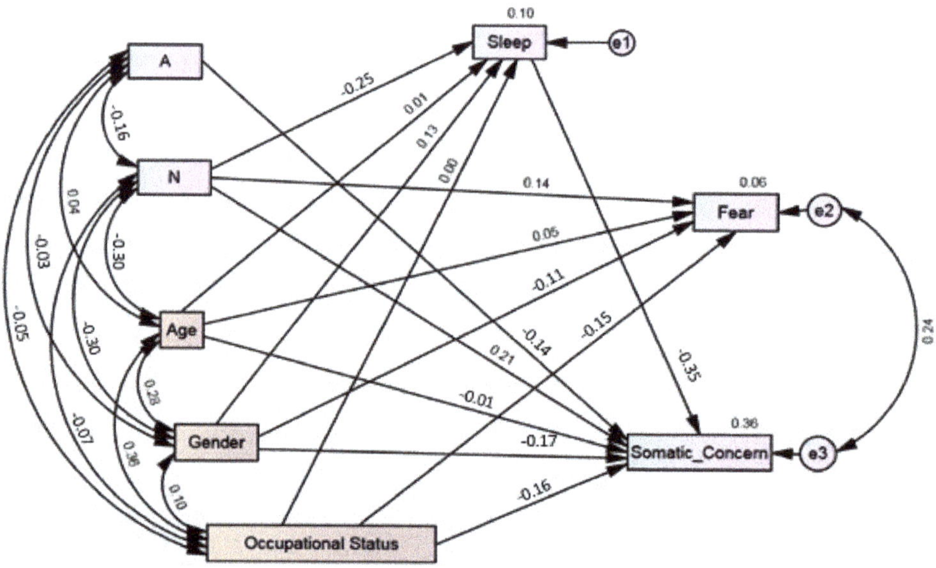

Figure 2. Path analysis model (M2) demonstrating the relationship between personality traits (A: Agreeableness; N: Neuroticism) and COVID-19 pandemic anxiety mediated through sleep quality. Note: The covariance between personality traits was assumed. Age, gender, and occupational status were included as control variables in the model.

4. Discussion

The purpose of the current study was to explore the relationship between the big five personality traits and the factors of COVID-19 anxiety, i.e., fear and somatic concern. The study also explored whether sleep quality acts as a mediator determining the relationship between personality traits and COVID-19 anxiety. Our findings provide a preliminary indication regarding the relationship between these associations. The findings partially support the hypothesis that personality traits have a relationship with the factors of COVID-19 pandemic anxiety, and that quality of sleep has a mediator effect on mediating certain relationships.

As hypothesized in the conceptual model, neuroticism indicated significant effects on COVID-19 anxiety components of fear and somatic concerns. The personality trait of neuroticism is characterized by emotional instability, moodiness, irritability, and sadness. Thus, the results indicated that as these tendencies increased in individuals, COVID-19 anxiety components, i.e., fear and somatic concerns, also increased. COVID-19 anxiety in individuals is driven by the fear of getting infected by COVID-19, leading to a painful death. Thus, interacting with people and going to public places evokes fear. However, sleep quality only partially mediated the relationship between neuroticism and somatic concern. Expressly, the results indicated that the individuals who are higher on emotional instability report poor sleep quality and report more somatic concerns. Thus, it can also be mentioned that if the sleep quality enhances, somatic concern in the individuals can reduce. Somatic concern has been marked by excessive focus on physiological discomfort. Any slight physiological symptoms like palpitations, shortness of breath, fatigue, giddiness, or change in eating patterns make people hyper-vigilant. Thus, these individuals are forced to check and recheck to confirm the absence of perceived symptoms. Over-indulgence in safety behaviors has also created pressure in the daily life of individuals and disrupted daily functioning. Further fear of lockdowns has also enhanced fear and insecurity due to the lack of control over the situation.

In the current study, neuroticism is the only big five traits related to the COVID-19 pandemic anxiety factors, i.e., fear and somatic concern. Therefore, it aligns with the expected results as neuroticism is considered a risk factor for heightened anxiety. The current results are further corroborated by findings of the other previous research on general anxiety [8,17,21]. However, the other personality traits, except agreeableness, have not shown any significant relationship with pandemic anxiety, indicating that COVID-19 pandemic anxiety may be slightly different in its form and impact from the general anxiety.

The trait of agreeableness has shown a significant negative relationship with somatic concern. This indicates that individuals with agreeableness demonstrate less somatic concerns. In addition, agreeableness enables individuals to demonstrate higher trust, modesty, cooperation, and sympathy with others. These relationships possibly indicate that agreeableness functions as a protective personality trait that can buffer the impact of COVID-19 pandemic anxiety related to somatic concerns. Earlier research has also indicated that agreeableness makes people more adaptable to the new and changing environment [8].

The individuals scoring high on agreeableness tend to be more trusting and plausibly have faith that preventive measures will control the spread of the virus. Their faith and trust in others enhance their ability to deal with anxiety. Thus, they are better equipped to deal with the required changes in their lifestyle to match the sudden changes and the new normal created due to the COVID-19. The path diagram also indicates that sleep quality did not mediate the relationship with somatic concern for agreeableness trait. Similarly, agreeableness did not significantly affect fear directly or indirectly through the mediator of sleep quality.

Other personality traits, namely, extraversion, openness to experience, and conscientiousness, have not significantly influenced the factors of COVID-19 pandemic anxiety, namely fear and somatic concerns. This may be due to the different nature of the pandemic anxiety compared to general anxiety. The possible difference in both could be attributed to the definitive known source of pandemic anxiety compared to the unknown in the case of anxiety experienced by individuals diagnosed with anxiety disorders. People are anxious only when they fear getting infected by being in unknown places outside their secure bio-bubble. Anxiety is usually pervasive and cannot be zeroed down to any specific source. In the case of pandemic anxiety, there is a known source of the infection from the coronavirus (SARS-COV-2). Thus, due to this discrete nature of anxiety, the other personality traits may not have influenced the experience of pandemic anxiety. People who are high on neuroticism are more inclined to be negatively influenced by anxiety arising from the two factors. Other individuals can handle the pandemic anxiety as they are only required to follow the protective measures, and the fear and related somatic concern can be managed.

The present study results further revealed that of the big five personality traits, the factor of fear had been predicted only by neuroticism out of the four traits. A pandemic like COVID-19, which affects various parts of the world with differing intensities across time, spreads in waves regarding the number of people infected with the virus. Thus, the fear component may vary across time. As the number of COVID-19 cases rises, the fear also rises. There are often restrictions, like lockdown which enhance fear among people. However, lockdown cannot be imposed indefinitely. The adverse economic impact on nations and individuals can be immense. Thus, we have seen that as the number of COVID-19 infections goes down, the restrictions are lifted. With the easing of restriction, the fear component also reduces. However, as the virus has frequently mutated, the world needs to be vigilant.

The current data was collected during July-September 2021 when the cases were waning in India after reaching peaks during the devastating second wave of infections during May 2021. Therefore, the fear may have probably waned due to the decrease in the positivity rate of COVID-19. Thus, the study's findings can be explained considering the changed scenario. Another plausible reason could be that as the pandemic has become so pervasive, people have started to accept it as a part of their life, and thus, it may be ignored consciously. Furthermore, the coverage of news related to the status of COVID-19 in media has also reduced a bit. Thus, it may not arouse anxiety in people compared to earlier times when there was a continuous bombardment of coronavirus-related news. Thus, it may be presumed that these factors may have reduced fear in people. However, longitudinal studies are needed to assess these plausible explanations.

5. Limitations

The study has some limitations, and the conclusions should be considered in light of these limitations. Firstly, there are methodological limitations that are prevalent in the field of psychology as a whole. Non-probability sampling and a cross-sectional design were used in this study which restricts causal inferences. In addition, the variables like age, gender, and occupational status (covariates) were controlled. However, theoretical evidence suggests that results may be influenced. Similarly, only the role of sleep quality as a mediator was investigated in the study. However, the role of other potential mediators like coping, resilience, and spirituality have not been assessed. Secondly, the participants in this study may not have been truly representative of the general population as more than 50% were females, and a more equally numbered male sample may have been better. Further, separate models for males and females were not assessed. Thirdly, the data collected using self-report measures may be subjected to social desirability and self-report errors.

Additionally, the data was collected when cases were on the decline. Thus, there is a need for testing the conclusions again as the sample was also not very large. Lastly, the BFI-10 personality measure was used in the study whose perceived reliability is considered low compared to the available similar longer measures. Thus, future studies may be needed to validate further and confirm these findings.

6. Conclusions

Despite the above limitations, the current study expands our understanding of vulnerability and protective factors regarding COVID-19 anxiety. Contrary to our perception, the path analysis results showed that sleep quality emerged as a partial mediator for neuroticism's influence on the somatic concern. Similarly, only the trait of neuroticism, whether directly and indirectly, affected the COVID-19 pandemic anxiety factors, i.e., fear and somatic concern. Additionally, only agreeableness has emerged as a protective factor in the case of COVID-19 pandemic anxiety. The present study findings may have important implications for dealing with pandemic anxiety. The derived model indicates that good sleep quality can reduce somatic concern in people experiencing anxiety, particularly those who are higher on neuroticism. Notably, it seems that people high on neuroticism are predisposed to experience more fear and somatic concerns. However, people high on agreeableness seem to have fewer somatic concerns. Thus, the current study's findings also provide a preliminary indication that the relationship of big five personality traits with pandemic anxiety might be quite different from the existing relationship with general anxiety. Thus, the findings of the COVID-19 anxiety studies using general anxiety instruments have to be cautiously interpreted when used for assessing pandemic anxiety.

Further, the current COVID-19 pandemic has ravaged the planet for two years. As the virus SARS-COV-2 is constantly mutating and with the emergence of mutations like Omicron predicted to be highly transmissible, pandemic anxiety may remain high even in the coming times. With no sign of an early end to the pandemic, mental health professionals should develop intervention programs to enhance sleep quality so that the somatic concerns arising from pandemic anxiety can be better managed. Thus, the intensity of anxiety perceived by individuals may be managed with sleep-based intervention programs. Intervention strategies for improvement in sleep quality can prepare individuals for combating pandemic anxiety and fatigue developed and driven environment by the persistent long-term nature of the pandemic. However, the current findings are based on a single male and female model. As gender can play a significant role in determining these relationships, future studies using larger samples are recommended to develop separate models for males and females to explore the relationships further.

Nevertheless, the current study presents preliminary evidence demonstrating the model explaining the relationship between personality traits, sleep quality, and COVID-19 pandemic anxiety. The current study helps mental health professionals better understand the role of personality traits in determining COVID-19 anxiety and demonstrates how sleep quality mediates the relationship, and enables them to develop psychological interventions to reduce anxiety and distress among individuals for the current and future pandemics.

Supplementary Materials: The following are available online at https://www.mdpi.com/article/10.3390/bs12020024/s1; Figure S1: Results of mediation path analysis (Model M1) showing the relationship among the Big Five personality domains and COVID-19 anxiety components; Figure S2: Confirmatory Factor analysis for the two factor COVID-19 pandemic anxiety scale; Table S1: Herman single factor test results, Table S2: Assessment of normality; Table S3: Standardized total effects for Model 1; Table S4: Standardized direct effects for Model 1; Table S5: Standardized indirect effects for Model 1; Table S6: Model Fit Summary for Model 1; Table S7: Standardized total effects for Model 2; Table S8: Standardized direct effects for Model 2; Table S9: Standardized indirect effects for Model 2; Table S10: Model fit summary for Model 2.

Author Contributions: Conceptualization and methodology, V.V.K.; formal analysis, V.V.K. and G.T.; writing—original draft preparation, V.V.K.; writing—review and editing, V.V.K. and G.T.; supervision, V.V.K. All authors have read and agreed to the published version of the manuscript.

Funding: This research received no external funding.

Institutional Review Board Statement: The study was conducted according to the guidelines of the Declaration of Helsinki.

Informed Consent Statement: Participation in this study was voluntary. Informed consent was obtained from the participants. Those who agreed to participate were assured that their information and responses would be kept confidential and solely used for research purposes.

Data Availability Statement: Data available upon request from the corresponding author.

Conflicts of Interest: The authors declare no conflict of interest.

References

1. Kumar, V.V.; Tankha, G.; Seth, S.; Timple, T.S. Construction and preliminary validation of the COVID-19 Pandemic Anxiety Scale. *Syst. Rev. Pharm.* **2020**, *11*, 1019–1024.
2. Xiong, J.; Lipsitz, O.; Nasri, F.; Lui, L.M.W.; Gill, H.; Phan, L.; Chen-Li, D.; Iacobucci, M.; Ho, R.; Majeed, A.; et al. Impact of COVID-19 pandemic on mental health in the general population: A systematic review. *J. Affect. Disord.* **2020**, *1*, 55–64. [CrossRef] [PubMed]
3. Luo, M.; Guo, L.; Yu, M.; Jiang, W.; Wang, H. The psychological and mental impact of coronavirus disease 2019 (COVID-19) on medical staff and general public—A systematic review and meta-analysis. *Psychiatry Res.* **2020**, *291*, 113190. [CrossRef] [PubMed]
4. Afshar, H.; Roohafza, H.R.; Keshteli, A.H.; Mazaheri, M.; Feizi, A.; Adibi, P. The association of personality traits and coping styles according to stress level. *J. Res. Med. Sci.* **2015**, *20*, 353–358. [PubMed]

5. McCrae, R.R.; Costa, P.T. *Personality in Adulthood: A Five-Factor Theory Perspective*, 2nd ed.; Guilford Press: New York, NY, USA, 2006.
6. Komulainen, E.; Meskanen, K.; Lipsanen, J.; Lahti, J.M.; Jylha, P.; Melartin, T.; Wichers, M.; Isometsa, E.; Ekelund, J. The effect of personality on daily life emotional processes. *PLoS ONE* **2014**, *9*, e110907. [CrossRef] [PubMed]
7. Ranieri, J.; Guerra, F.; Cilli, E.; Caiazza, I.; Gentili, N.; Ripani, B.; Di Giacomo, D. Buffering effect of e-learning on Generation Z undergraduate students: A cross-sectional study during the second COVID-19 lockdown in Italy. *Mediterr. J. Clin. Psychol.* **2021**, *9*. [CrossRef]
8. Nikcevic, A.V.; Marino, C.; Kolubinski, D.C.; Leach, D.; Spada, M.M. Modelling the contribution of the Big Five personality traits, health anxiety, and COVID-19 psychological distress to generalised anxiety and depressive symptoms during the COVID-19 pandemic. *J. Affect. Disord.* **2021**, *15*, 578–584. [CrossRef] [PubMed]
9. Khosravi, M. Neuroticism as a marker of vulnerability to COVID-19 infection. *Psychiatry Investig.* **2020**, *17*, 710–711. [CrossRef] [PubMed]
10. Shokrkon, A.; Nicoladis, E. How personality traits of neuroticism and extroversion predict the effects of the COVID-19 on the mental health of Canadians. *PLoS ONE* **2021**, *16*, e0251097. [CrossRef] [PubMed]
11. Brooks, S.K.; Webster, R.K.; Smith, L.E.; Woodland, L.; Wessely, S.; Greenberg, N.; Rubin, G.J. The psychological impact of quarantine and how to reduce it: Rapid review of the evidence. *Lancet* **2020**, *14*, 912–920. [CrossRef]
12. Kotov, R.; Gamez, W.; Schmidt, F.; Watson, D. Linking "big" personality traits to anxiety, depressive, and substance use disorders: A meta-analysis. *Psychol. Bull.* **2010**, *136*, 768–821. [CrossRef] [PubMed]
13. Otonari, J.; Nagano, J.; Morita, M.; Budhathoki, S.; Tashiro, N.; Toyomura, K.; Kono, S.; Imai, K.; Ohnaka, K.; Takayanagi, R. Neuroticism and extraversion personality traits, health behaviours, and subjective well-being: The Fukuoka Study (Japan). *Qual. Life Res.* **2012**, *21*, 1847–1855. [CrossRef]
14. Barrick, M.R.; Mount, M.K.; Judge, T.A. Personality and performance at the beginning of the new millennium: What do we know and where do we go next? *Int. J. Sel. Assess.* **2001**, *9*, 9–30. [CrossRef]
15. Costa, P.T.; McCrae, R.R. Normal personality assessment in clinical practice: The NEO Personality Inventory. *Psychol. Assess.* **1992**, *4*, 5–13. [CrossRef]
16. Mitchell, L.L.; Zmora, R.; Finlay, J.M.; Jutkowitz, E.; Gaugler, J.E. Do big five personality traits moderate the effects of stressful life events on health trajectories? Evidence from the health and retirement study. *J. Gerontol. B Psychol. Sci. Soc. Sci.* **2021**, *76*, 44–55. [CrossRef]
17. Lee, S.A.; Jobe, M.C.; Mathis, A.A.; Gibbons, J.A. Incremental validity of coronaphobia: Coronavirus anxiety explains depression, generalized anxiety, and death anxiety. *J. Anxiety Disord.* **2020**, *74*, 102268. [CrossRef]
18. Liu, N.; Zhang, F.; Wei, C.; Jia, Y.; Shang, Z.; Sun, L.; Wu, L.; Sun, Z.; Zhou, Y.; Wang, Y.; et al. Personality and perceived stress during COVID-19 pandemic: Testing the mediating role of perceived threat and efficacy. *Pers. Individ. Differ.* **2020**, *168*, 110351. [CrossRef]
19. Kroencke, L.; Geukes, K.; Utesch, T.; Kuper, N.; Back, M.D. Neuroticism and emotional risk during the COVID-19 pandemic. *J. Res. Pers.* **2020**, *89*, 104038. [CrossRef]
20. Modersitzki, N.; Phan, L.V.; Kuper, N.; Rauthmann, J.F. Who is impacted? Personality predicts individual differences in psychological consequences of the COVID-19 Pandemic in Germany. *Soc. Psychol. Personal. Sci.* **2021**, *12*, 1110–1130. [CrossRef]
21. Mengual, N.P.; Aragones-Barbera, I.; Moret-Tatay, C.; Moliner-Albero, A.R. The relationship of fear of death between neuroticism and anxiety during the Covid-19 Pandemic. *Front. Psychiatry* **2021**, *12*, 648498. [CrossRef]
22. Albuquerque, I.; de Lima, M.P.; Matos, M.; Figueiredo, C. Personality and subjective well-being: What hides behind global analyses? *Soc. Indic. Res.* **2012**, *105*, 447–460. [CrossRef]
23. Woodcock, A.; Graziano, W.G.; Branch, S.E.; Habashi, M.M.; Ngambeki, I.; Evangelou, D. Person and thing orientations: Psychological correlates and predictive utility. *Soc. Psychol. Personal. Sci.* **2013**, *4*, 116–123. [CrossRef]
24. Wijngaards, I.; de Zilwa, S.C.M.; Burger, M.J. Extraversion moderates the relationship between the stringency of COVID-19 protective measures and depressive symptoms. *Front. Psychol.* **2020**, *11*, 568907. [CrossRef]
25. Mendoza, J.F.; Vgontzas, A.N. Insomnia and its impact on physical and mental health. *Curr. Psychiatry Rep.* **2013**, *15*, 418. [CrossRef]
26. Li, L.; Wu, C.; Gan, Y.; Qu, X.; Lu, Z. Insomnia and the risk of depression: A meta-analysis of prospective cohort studies. *BMC Psychiatry* **2016**, *16*, 375. [CrossRef] [PubMed]
27. Potvin, O.; Lorrain, D.; Belleville, G.; Grenier, S.; Préville, M. Subjective sleep characteristics associated with anxiety and depression in older adults: A population-based study. *Int. J. Geriatr. Psychiatry* **2014**, *29*, 1262–1270. [CrossRef] [PubMed]
28. Sofi, F.; Cesari, F.; Casini, A.; Macchi, C.; Abbate, R.; Gensini, G.F. Insomnia and risk of cardiovascular disease: A meta-analysis. *Eur. J. Prev. Cardiol.* **2014**, *21*, 57–64. [CrossRef]
29. Allen, M.S.; Magee, C.A.; Vella, S.A. Personality, hedonic balance and the quality and quantity of sleep in adulthood. *Psychol. Health* **2016**, *31*, 1091–1107. [CrossRef]
30. Cellini, N.; Duggan, K.A.; Sarlo, M. Perceived sleep quality: The interplay of neuroticism, affect, and hyperarousal. *Sleep Health* **2017**, *3*, 184–189. [CrossRef]
31. Duggan, K.A.; Friedman, H.S.; McDevitt, E.A.; Mednick, S.C. Personality and healthy sleep: The importance of conscientiousness and neuroticism. *PLoS ONE* **2014**, *9*, e90628. [CrossRef]

32. Gray, E.K.; Watson, D. General and specific traits of personality and their relation to sleep and academic performance. *J. Pers.* **2002**, *70*, 177–206. [CrossRef] [PubMed]
33. Hintsanen, M.; Puttonen, S.; Smith, K.; Tornroos, M.; Jokela, M.; Pulkki-Raback, L.; Hintsa, T.; Merjonen, P.; Dwyer, T.; Raitakari, O.T.; et al. Five-factor personality traits and sleep: Evidence from two population-based cohort studies. *Health Psychol.* **2014**, *33*, 1214–1223. [CrossRef] [PubMed]
34. Huang, V.; Peck, K.; Mallya, S.; Lupien, S.J.; Fiocco, A.J. Subjective sleep quality as a possible mediator in the relationship between personality traits and depressive symptoms in middle-aged adults. *PLoS ONE* **2016**, *11*, e0157238. [CrossRef]
35. Williams, P.G.; Moroz, T.L. Personality vulnerability to stress-related sleep disruption: Pathways to adverse mental and physical health outcomes. *Pers. Individ. Differ.* **2009**, *46*, 598–603. [CrossRef]
36. Kim, H.N.; Cho, J.; Chang, Y.; Ryu, S.; Shin, H.; Kim, H.L. Association between personality traits and sleep quality in young Korean women. *PLoS ONE* **2015**, *10*, e0129599. [CrossRef]
37. Stephan, Y.; Sutin, A.R.; Bayard, S.; Križan, Z.; Terracciano, A. Personality and sleep quality: Evidence from four prospective studies. *Health Psychol.* **2018**, *37*, 271–281. [CrossRef]
38. Butkovic, A.; Vukasovic, T.; Bratko, D. Sleep duration and personality in Croatian twins. *J. Sleep Res.* **2014**, *23*, 153–158. [CrossRef]
39. Cankurtaran, D.; Tezel, N.; Ercan, B.; Yildiz, S.Y.; Akyuz, E.U. The effects of COVID-19 fear and anxiety on symptom severity, sleep quality, and mood in patients with fibromyalgia: A pilot study. *Adv. Rheumatol.* **2021**, *61*, 41. [CrossRef]
40. Yue, L.; Zhao, R.; Xiao, Q.; Zhuo, Y.; Yu, J.; Meng, X. The effect of mental health on sleep quality of frontline medical staff during the COVID-19 outbreak in China: A cross-sectional study. *PLoS ONE* **2021**, *16*, e0253753. [CrossRef]
41. Bower, B.; Bylsma, L.M.; Morris, B.H.; Rottenberg, J. Poor reported sleep quality predicts low positive affect in daily life among healthy and mood-disordered persons. *J. Sleep Res.* **2010**, *19*, 323–332. [CrossRef]
42. Lund, H.G.; Reider, B.D.; Whiting, A.B.; Prichard, J.R. Sleep patterns and predictors of disturbed sleep in a large population of college students. *J. Adolesc. Health* **2010**, *46*, 124–132. [CrossRef] [PubMed]
43. McCrae, C.S.; McNamara, J.P.; Rowe, M.A.; Dzierzewski, J.M.; Dirk, J.; Marsiske, M.; Craggs, J.G. Sleep and affect in older adults: Using multilevel modeling to examine daily associations. *J. Sleep Res.* **2008**, *17*, 42–53. [CrossRef] [PubMed]
44. Nyer, M.; Farabaugh, A.; Fehling, K.; Soskin, D.; Holt, D.; Papakostas, G.I.; Pedrelli, P.; Fava, M.; Pisoni, A.; Vitolo, O.; et al. Relationship between sleep disturbance and depression, anxiety, and functioning in college students. *Depress. Anxiety* **2013**, *30*, 873–880. [CrossRef] [PubMed]
45. Fuligni, A.J.; Hardway, C. Daily variation in adolescents' sleep, activities, and psychological well-being. *J. Res. Adolesc.* **2006**, *16*, 353–378. [CrossRef]
46. Kaneita, Y.; Yokoyama, E.; Harano, S.; Tamaki, T.; Suzuki, H.; Munezawa, T.; Nakajima, H.; Asai, T.; Ohida, T. Associations between sleep disturbance and mental health status: A longitudinal study of Japanese junior high school students. *Sleep Med.* **2009**, *10*, 780–786. [CrossRef]
47. Meijer, A.M.; Reitz, E.; Dekovic, M.; van den Wittenboer, G.L.; Stoel, R.D. Longitudinal relations between sleep quality, time in bed and adolescent problem behaviour. *J. Child Psychol. Psychiatry* **2010**, *51*, 1278–1286. [CrossRef]
48. Du, C.; Zan, M.C.H.; Cho, M.J.; Fenton, J.I.; Hsiao, P.Y.; Hsiao, R.; Keaver, L.; Lai, C.C.; Lee, H.; Ludy, M.J.; et al. Increased resilience weakens the relationship between perceived stress and anxiety on sleep quality: A moderated mediation analysis of higher education students from 7 countries. *Clocks Sleep* **2020**, *2*, 334–353. [CrossRef]
49. Scott, A.J.; Webb, T.L.; Martyn-St James, M.; Rowse, G.; Weich, S. Improving sleep quality leads to better mental health: A meta-analysis of randomised controlled trials. *Sleep Med. Rev.* **2021**, *60*, 101556. [CrossRef]
50. Peltz, J.S.; Rogge, R.D.; Pugach, C.P.; Strang, K. Bidirectional associations between sleep and anxiety symptoms in emerging adults in a residential college setting. *Emerg. Adulthood* **2017**, *5*, 204–215. [CrossRef]
51. Alvaro, P.K.; Roberts, R.M.; Harris, J.K. A systematic review assessing bidirectionality between sleep disturbances, anxiety, and depression. *Sleep* **2013**, *36*, 1059–1068. [CrossRef]
52. Lovibond, S.H.; Lovibond, P.F. *Manual for the Depression Anxiety Stress Scales*, 2nd ed.; Psychology Foundation: Sydney, Australia, 1995.
53. Zung, W.W. A rating instrument for anxiety disorders. *Psychosomatics* **1971**, *12*, 371–379. [CrossRef]
54. Spitzer, R.L.; Kroenke, K.; Williams, J.B.; Lowe, B. A brief measure for assessing generalized anxiety disorder: The GAD-7. *Arch. Intern. Med.* **2006**, *166*, 1092–1097. [CrossRef] [PubMed]
55. Rammstedt, B.; John, O.P. Measuring personality in one minute or less: A 10-item short version of the Big Five Inventory in English and German. *J. Res. Pers.* **2007**, *41*, 203–212. [CrossRef]
56. Soto, C.J.; John, O.P. Short and extra-short forms of the Big Five Inventory–2: The BFI-2-S and BFI-2-XS. *J. Res. Pers.* **2017**, *68*, 69–81. [CrossRef]
57. Kumar, V.V.; Tankha, G.; Shelly; Seth, S.; Apeksha; Timple, T.S. COVID-19 Pandemic Anxiety Scale. [PsycTESTS. Database record] 2020. Available online: https://www.researchgate.net/publication/353701992_COVID_19_Pandemic_Anxiety_Scale_COVID-19_PAS-10 (accessed on 1 December 2021).
58. Snyder, E.; Cai, B.; DeMuro, C.; Morrison, M.F.; Ball, W.A. New single-item Sleep Quality Scale: Results of psychometric evaluation in patients with chronic primary insomnia and depression. *J. Clin. Sleep Med.* **2018**, *14*, 1849–1857. [CrossRef]
59. Cohen, J. *Statistical Power Analysis for the Behavioral Sciences;* Routledge Academic: New York, NY, USA, 1988.
60. Mardia, K.V. Measures of multivariate skewness and kurtosis with applications. *Biometrika* **1970**, *57*, 519–530. [CrossRef]

61. Bentler, P.M.; Wu, E.J.C. *EQS 6.1 for Windows User's Guide*; Multivariate Software: Los Angeles, CA, USA, 2005.
62. Byrne, B.M. *Structural Equation Modeling with AMOS: Basic Concepts, Applications, and Programming*; Routledge: New York, NY, USA, 2010.
63. Nevitt, J.; Hancock, G.R. Performance of bootstrapping approaches to model test statistics and parameter standard error estimation in structural equation modeling. *Struct. Equ. Modeling* **2001**, *8*, 353–377. [CrossRef]
64. Bollen, K.A.; Stine, R.A. Bootstrapping goodness-of-fit measures in structural equation models. *Sociol. Methods Res.* **1992**, *21*, 205–229. [CrossRef]
65. Hu, L.; Bentler, P.M. Cutoff criteria for fit indexes in covariance structure analysis: Conventional criteria versus new alternatives. *Struct. Equ. Modeling* **1999**, *6*, 1–55. [CrossRef]
66. Kline, R.B. *Principles and Practice of Structural Equation Modeling*, 3rd ed.; The Guilford Press: New York, NY, USA, 2011.

behavioral sciences

MDPI

Communication

Obsessive-Compulsive Disorders and Functional Urinary Disorders: A Fortuitous Association?

Qin Xiang Ng [1,*], Yu Liang Lim [1], Wayren Loke [1], Wee Song Yeo [2] and Kuan Tsee Chee [3]

1 MOH Holdings Pte Ltd., 1 Maritime Square, Singapore 099253, Singapore; yulianglim95@gmail.com (Y.L.L.); wayren.loke@mohh.com.sg (W.L.)
2 Mount Elizabeth Hospital, 3 Mount Elizabeth, Singapore 228510, Singapore; corneliuslionel@gmail.com
3 Department of General and Community Psychiatry, Institute of Mental Health, 10 Buangkok View, Buangkok Green, Medical Park, Singapore 539747, Singapore; kuan_tsee_chee@imh.com.sg
* Correspondence: ng.qin.xiang@u.nus.edu; Tel.: +65-6638-6979

Abstract: Although psychological factors are known to affect bladder and bowel control, the occurrence of functional urinary disorders in patients with psychiatric disorders has not been well-studied or described. A higher prevalence of functional lower urinary tract disorders have also been reported amongst patients with obsessive-compulsive (OC) disorders. A systematic literature search of PubMed, EMBASE, OVID Medline, PsycINFO, Clinical Trials Register of the Cochrane Collaboration Depression, Anxiety and Neurosis Group (CCDANTR), Clinicaltrials.gov and Google Scholar databases found five observational studies on the topic. Unfortunately, as only one study had a (healthy) control group, a meta-analytic approach was not possible. Overall, patients with OC symptoms appeared to have increased occurrence of functional urinary symptoms, e.g., overactive bladder, increase in urgency, frequency, incontinence and enuresis. This was even more common amongst patients with Pediatric Autoimmune Neuropsychiatric Disorder Associated with Streptococcal Infections (PANDAS) or Pediatric Acute-onset Neuropsychiatric Syndrome (PANS) as opposed to patients with OCD alone. Several biological and behavioural mechanisms and treatment approaches were discussed. However, as the current evidence base was significantly limited and had moderate to serious risk of bias, no strong inferences could be drawn. Further well-designed cohort studies are necessary to better elucidate the observed associations and their management.

Keywords: urinary incontinence; functional; enuresis; obsessive-compulsive; rituals

1. Introduction

Urinary incontinence is a common and often impairing and socially embarrassing occurrence [1]. It is increasingly recognized as a potential symptom in patients with psychiatric disorders [2]. Although psychological factors (including depression and anxiety) are known to affect bladder and bowel control [3], the occurrence of functional urinary disorders in patients with psychiatric disorders has not been well-studied or described.

Functional lower urinary tract disorders comprise a diverse group of disorders, for which there is no apparent neurological disease and the structural aspect remains unknown [4]. They are frequently comorbid in children with attentional and obsessive-compulsive (OC) disorders [5–7]. Some case reports have suggested that urination could be a form of compulsion [8,9]; cognitive behavioural therapy (CBT) has long been applied in the treatment of functional urinary disorders [10]. It has also been hypothesized that these conditions may at least share some common neuropharmacological pathways involving stress-related peptide corticotropin-releasing factor (CRF) and CRF-related peptides [11], and the treatment of one may improve the other.

It is important for clinicians to promptly recognize and manage these conditions as the experience of incontinence in children and adolescents can perpetuate poor mental health and increase one's risk of social isolation, bullying and self-esteem issues [12]. However, understanding of the potential Psyche–Soma relationship and its interactions remains underdeveloped.

To the best of our knowledge, no systematic review or meta-analysis has been done hitherto to investigate the extent of the association between OC disorders and functional urinary disorders in either adults or children. It was hypothesized that patients with OC symptoms would also have an increased occurrence of functional urinary symptoms. This study aimed to investigate this a priori hypothesis, summarize current evidence and suggest areas for future research.

2. Methods

A systematic literature search was performed in accordance with the latest Preferred Reporting Items for Systematic Reviews and Meta-Analyses (PRISMA) guidelines [13]. By using the following combinations of broad Major Exploded Subject Headings (MesH) terms or text words [urinary OR incontinence OR enuresis OR overactive OR bladder] AND [obsess * OR compuls * OR OC OR OCD OR yale-brown], a comprehensive search of PubMed, EMBASE, OVID Medline, PsycINFO, Clinical Trials Register of the Cochrane Collaboration Depression, Anxiety and Neurosis Group (CCDANTR), Clinicaltrials.gov and Google Scholar databases yielded 2359 papers published in English between 1 January 1988 and 1 April 2021. Attempts were made to search grey literature using the Google search engine. Title/abstract screenings were performed independently by three study investigators (Q.X.N., Y.L.L. and W.L.) to identify articles of interest. All retrieved publications were manually reviewed and also checked for references of interest.

The inclusion criteria for this review were: (1) published clinical study, (2) study population with a diagnosis of OCD, and (3) reported occurrence or prevalence of functional urinary disorders (e.g., overactive bladder, functional urinary incontinence, etc.). Any disagreement on inclusion was resolved by consensus. Exclusion criteria included case reports, case series, conference abstracts and proceedings, which were not accepted for this systematic review.

Data were extracted using a standardized electronic form by one study investigator (Q.X.N.) and cross-checked by a second investigator (Y.L.L.) for accuracy. The quality and risk of bias of the studies were also assessed with the ROBINS-I (Risk of Bias in Non-randomized Studies-of Interventions) tool [14], graded based on consensus of three study investigators (Q.X.N., Y.L.L. and W.L.).

3. Results

The abstraction process (and reasons for exclusion) is summarized in Figure 1.

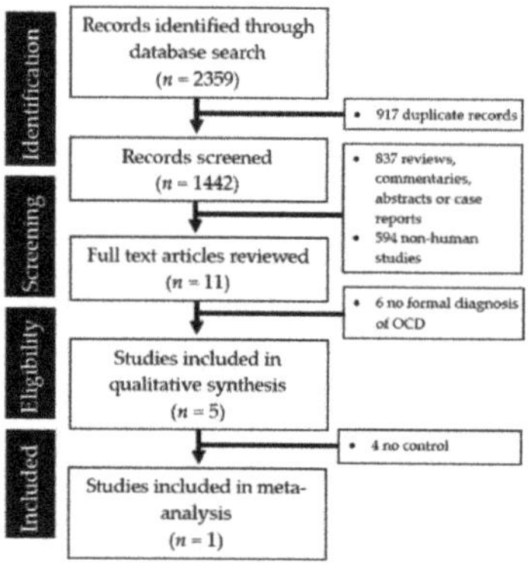

Figure 1. PRISMA flow diagram summarizing the studies identified during the literature search and abstraction process.

A total of five observational studies were systematically reviewed. The details of the studies, including the study demographics, are summarized in Table 1. Unfortunately, as only one study had a (healthy) control group, a meta-analytic approach was not possible. For the same reasons, a sensitivity analysis was not performed.

Table 1. Clinical studies reporting the occurrence of functional urinary disorders in patients with OC symptoms.

Author, Year	Country of Origin	Study Design and Study Population	Key Findings
Ahn et al., 2016 [15]	Korea	Case-control; n = 114 (57 women with OAB and 57 healthy female controls); Average age 50.65 ± 14.72 years	- Significant association between OAB and OC symptoms (OR 5.47 (95% CI: 1.99 to 15.04, p = 0.001) compared to control group - Consider screening for OCD and appropriate psychiatric referral for female patients with OAB
Arlen et al., 2014 [16]	United States	Retrospective chart review; n = 20 (2 boys and 18 girls); Average age 6.9 (range: 4 to 12 years)	- All children presented with the sensation of urinary leakage despite being completely dry and had normal physical examination and investigations. - Most children (75%) also experienced urinary urgency and half (50%) had increased urinary frequency (voiding more than eight times a day). - 70% (n = 14) had a prior diagnosis of OCD or OCD traits, as reported by their parents.
Bernstein et al., 2010 [17]	United States	Case-control; n = 39 (24 boys and 15 girls); Average age 10.66 years	- Urinary symptoms (including increase in urgency, frequency and enuresis) were much more common in children with PANDAS as opposed to non-PANDAS OCD. - There were no significant differences between the two groups of children in terms of demographics or OCD severity rating.
Jaspers-Fayer et al., 2017 [18]	Canada	Prospective cohort; n = 136 (54% males); Age range 6 to 19 years	- Parents of children with PANDAS/PANS were more likely than parents of children with OCD to report a history of urinary incontinence (57%, n = 4 out of 7 vs. 18%, n = 17 out of 92, p = 0.035).
Murphy & Pichichero, 2002 [19]	United States	Prospective case identification and followup; n = 12 (7 boys and 5 girls); Average age 5 years (range: 5 years 4 months to 10 years 11 months)	- Of the 12 children with PANDAS, 7 (58%) had compulsive daytime urinary urgency, frequency, and wiping, without fever, dysuria, nighttime symptoms or evidence of UTI.

Abbreviations: CI, confidence intervals; OAB, overactive bladder; OCD, obsessive-compulsive disorder; OR, odds ratio; PANDAS, pediatric autoimmune neuropsychiatric disorders associated with streptococcal infections; PANS, pediatric acute-onset neuropsychiatric syndrome; UTI, urinary tract infection.

In terms of the quality of the available studies, most were observational in nature, had relatively small sample sizes and overall moderate to serious risk of bias, due to the lack of control for potential confounding factors and selection bias, as seen in Table 2.

Table 2. Risk of bias assessment with ROBINS-I tool.

Study	Confounding	Selection	Measurement of Intervention	Missing Data	Measurement of Outcomes	Reported Result	Overall
Ahn et al., 2016 [15]	Serious	Serious	N/A	?	Moderate	Moderate	Serious
Arlen et al., 2014 [16]	Serious	Serious	N/A	?	Serious	Serious	Serious
Bernstein et al., 2010 [17]	Serious	Serious	N/A	?	Moderate	Moderate	Serious
Jaspers-Fayer et al., 2017 [18]	Moderate	Serious	N/A	?	Moderate	Moderate	Serious
Murphy & Pichichero, 2002 [19]	Serious	Serious	N/A	Moderate	Serious	Moderate	Serious

Abbreviations: ?, insufficient information to determine risk of bias; N/A, not applicable.

4. Discussion

Overall, patients with OC symptoms appeared to have increased occurrence of functional urinary symptoms, e.g., an increase in urgency, frequency, incontinence and enuresis. This appeared to be even more common amongst patients with PANDAS/PANS as opposed to patients with OCD alone [17–19].

There are many causes of urinary incontinence and they can be broadly classified as stress incontinence (related to weakness of the pelvic floor support and increases in intraabdominal pressure), urge incontinence (believed to be due to detrusor overactivity), overflow incontinence, mixed incontinence, or functional incontinence (thought to be caused by non-genitourinary factors, such as cognitive or physical impairments, affecting one's ability to void independently) [20]. Psychogenic polydipsia is more common in patients with schizophrenia than patients with OCD [21]. It is thought that some patients with OCD may have delayed voiding of the bladder because of certain contamination fears or OC rituals, resulting in functional incontinence. To remedy this, adherence to a strict bowel program and timed voiding regimen may be helpful [16]. Clinicians may schedule for them to urinate every two to four hours.

There is also a proposed subtype of OCD patients who have urinary obsessions and they may report predominant fear of urinary incontinence and urinary frequency without organic etiology [22]. These patients appear to respond to antidepressants. The treatment of OCD may be very complex and refractory in some cases and could require add-on atypical antipsychotic medication and psychotherapies [23].

Another potential contributory factor include the psychotropic medications themselves. The lower urinary tract is influenced by various neurotransmitter pathways. In literature, there have been several case reports of urinary incontinence associated with the use of selective serotonin reuptake inhibitor (SSRI) antidepressants [24] and antipsychotics over a broad range of doses [25]. In terms of biological mechanisms, SSRIs may have agonist effects on 5-HT4 receptors, which are also found in the urinary tract and could evoke responses in the bladder and urethra [26]. In isolated detrusor muscle strips from guinea pigs, 5-HT4 receptors were found to potentiate purinergic transmission and thus initiate the voiding reflex [27]. A retrospective chart analysis of 13,531 first-time users of an SSRI also found that the adjusted relative risk of urinary incontinence with SSRI exposure (compared to non-exposure) was 1.61 (with a 95% confidence interval of 1.42 to 1.82) [28]. This risk was higher amongst females, the elderly and patients prescribed sertraline compared to the other SSRI antidepressants. As for both typical and atypical antipsychotics, they may affect detrusor overactivity and reduce bladder compliance [29]. However, the mechanisms remain unclear and individual susceptibility may differ.

In addition to the serotonergic and antipsychotic drugs, clomipramine could also induce urinary symptoms in patients with OCD [30], as can happen with benzodiazepines and other drugs [31].

Unfortunately, the current evidence base was significantly limited and a meta-analytic approach was not possible. The studies were also observational in nature, had relatively small sample sizes and overall moderate to serious risk of bias. This also meant that we were unable to prove causation and the observations could indeed be fortuitous. There was also the possibility of ascertainment bias with case collection studies. The conclusions must thus be interpreted in light of these shortcomings.

Further well-designed cohort studies on the subject are necessary to clarify these observed associations and their management.

5. Conclusions

In conclusion, our systematic review found five observational studies, which all showed increased occurrence of functional urinary symptoms in patients with OC symptoms. In clinical practice, it is known that patients with OCD may manifest with various symptoms, however, it remains unclear if the observed functional urinary symptoms are fortuitous, biological or even behavioral in nature. Nonetheless, as urinary incontinence can be particularly distressing and socially embarrassing for the individual, this should be sensitively elicited in the clinical history and approach to these patients. The importance of a good history and a holistic understanding of the patient's psychiatric phenomenology cannot be overstated. There are still significant gaps in our present understanding of this Psyche–Soma relationship, which could be the result of biological feedback, medications or other neural pathways. Further well-designed cohort studies on the subject would help shed light on these associations and their management.

Author Contributions: Conceptualization, Q.X.N. and K.T.C.; methodology, Q.X.N., Y.L.L., W.L. and W.S.Y.; formal analysis, Q.X.N., Y.L.L., W.L., W.S.Y. and K.T.C.; investigation, Q.X.N., Y.L.L., W.L., W.S.Y. and K.T.C.; resources, Q.X.N., W.L. and K.T.C.; writing—original draft preparation, Q.X.N., Y.L.L., W.L., W.S.Y. and K.T.C.; writing—review and editing, Q.X.N., Y.L.L., W.L., W.S.Y. and K.T.C.; supervision, W.S.Y. and K.T.C. All authors have read and agreed to the published version of the manuscript.

Funding: This research received no external funding.

Institutional Review Board Statement: Not applicable.

Informed Consent Statement: Not applicable.

Data Availability Statement: The datasets generated during and/or analysed during the current study are available from the corresponding author on reasonable request.

Conflicts of Interest: The authors declare no conflict of interest.

References

1. Elenskaia, K.; Haidvogel, K.; Heidinger, C.; Doerfler, D.; Umek, W.; Hanzal, E. The greatest taboo: Urinary incontinence as a source of shame and embarrassment. *Wien. Klin. Wochenschr.* **2011**, *123*, 607–610. [CrossRef]
2. Carvalhais, A.; Araújo, J.; Jorge, R.N.; Bø, K. Urinary incontinence and disordered eating in female elite athletes. *J. Sci. Med. Sport* **2019**, *22*, 140–144. [CrossRef]
3. Vasudev, K.; Gupta, A.K. Incontinence and mood disorder: Is there an association? *Case Rep.* **2010**, *2010*, bcr0720092118. [CrossRef]
4. Leue, C.; Kruimel, J.; Vrijens, D.; Masclee, A.; Van Os, J.; Van Koeveringe, G. Functional urological disorders: A sensitized defence response in the bladder–gut–brain axis. *Nat. Rev. Urol.* **2017**, *14*, 153–163. [CrossRef] [PubMed]
5. Von Gontard, A.; Hollmann, E. Comorbidity of functional urinary incontinence and encopresis: Somatic and behavioral associations. *J. Urol.* **2004**, *171*, 2644–2647. [CrossRef] [PubMed]
6. Yang, T.K.; Huang, K.H.; Chen, S.C.; Chang, H.C.; Yang, H.J.; Guo, Y.J. Correlation between clinical manifestations of nocturnal enuresis and attentional performance in children with attention deficit hyperactivity disorder (ADHD). *J. Formos. Med. Assoc.* **2013**, *112*, 41–47. [CrossRef]
7. Gulisano, M.; Domini, C.; Capelli, M.; Pellico, A.; Rizzo, R. Importance of neuropsychiatric evaluation in children with primary monosymptomatic enuresis. *J. Pediatric Urol.* **2017**, *13*, 36.e1–36.e6. [CrossRef]
8. Jiwanmall, S.A.; Kattula, D. Obsessive-Compulsive Disorder Presenting with Compulsions to Urinate Frequently. *Indian J. Psychol. Med.* **2016**, *38*, 364–365. [CrossRef]
9. Rahmat, R. Urinary frequency: Going beyond the tract. *Malays Fam. Physician* **2020**, *15*, 58–60. [PubMed]
10. Mowrer, O.H.; Mowrer, W.M. Enuresis—A method for its study and treatment. *Am. J. Orthopsychiatry* **1938**, *8*, 436–459. [CrossRef]
11. Seki, M.; Zha, X.M.; Inamura, S.; Taga, M.; Matsuta, Y.; Aoki, Y.; Ito, H.; Yokoyama, O. Role of corticotropin-releasing factor on bladder function in rats with psychological stress. *Sci. Rep.* **2019**, *9*, 9828. [CrossRef]
12. Ikeda, H.; Oyake, C.; Oonuki, Y.; Fuyama, M.; Watanabe, T.; Kyoda, T.; Tamura, S. Complete resolution of urinary incontinence with treatment improved the health-related quality of life of children with functional daytime urinary incontinence: A prospective study. *Health Qual. Life Outcomes* **2020**, *18*, 14. [CrossRef]

13. Page, M.J.; McKenzie, J.E.; Bossuyt, P.M.; Boutron, I.; Hoffmann, T.C.; Mulrow, C.D. The PRISMA 2020 statement: An updated guideline for reporting systematic reviews. *BMJ* **2021**, *372*, n71. [CrossRef] [PubMed]
14. Sterne, J.A.; Hernán, M.A.; Reeves, B.C.; Savović, J.; Berkman, N.D.; Viswanathan, M.; Higgins, J.P. ROBINS-I: A tool for assessing risk of bias in non-randomised studies of interventions. *BMJ* **2016**, *355*, i4919. [CrossRef]
15. Ahn, K.S.; Hong, H.P.; Kweon, H.J.; Ahn, A.L.; Oh, E.J.; Choi, J.K.; Cho, D.Y. Correlation between overactive bladder syndrome and obsessive compulsive disorder in women. *Korean J. Fam. Med.* **2016**, *37*, 25–30. [CrossRef] [PubMed]
16. Arlen, A.M.; Dewhurst, L.L.; Kirsch, S.S.; Dingle, A.D.; Scherz, H.C.; Kirsch, A.J. Phantom urinary incontinence in children with bladder-bowel dysfunction. *Urology* **2014**, *84*, 685–688. [CrossRef]
17. Bernstein, G.A.; Victor, A.M.; Pipal, A.J.; Williams, K.A. Comparison of clinical characteristics of pediatric autoimmune neuropsychiatric disorders associated with streptococcal infections and childhood obsessive-compulsive disorder. *J. Child Adolesc. Psychopharmacol.* **2010**, *20*, 333–340. [CrossRef] [PubMed]
18. Jaspers-Fayer, F.; Han SH, J.; Chan, E.; McKenney, K.; Simpson, A.; Boyle, A.; Stewart, S.E. Prevalence of acute-onset subtypes in pediatric obsessive-compulsive disorder. *J. Child Adolesc. Psychopharmacol.* **2017**, *27*, 332–341. [CrossRef]
19. Murphy, M.L.; Pichichero, M.E. Prospective identification and treatment of children with pediatric autoimmune neuropsychiatric disorder associated with group A streptococcal infection (PANDAS). *Arch. Pediatrics Adolesc. Med.* **2002**, *156*, 356–361. [CrossRef] [PubMed]
20. Holroyd-Leduc, J.M.; Tannenbaum, C.; Thorpe, K.E.; Straus, S.E. What type of urinary incontinence does this woman have? *JAMA* **2008**, *299*, 1446–1456. [CrossRef] [PubMed]
21. Oades, R.D.; Daniels, R. Subclinical polydipsia and polyuria in young patients with schizophrenia or obsessive-compulsive disorder vs normal controls. *Prog. Neuro-Psychopharmacol. Biol. Psychiatry* **1999**, *23*, 1329–1344. [CrossRef]
22. Epstein, S.; Jenike, M.A. Disabling urinary obsessions: An uncommon variant of obsessive-compulsive disorder. *Psychosomatics* **1990**, *31*, 450–452. [CrossRef]
23. Del Casale, A.; Sorice, S.; Padovano, A.; Simmaco, M.; Ferracuti, S.; Lamis, D.A.; Rapinesi, C.; Sani, G.; Girardi, P.; Kotzalidis, G.D.; et al. Psychopharmacological treatment of obsessive-compulsive disorder (OCD). *Curr. Neuropharmacol.* **2019**, *17*, 710–736. [CrossRef] [PubMed]
24. Maalouf, F.T.; Gilbert, A.R. Sertraline-Induced enuresis in a prepubertal child resolves after switching to fluoxetine. *J. Child Adolesc. Psychopharmacol.* **2010**, *20*, 161–162. [CrossRef] [PubMed]
25. Barnes, T.R.; Drake, M.J.; Paton, C. Nocturnal enuresis with antipsychotic medication. *Br. J. Psychiatry* **2012**, *200*, 7–9. [CrossRef]
26. Bockaert, J.; Claeysen, S.; Compan, V.; Dumuis, A. 5-HT4 receptors: History, molecular pharmacology and brain functions. *Neuropharmacology* **2008**, *55*, 922–931. [CrossRef]
27. Messori, E.; Rizzi, C.A.; Candura, S.M.; Lucchelli, A.; Balestra, B.; Tonini, M. 5-Hydroxytryptamine receptors that facilitate excitatory neuromuscular transmission in the guinea-pig isolated detrusor muscle. *Br. J. Pharmacol.* **1995**, *115*, 677–683. [CrossRef]
28. Movig, K.L.L.; Leufkens, H.G.M.; Belitser, S.V.; Lenderink, A.W.; Egberts, A.C.G. Selective serotonin reuptake inhibitor-induced urinary incontinence. *Pharmacoepidemiol. Drug Saf.* **2002**, *11*, 271–279. [CrossRef]
29. Torre, D.L.; Isgrò, S.; Muscatello, M.R.A.; Magno, C.; Melloni, D.; Meduri, M. Urinary incontinence in schizophrenic patients treated with atypical antipsychotics: Urodynamic findings and therapeutic perspectives. *Int. J. Psychiatry Clin. Pract.* **2005**, *9*, 116–119. [CrossRef] [PubMed]
30. Hermesh, H.; Aizenberg, D.; Weizman, A.; Lapidot, M.; Munitz, H.; Rivera, G.C.; Dion, P. Clomipramine-induced urinary dysfunction in an obsessive-compulsive adolescent. *Drug Intell. Clin. Pharm.* **1987**, *21*, 877–879. [CrossRef]
31. Verhamme, K.M.; Sturkenboom, M.C.; Stricker, B.H.C.; Bosch, R. Drug-induced urinary retention. *Drug Saf.* **2008**, *31*, 373–388. [CrossRef] [PubMed]

behavioral sciences

MDPI

Article

DAT1 and Its Psychological Correlates in Children with Avoidant/Restrictive Food Intake Disorder: A Cross-Sectional Pilot Study

Silvia Cimino [1], Eleonora Marzilli [1], Alessandra Babore [2], Carmen Trumello [2] and Luca Cerniglia [3,*]

1 Department of Dynamic and Clinical Psychology, Sapienza, University of Rome, 00185 Roma, Italy; silvia.cimino@uniroma1.it (S.C.); eleonora.marzilli@uniroma1.it (E.M.)
2 Department of Psychological, Health and Territorial Sciences, University "G. d'Annunzio", 66100 Chieti, Italy; a.babore@unich.it (A.B.); c.trumello@unich.it (C.T.)
3 Faculty of Psychology, International Telematic University Uninettuno, 00186 Roma, Italy
* Correspondence: l.cerniglia@uninettunouniversity.net; Tel.: +39-066920761

Abstract: International research has underlined the role played by children's and maternal psychopathological symptoms on the onset of avoidant/restrictive food intake disorder (ARFID) in early childhood. No study has considered the possible interplay between children's dopamine transporter (DAT1) genotype and methylation, dysregulation problems and maternal psychopathological risk. This study aimed to investigate the complex relationship between these variables, considering the possible mediation role played by children's DAT1 methylation on the relationship between mothers' psychopathological risk and children's dysregulation problems, moderated by children's DAT1 genotype. Our sample consisted of 94 early children and their mothers, divided into four subgroups, based on children's ARFID subtypes (irritable/impulsive (I/I), sensory food aversions (SFA), post-traumatic feeding disorders subtypes (PTFD), and a non-clinical group (NC)). We addressed children's dysregulation problems and maternal psychopathological risk, and collected children's DNA through buccal swabs. Results showed that children's 9/x genotype was associated with PTFD and NC groups, whereas the 10/10 genotype was associated with the SFA group, with large effect size. There were significant large differences in the study groups on children's DAT1 total methylation, children's dysregulation problems, and maternal psychopathological risk. Children's DAT1 methylation did not mediate the relationship between mother's psychopathological risk and children's dysregulation problems, but there was a significant large direct effect. Children's 9/x genotype moderated the relationship between maternal psychopathological risk and children's DAT1 methylation but, respectively, with a large and small effect. Our pilot study suggested that the relationship between children's DAT1 genotype and methylation, dysregulation problems, and maternal psychopathological risk has a crucial contribution to ARFID.

Keywords: avoidant/restrictive food intake disorder; diagnostic subtypes; dopamine transporter; genotype; methylation; gene-environment interaction; psychopathological symptoms

1. Introduction

1.1. Dopamine Transporter Gene and Feeding Disorders

Central dopaminergic mechanisms play a major role in reward-motivated behavior involved in eating and food choices [1,2], and are associated with positive hedonic processes related to food [3–5]. Dopamine (DA) neurotransmission is regulated primarily by DA transporter (DAT), which removes DA from the synaptic cleft back into the presynaptic neurons. The gene that encodes the DAT protein, known as DAT1, has a variable number of tandem repeats (VNTR) of 40 bp (3–11 repeats) in the 3′ untranslated region (UTR). A greater gene expression has been shown associated with DAT1 10/10 genotype [6,7]. Thus, DAT1 is implicated in a number of DA-related disorders (including attention-deficit/hyperactivity disorder (ADHD), bipolar disorder, depression, and substance dependence) [8–10]. Dysregulation of DA signaling (ascribable to either DAT1 polymorphisms or hyper/hypomethylation of DAT1 promoter) is also likely to be involved in eating disorders (EDs), including bulimia nervosa and binge eating disorder [11,12]. The higher frequency of the short allele (i.e., 7 or 9 repeats, in comparison to the long allele, 10 or 11 repeats) in the DAT1 gene reported by Shinohara and colleagues [13] suggests decreased DAT function in patients who have EDs with binge-eating behaviors. Moreover, increased DAT mRNA levels have been reported by Frieling and colleagues [14] on bulimic patients. Despite the above literature, no studies to our best knowledge focused on samples of young children. Interestingly, however, one study [15] found an association between ADHD symptoms and disordered eating in young children, suggesting that the DA path could be involved in the underpinning mechanism explaining both difficulties. Previous research has shown associations between ADHD in children and DAT1 polymorphism and methylation [16–19]. Moreover, undernutrition has been shown to be associated with epigenetic changes in humans and DNA polymorphisms [20,21].

1.2. Bio-Psycho-Social Correlates of Avoidant/Restrictive Food Intake Disorder in Early Childhood

Recent studies, rooted in the developmental psychopathology framework [22], have employed complex bio-psycho-social approaches evaluating the interaction of environmental (maternal psychopathology) and individual factors (bio/genetic characteristics of offspring), especially in samples of early children [23,24], also reporting significant associations between children's DAT1 methylation and polymorphism with maternal psychopathology [18,19,25]. Notwithstanding these important results, no previous study evaluated DAT1 polymorphism and methylation status in children with avoidant/restrictive food intake disorder (ARFID), a new diagnostic category included in the section of Feeding and Eating Disorders of the Fifth Edition of the Diagnostic and Statistical Manual of Mental Disorders (DSM-5) [26]. Children with ARFID fail to eat adequate intake of food and required nutrients manifesting impaired social and psychological functioning [26,27]. Very importantly, ARFID encompasses different clinical manifestations, and some studies have used the term subtypes [28–31], according to the nature of their eating restrictions. One possibility is that children may be highly selective and avoid specific foods due to their smell, texture, or appearance, a subtype named sensory food aversion (SFA) [27,32]. Other patients, named with the clinical labels of post-traumatic feeding disorder (PTFD) subtype [30,32], may show food avoidance after distressing experiences involving oropharyngeal and gastrointestinal tract. Moreover, some children with ARFID may show characteristics of impulsiveness, irritability, and difficult to console and to engage during meals [26,27,33]. It has also been reported significant association between impulsive/hyperactive difficulties and food refusal behaviors among preschooler children [15,34], as well a history of selective eating during the early childhood of children with ADHD [35]. Although difficulties in emotional/behavioral regulation have been posited as correlated with EDs in adolescents and adults, very few studies have focused on children with ARFID [36–38], considering its subtypes [31,39]. Maternal psychopathology is also frequently associated with internalizing and externalizing, emotional/behavioral dysregulation, and eating/feeding disorders in children [28,39,40]. Moreover, although it has been suggested that the influence of the quality of the emotional environment provided by parents on children's psychological well-being could be mediated by DNA methylation mechanisms [41,42] that, in turn, could be moderated by the child's genotype [43,44], no study to date has assessed the role played by DAT1 in these processes.

1.3. The Present Study

Based on the above premises, this pilot study aimed at increasing knowledge of these processes among children with three specific ARFID sub-groups (impulsive/irritable (I/I), SFA, PTFD), compared with a control group. In accordance with previous literature [28–

31], we have chosen to focus on three specific clinical manifestations of ARFID, defining them in terms of subtypes. In particular, we wanted to explore: (a) the possible association between children's DAT1 genotype and ARFID diagnosis; (b) the possible significant differences on children's DAT1 total methylation, their dysregulation problems, and maternal psychopathological risk; and (c) the possible mediation role played by children's DAT1 methylation on the relationship between mothers' psychopathological risk on children's dysregulation problems, moderated by children's DAT1 genotype.

2. Materials and Methods

2.1. Study Design

A cross-sectional study was carried out involving N = 191 children and their mothers, recruited through public and private kindergartens, mental health clinics, and pediatric hospitals in central Italy. Mothers were contacted by expert psychologists who explained the phases and the scope of the study. All mothers who decided to participate in the study signed an informed consent form, in which the aims of the study were explained in detail. The study was approved by the Ethical Committee of the Psychology Faculty at the International Telematic University Uninettuno (n. 2018/3), and it is in line with the Declaration of Helsinki (see Supplementary Materials).

2.2. Procedure

Children's biological samples were collected through buccal swabs (Isohelix Swab Pack) from which it is possible to extract the DNA present in the epithelial cells and subsequently examine genetic polymorphism and methylation status of DAT1. Mothers were previously informed that, for at least 1 h before collecting children's salivary sample, they should not have eaten (including chewing gum, sweets, etc.), drunk (with the exception of water), or brushed their teeth. Once the buccal swabs were collected, they were slightly chilled by normal ice (+4 °C). After the administration of tampons, mothers filled out self-report and report-form questionnaires (described below), for the assessment of children's emotional-behavioral functioning and their own psychopathological symptoms. The administration of buccal swabs and questionnaires was made by expert psychologists inside a room made available, respectively, by kindergartens and mental health clinics.

2.3. Participants

To recruit clinical cases we used consecutive sampling, whereas children of the control group were randomly selected from each kindergartens. Inclusion criteria for the clinical groups were the presence of a diagnosis of one of the three ARFID subtypes (I/I, SFA, PTFD), without a comorbid disorder. The diagnosis subtypes were made by two clinicians, independently (Cohen's k = 0.81), on the basis of the clinical presentations outlined in the DSM-5 [26,33] and in DC 0-3R [27]. The inclusion criteria of the control group were: age range of children from 24 to 36 months; absence of physical or mental disorders in children and/or their mothers; mothers were biological parents of the child.

2.4. Measures

For the assessment of children's emotional-behavioral self-dysregulation, mothers were administered the Child Behavior Check-List/$1\frac{1}{2}$–5 (CBCL $1\frac{1}{2}$–5) [45,46]. The CBCL $1\frac{1}{2}$–5 is a 99-item informant-report questionnaire through which the parent is asked to answer on a three-point Likert scale (from 0 = "not true" to 2 = "very true or often true"). The scores of items were grouped on seven syndrome scales: Emotionally Reactive, Anxious/Depressed, Somatic Complaints, Withdrawn, Attention Problems, Aggressive Behavior, and Sleep Problems. The CBCL Dysregulation Profile (DP) is composed of the sum of the raw scores of the following syndrome scales: Anxious/Depressed, Attention Problems, and Aggressive Behavior [47]. The scale showed very good internal consistency, with a Cronbach's α value of 0.79 in this study. For the assessment of maternal psychopathological risk, mothers filled out the Symptom Check-List-90 item-Revised

(SCL-90-R) [48]. The SCL-90-R is a 90-item self-report questionnaire aimed at evaluating psychological symptoms and psychological distress in adults. Items are measured on a Likert scale ranging from 0 (not at all) to 4 (extremely). It is composed of nine primary dimensions (Somatization, Obsessive-Compulsivity, Interpersonal Sensitivity, Depression, Anxiety, Hostility, Phobic Anxiety, Paranoid Ideation, and Psychoticism), and to provide the severity and degree of psychological distress, it is possible to calculate a Global Severity Index (GSI), used for the aim of this study. The Italian validation [49] showed good reliability in terms of internal consistency (Cronbach's $\alpha = 0.70$–0.96), that in this study was also adequate (Cronbach $\alpha = 0.83$).

2.5. DNA Isolation and Genotyping

DNA extraction from the buccal wall cells was performed using the Buccal-Prep Plus DNA isolation (Isohelix), following the manufacturer's instructions. Information of the DAT1 gene was determined from the DAT1 gene sequence (NG_015885.1). Specifically, to identify the DAT1 polymorphism we amplified the repeated sequence of the 3 'untranslated (3′-UTR) region, by the polymerase chain reaction (PCR) technique [50]. Based on previous studies in the field of developmental psychopathology, which compared children with at least one allele 9-repeated ($9/x$; $9/9, 9/10$) [17–19,51,52], results are reported considering the absence or presence of the $9/x$ allele ($10/10$ vs. $9/9, 9/10$). Allelic distributions were consistent with Hardy–Weinberg equilibrium for each group (I/I, $\chi^2 = 2.13$, $p = 0.14$; SFA, $\chi^2 = 0.57$, $p = 0.45$; PTFD, $\chi^2 = 2.68$, $p = 0.10$; NC, $\chi^2 = 2.83$, $p = 0.09$).

2.6. Analysis of DNA Methylation

The DNA extracted from the buccal swabs was further processed to evaluate the amount of methylation in the 5′-UTR sequence of DAT1. The amount of methylation was determined in six specific CpG sites (named M1, M2, M3, M5, M6 and M7), as suggested by previous studies in the field of developmental psychopathology [17–19]. The following primers (5′-3′) were used to amplify the gene: Fwd, AGCTACCATGCCCATCCCTA TGTGGG; Rev, ATCAGCACTCCAACCCAACCCAAC. The DNA was amplified with the PyroMark PCR kit (Qiagen, Hilden, Germany) according to the manufacturer's protocol. The PCR conditions were as follows: 95 °C for 15 min, followed by 45 cycles of 94 °C for 30 s, 56 °C for 30 s, 72 °C for 30 s, and 72 °C for 10 min. PCR products were verified by agarose electrophoresis. The methylation level was analyzed using the PyroMark Q24 software (Qiagen, Hilden, Germany), which calculates the methylation percentage using the formula mC/(mC + C) for each CpG site, allowing quantitative comparisons (mC is the methylated cytosine and C is unmethylated cytosine). Finally, we calculated the Total DNA methylation (overall 6 CpG sites) of this promoter region, used for statistical analyses. Details on the sequence and the pyrosequencing assay (PM00022064) are available on the Qiagen web site (www.qiagen.com).

2.7. Statistical Analyses

Preliminary analyses were performed using descriptive statistics (frequencies, percentages, and mean scores). The association between children's DAT1 genotype and children's diagnoses was examined using chi-square analysis, with the effect size represented using Cramer's V. Information about the frequency distribution of the variables was reported in contingency table. If the value of an adjusted residual was more than 1.96, the number of cases in that cell was significantly larger than expected. Differences between the four subgroups on children's levels of DAT1 total methylation, their emotional-behavioral self-dysregulation, and mothers' psychopathological risk were examined using univariate analyses of variance (ANOVAs), and partial eta squared (ηp^2) were reported as a measure of effect size. Finally, on the total sample, we explored possible mediation effects of children's DAT1 total methylation on the relationship between maternal GSI and children's score of CBCL DP, moderated by children's DAT1 genotype.

We reported R^2 as a measure of effect size. Moderated mediation analyses were performed using Hayes's [53] PROCESS macro (Model 59). Indirect (i.e., mediating) effects were evaluated with 95% bias-corrected confidence intervals based on 10,000 bootstrap samples. Confidence intervals (CI) that do not include zero indicate effects that are significant at α = 05. All analyses were performed using SPSS software, Version 25.0.

3. Results

3.1. Sample Characteristics

From the total sample, N = 39 families refused to participate in the study. Moreover, were excluded families in which children had comorbidity between SFA and infantile anorexia (N = 9) and/or had comorbidity between PTFD and SFA (N = 2), and/or in which a member (the child and/or the mother) was under pharmacological or psychological treatment (N = 14), or suffering from cognitive, neurological, and/or physical problems (N = 21). Moreover, N = 8 families were excluded because mothers did not complete all measures, and N = 4 because it was not possible to analyze DAT1 due to errors in gathering biological samples.

The final sample consisted of N = 94 children aged from 24 to 36 months (M = 29 months, SD = 3.14; 51.1% males) and their mothers (M = 32.3; SD = 4.2), divided into four subgroups, based on children's diagnosis: (i) I/I group, composed by children with ARFID I/I subtype diagnosis, and their mothers (N = 23); (ii) SFA group, composed by children with ARFID SFA subtype diagnosis, and their mothers (N = 23); (iii) PTFD group, composed by children with ARFID PTFD subtype diagnosis, and their mothers (N = 23); and (iv) NC group, composed by children with no diagnosis, and their mothers (N = 25). Most mothers had high school (78.5%) or university (20.1%) education, and only 1.4% of mothers had only middle school education. The vast majority of mothers had average socioeconomic status (94% had an average income of 25,000–30,000 Euros per year). All mothers were the biological parent of the children and were Caucasian.

3.2. Association between Children's Dopamine Trasnporter Genotype and Children's Diagnoses

Chi-square analysis showed a significant association between children's DAT1 genotype and children's diagnoses, $\chi^2(3, N = 94) = 40.05$, $p < 0.0001$, with a large effect size (Cramer's V = 0.70). ARFID I/I subtype was not associated with any specific DAT1 genotype. SFA subtype was associated with 10/10 genotype, whereas PTFD and NC groups were associated with 9/x genotype (Table 1).

Table 1. Association between children's dopamine transporter (DAT1) genotype and children's diagnoses.

		Children's Diagnoses				
DAT1 Genotype		**I/I**	**SFA**	**PTFD**	**NC**	**Total**
9/x	N (%)	19 (82.6)	4 (17.4)	21 (91.3)	24 (96)	68
	Exp. Val.	16.6	16.6	16.6	18.1	68.0
	St. R	1.3	−6.8	**2.3**	**3.1**	
10/10	N (%)	4 (17.4)	19 (82.6)	2 (8.7)	1 (4)	26
	Exp. Val.	6.4	6.4	6.4	6.9	26.0
	St. R	−1.3	**6.8**	−2.3	−3.1	
Total	N	23	23	23	25	94

9/x = 9/9, 9/10 genotypes; I/I = Avoidant/restrictive food intake disorder (ARFID) irritable/impulsive subtype group; SFA = ARFID sensory food aversions subtype group; PTFD= ARFID post-traumatic feeding disorder group; NC = Non-clinical group; Exp. Val = Expected values; St. R = Standardized adjusted residuals. All bold values are statistically significant.

3.3. Children's Dopamine Transporter Methylation, Emotional-Behavioral Dysregulation, and Maternal Psychopathological Risk in the Four Groups

Possible differences in the children's DAT1 total methylation levels, children's dysregulation (CBCL DP), and maternal psychopathological risk (SCL-90/R GSI) were examined using ANOVAs, considering the group (I/I, SFA, PTFD, NC) as independent variables. Levene's test showed the presence of a non-homogeneity of variance (Levene test, $p < 0.05$) for all dimensions considered. Thus, Welch's test was conducted. The results showed that the four groups were significantly different on children's levels of DAT1 total methylation ($F(3,46) = 52.76$, $p < 0.0001$, $\eta p^2 = 0.71$), the score of CBCL DP ($F(3,46) = 266.06$, $p < 0.0001$, $\eta p^2 = 0.85$), and mothers score on GSI ($F(3,44) = 791.57$, $p < 0.0001$, $\eta p^2 = 0.95$), with large effect sizes. In particular, Dunnett T3 post-hoc test showed that children of the I/I group had higher levels of DAT1 total methylation than other groups ($p < 0.0001$). Moreover, children with an SFA diagnosis and with no diagnosis had higher levels of DAT1 methylation than children with PTFD diagnosis ($p < 0.0001$). Finally, children with PTFD had lower levels of DAT1 total methylation than other groups ($p < 0.0001$). As regards children's emotional and behavioral self-dysregulation, children of the NC group had lower scores than other groups in CBCL DP ($p < 0.0001$). Moreover, children with I/I and with a PTFD diagnosis had higher levels of DP than the SFA and NC groups ($p < 0.0001$). There were no significant differences between children of the I/I and PTFD groups ($p > 0.05$). Finally, mothers of children with no diagnosis reported lower scores on GSI than other groups ($p < 0.0001$), whereas mothers of children with a I/I diagnosis reported higher scores compared to mothers of other groups ($p < 0.0001$). Mothers of the PTFD group had higher scores of GSI than mothers of the SFA group ($p < 0.0001$) (Table 2).

Table 2. Means (M) and standard deviations (SD) in the four groups.

	Children's Diagnosis							
	I/I		SFA		PTFD		NC	
Variable	M	SD	M	SD	M	SD	M	SD
DAT1 Total methylation	8.29 [a]	1.07	6.01 [b]	0.93	4.08 [c]	1.18	6.08 [b]	0.54
CBCL DP	33.69 [a]	5.53	18.39 [b]	5.67	35.43 [a]	5.05	7.12 [c]	2.83
SCL-90/R GSI	1.95 [a]	0.22	0.60 [b]	0.10	1.54 [c]	0.17	0.18 [d]	0.06

[a,b,c,d] Means that do not share a letter are significantly different. I/I = ARFID irritable/impulsive subtype group, SFA = ARFID sensory food aversions subtype group, PTFD = ARFID post-traumatic feeding disorder group, NC = Non-clinical group.

3.4. Children's Dopamine Transporter Methylation as a Mediator of the Association between Maternal Psychopathological Risk and Children's Dysregulation, Moderated by Children's Genotype

Finally, in order to verify whether children's DAT1 total methylation mediates the effect of mothers' GSI on children's DP by children's DAT1 genotype we conducted moderated mediation analysis. For this aim, we considered the total sample. Figure 1 shows the proposed moderated mediation model.

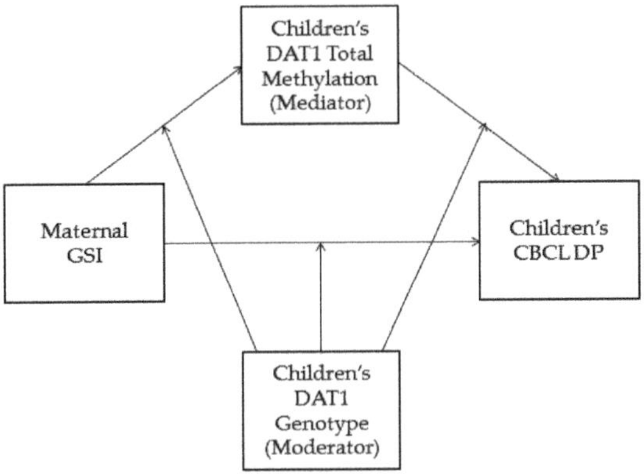

Figure 1. Diagram of moderated mediation model with children's DAT1 total methylation as the mediator of the relationship between maternal global severity index (GSI) and Children CBCL/1$\frac{1}{2}$-5 Dysregulation Profile (CBCL DP), with children's DAT1 genotype as the moderator.

Results showed that the significant direct effect of GSI on children's DAT1 total methylation was significant. Moreover, there were significant direct effects of mothers' psychopathological risk and children's DAT1 genotype on children's CBCL DP. The interaction effect of children's DAT1 genotype with children's DAT1 total methylation was also significant. To probe this significant interaction, conditional effects were evaluated using the PROCESS macro [53]. Results showed that the level of children's DAT1 total methylation was a significant negative predictor of the score of CBCL DP, but only for children with 9/x genotype (B = −2.57, SE = 0.64, $p < 0.0001$; 10/10, B = 3.90, SE = 2.78, $p = 0.16$), but with a low effect size ($F(1,88) = 5.14$, $p = 0.02$, R^2-chng = 0.01). Moreover, results of conditional direct effect of maternal GSI on CBCL DP showed that mother's psychopathological risk significantly predicted children's CBCL DP for both children's genotypes ($p < 0.0001$), with a large effect size. Finally, the indirect effect of mothers' GSI on children's DP through levels of children's DAT1 total methylation was not significant (the CI included zero) (Table 3).

Table 3. Results of moderated mediation analyses.

	Variable	B(SE)	LLCI	ULCI
DAT methyl.				
	GSI	0.23 (0.11) *	**0.01**	**0.45**
	DAT1 genotype †	−0.14 (0.26)	−0.66	0.38
	GSI x DAT1 genotype †	−0.31 (0.32)	−0.96	0.33
			$R^2 = 0.04$ F (3,90) = 1.51	
CBCL DP				
	GSI	11.26 (0.73) **	**9.80**	**12.71**
	DAT methylation	−1.06 (0.81)	−2.68	0.56
	DAT1 genotype †	−3.39 (1.61) *	**−6.60**	**−0.19**
	GSI x DAT1 genotype †	0.84 (2.35)	−3.83	5.52
	DAT methyl x DAT1 genotype †	−6.48 (2.85) *	**−12.15**	**−0.80**
			$R^2 = 0.79$ F (5,88) = 69.98 ***	

Table 3. *Cont.*

Conditional Direct Effect at Specific Levels of Moderator				
Predictor	**Moderator**	**Direct Effect (SE)**	**LLCI**	**ULCI**
GSI	10/10	10.61 (2.25) **	**6.12**	**15.10**
	9/9, 9/10	11.45 (0.66) **	**10.13**	**12.77**
		R^2 = 0.75F (3,90) = 93.75 **		
Conditional Indirect Effect at Specific Levels of Moderator				
Mediator	**Moderator**	**Indirect Effect (BootSE)**	**LLCI**	**ULCI**
DAT methyl.	10/10	1.85 (2.52)	−3.20	6.74
	9/9, 9/10	−0.41 (0.33)	−1.17	0.14

† The contrast group is 10/10 genotype. * $p < 0.05$, ** $p < 0.0001$. SE = Standard error; LLCI = Lower level confidence interval; ULCI = Upper level confidence interval; BootSE = Boot-strapped standard error. All bold values are statistically significant.

4. Discussion

This pilot study aimed to investigate children's levels of DAT1 methylation, their emotional and behavioral dysregulation, and psychopathological risk of their mothers, in a sample of young children with three different ARFID subtypes (i.e., I/I, SFA, PTFD). Our preliminary analyses, focused on the specific characteristics of the three ARFID subtypes, have underlined peculiar features associated with each diagnosis.

4.1. Impulsive/Irritable Subtype

Regarding the I/I subtype, results showed no significant association with children's DAT1 genotype, although the majority of this group (82.6%) had 9/x genotype. Moreover, children with I/I had the highest levels of DAT1 methylation, which are generally associated with reduced levels of transcription and gene expression, resulting in lower availability of DAT and greater levels of extracellular DA [54,55]. Consequently, our results suggested that children with I/I may have dopaminergic hyperfunctioning that, in turn, have been associated with children's impulsive behaviors [56], as well as with adolescent's and adults' restraint eating and bulimic behaviors [57,58]. They also showed high levels of emotional-behavioral dysregulation, and their mothers showed the greatest psychopathological risk. Previous studies have shown that early food avoidant behaviors may be associated with impulsivity behaviors in preschooler children [15] and hyperactive symptoms over time [34,35], and recent studies by Peyre and colleagues [59] and by Katsuki and colleagues [60] have evidenced a key role played by CBCL DP in ADHD. The present study also suggested that the I/I subtype may be a higher risk for dysregulation problems, in line with recent literature [31].

4.2. Sensory Food Aversions Subtype

With regard to SFA diagnosis, we found a significant association with 10/10 genotype, with large effect size, and DAT1 methylation was at a medium level (higher than PTFD, lower than I/I, and similar to NC). In addition, these children reported the lowest dysregulation problems compared to other clinical groups and, in turn, their mothers' showed the lowest psychopathological risk than mothers of other ARFID groups. These results are in line with the study by Lucarelli and colleagues [28] and Cerniglia and colleagues [31] that have evidenced lower psychopathological problems in children with SFA and among their mothers, compared to other ARFID subtypes.

4.3. Post Traumatic Feeding Disorder Subtype

Finally, PTFD diagnosis was associated with 9/x genotype, as well as the NC group, with a large effect size. In this context, it is important to note that although previous studies have reported significant association between DAT1 and a wide range of children's psychopathologies [8,17,61–63], only few studies have focused on feeding disorders [13,64]. Our study is one of the first, supporting the recent evidence that individual genetic features could make the child more susceptible to both adverse and supportive influences [62,65,66], as a possible explanation of the associations found between genotype 9/x with both PTFD and NC group. Children with PTFD diagnosis also reported the lowest levels of DAT1 methylation, in line with previous studies on traumatized individuals that found low levels of DA in the brain among this population [67]. They also had the highest scores of CBCL DP, and their mothers had the highest psychopathological risk. The research on the impact of early traumatic experiences has evidenced a significant association with emotional and behavioral dysregulation difficulties [68,69]. This study suggests that even a child exposed to an early food-related trauma may be at higher risk to develop dysregulation problems. Moreover, our findings are in accordance with previous studies that have shown the highest psychopathological risk in children with PTFD and among their mothers compared to other ARFID diagnosis [28,31].

4.4. The Complex Interplay between the Variables

Our last aim was to verify the possible mediation role played by children's DAT1 methylation on the relationship between maternal psychopathological risk and children's dysregulation, and if these relationships were moderated by children's DAT1 genotype. To this end, we considered the total sample. However, our results showed no significant indirect effect of mothers' GSI on children's DP through levels of children's DAT1 total methylation. We found a significant association between maternal GSI and children' DAT1 methylation, as well as a direct and moderated association with children's DAT1 genotype, in accordance with previous studies [18,19]. Moreover, both maternal psychopathological risk and children's DAT1 genotype (i.e., 9/x genotype) were significantly and directly associated with children's emotional-behavioral self-dysregulation, but the interactive effect was not significant. At the same time, 9/x genotype was shown to have a positive contribution on the scores of CBCL DP. This result is in line with our preliminary results on the different ARFID subtypes, which evidenced high levels of dysregulation problems among children with PTFD and I/I subtypes, which in turn were carriers of 9/x genotype. Regarding the relationship between children's DAT1 methylation and children's levels of DP, only the moderated association by children's DAT1 genotype was significant, but with a low effect size. The level of children's DAT1 methylation was significantly and negatively associated with the score of CBCL DP, but only for children with 9/x genotype. Given that the literature and our previous findings have suggested that psychopathological symptoms are associated with hypo-methylation of DNA (the PTFD group reported the lowest methylation levels, the highest scores on CBCL DP, and association with 9/x genotype), it would seem that the 9/x genotype confers an additional risk with respect to the effects of methylation on dysregulation problems. A recent study by Cimino and colleagues [19] also showed a moderating effect of children's DAT1 genotype on the relationship between maternal psychological profiles and children's methylation of DAT1, considering a sample of school-aged children of the general population.

4.5. Limitations and Strengths

This pilot study has some limitations. First of all, the small sample size of each subgroup compared to the standards of genetic studies, which implies a limited statistical power and does not allow to generalize our results. Furthermore, due to the cross-sectional nature of the study design, it is suggested to take with caution the preliminary causal links found. Consequently, further studies with larger study populations and within longitudinal study design are needed to support our preliminary findings. In addition, we assessed maternal psychopathological risk and children's emotional-behavioral dysregulation, respectively, through self-report and report-form measures. Although the tools chosen are widely validated and used in the literature, information provided may be influenced by perception biases, and should be interpreted with caution. Further studies should evaluate these variables through more objective and robust methodologies, such as clinical interview and observational methodologies. Moreover, we didn't consider the possible role played by confounder variables, such as: father's psychopathological risk, which literature has evidenced to be implicated in children's emotional-behavioral dysregulation, offspring's feeding disorders [70–72], as well as children's DAT1 methylation [18,19], which may act as an additional moderator on the relationship between maternal psychopathological risk and children's outcomes; social support and marital adjustment, which are widely shown to be associated the psychological well-being of both parents and children [73,74]; the quality of feeding interactions, which may act as mediator on the relationship between mothers and children emotional-behavioral and feeding problems [71,75], with bidirectional effects [76]; finally, maternal DAT1 genotype, which in turn can influence maternal psychological profiles, as well as the quality of the relationship with their child, and the consequences on his/her adjustment [77,78]. Nonetheless, the present pilot study has several strengths. In fact, it was the first to explore the role played by DAT1 genotype, DAT1 methylation, and dysregulation problems among three different subtypes of ARFID, also considering the possible moderated mediation role played by levels of children's DAT1 methylation on the relationship between maternal psychopathological risk and emotional-adaptive functioning of the child. Furthermore, the study added to the previous literature new support on the risk and/or protective factors, in children and their mothers, at the basis of ARFID in early children, which can be evaluated for the planning of more targeted and effective intervention strategies. Interestingly, the significant associations that we found between ARFID diagnosis, children's DAT1 genotype and methylation, dysregulation problems, and maternal psychopathological risk had large effect sizes. The only one significant effect found in a low size was the moderated effect of children's genotype on the association between children's DAT1 methylations and their dysregulation problems. This finding may suggest that the influence of children's DAT1 genotype is higher by itself and in response to the risk exerted by maternal psychopathological risk.

5. Conclusions

Overall, our preliminary findings have supported the importance to considering the complex interaction between DAT1 gene and environment provided by mothers, both in terms of genotype-environment interactions and the possible methylation mechanisms involved. The link that has emerged between maternal psychopathological risk, children's DNA methylation, and their regulatory difficulties further suggests the importance of intervening also on the maternal difficulties of children with ARFID. In fact, recent evidence has shown that intervention strategies aimed at reducing risk factors and promoting protective factors can reverse the epigenetic signs, modifying that sequence of events called developmental cascade [79], in order to obtain the maximum effect on the change of a negative cascade in a positive one [80]. In contrast, epigenetic modifications resulting from exposure to environmental risk factors, and their effects on child's emotional-behavioral functioning, can last well beyond the end of exposure itself [42,81]. Our study is in line with these evidences, supporting the importance of an assessment and intervention approach that takes into account not only the child's feeding difficulties, but also their regulatory difficulties within the more complex family context [36,82].

Supplementary Materials: Supplementary Materials are available online at https://www.mdpi.com/2076-328X/11/1/9/s1.

Author Contributions: Conceptualization, S.C.; writing and supervision, L.C.; methodology, data curation and writing—original draft preparation, E.M., A.B. and C.T. All authors have read and agreed to the published version of the manuscript.

Funding: This research received no external funding.

Institutional Review Board Statement: The study was conducted according to the guidelines of the Declaration of Helsinki, and approved by the Ethics Committee of Sapienza, University of Rome number: 27/2016.

Informed Consent Statement: Informed consent was obtained from all subjects involved in the study.

Data Availability Statement: Data is available on request to the corresponding author.

Acknowledgments: We thank Claudio D'Addario (Faculty of Bioscience and Technology for Food, Agriculture and Environment, University of Teramo, Italy) for the DNA methylation analyses.

Conflicts of Interest: The authors declare no conflict of interest.

References

1. Bressan, R.; Crippa, J. The Role of Dopamine in Reward and Pleasure Behaviour—Review of Data from Preclinical Research. *Acta Psychiatr. Scand.* **2005**, *111*, 14–21. [CrossRef] [PubMed]
2. Bromberg-Martin, E.; Matsumoto, M.; Hikosaka, O. Dopamine in Motivational Control: Rewarding, Aversive, and Alerting. *Neuron* **2010**, *68*, 815–834. [CrossRef] [PubMed]
3. Erlanson-Albertsson, C. How Palatable Food Disrupts Appetite Regulation. *Basic Clin. Pharmacol. Toxicol.* **2005**, *97*, 61–73. [CrossRef] [PubMed]
4. Wang, G.-J.; Volkow, N.D.; Fowler, J.S. The Role of Dopamine in Motivation for Food in Humans: Implications for Obesity. *Expert Opin. Ther Targets* **2002**, *6*, 601–609. [CrossRef] [PubMed]

5. Cordeira, J.W.; Frank, L.; Sena-Esteves, M.; Pothos, E.N.; Rios, M. Brain-Derived Neurotrophic Factor Regulates Hedonic Feeding by Acting on the Mesolimbic Dopamine System. *J. Neurosci.* **2010**, *30*, 2533–2541. [CrossRef]
6. Heinz, A.; Goldman, D.; Jones, D.W.; Palmour, R.; Hommer, D.; Gorey, J.G.; Lee, K.S.; Linnoila, M.; Weinberger, D.R. Genotype influences in vivo dopamine transporter availability in human striatum. *Neuropsychopharmacology* **2000**, *22*, 133–139. [CrossRef]
7. Jacobsen, L.K.; Staley, J.K.; Zoghbi, S.S.; Seibyl, J.P.; Kosten, T.R.; Innis, R.B.; Gelernter, J. Prediction of dopamine transporter binding availability by genotype: A preliminary report. *Am. J. Psychiatry* **2000**, *157*, 1700–1703. [CrossRef]
8. Franke, B.; Vasquez, A.A.; Johansson, S.; Hoogman, M.; Romanos, J.; Boreatti-Hümmer, A.; Heine, M.; Jacob, C.P.; Lesch, K.-P.; Casas, M.; et al. Multicenter Analysis of the SLC6A3/DAT1 VNTR Haplotype in Persistent ADHD Suggests Differential Involvement of the Gene in Childhood and Persistent ADHD. *Neuropsychopharmacology* **2010**, *35*, 656–664. [CrossRef]
9. Pinsonneault, J.K.; Han, D.D.; Burdick, K.E.; Kataki, M.; Bertolino, A.; Malhotra, A.K.; Gu, H.H.; Sadee, W. Dopamine Transporter Gene Variant Affecting Expression in Human Brain Is Associated with Bipolar Disorder. *Neuropsychopharmacology* **2011**, *36*, 1644–1655. [CrossRef]
10. Blum, K.; Oscar-Berman, M.; Barh, D.; Giordano, J.; Genetics, G.M.D. Dopamine genetics and Function in Food and Substance Abuse. *J. Genet. Syndr. Gene. Ther.* **2013**, *4*, 121. [CrossRef]
11. Bello, N.T.; Dopamine, H.A. Dopamine and Binge Eating Behaviors. *Pharmacol. Biochem. Behav.* **2010**, *97*, 25–33. [CrossRef] [PubMed]
12. Brooks, S.J.; Rask-Andersen, M.; Benedict, C.; Schiöth, H.B. A Debate on Current Eating Disorder Diagnoses in Light of Neurobiological Findings: Is It Time for a Spectrum Model? *BMC Psychiatry* **2012**, *12*, 76. [CrossRef] [PubMed]
13. Shinohara, M.; Mizushima, H.; Hirano, M.; Shioe, K.; Nakazawa, M.; Hiejima, Y.; Ono, Y.; Kanba, S. Eating disorders with binge-eating behaviour are associated with the s allele of the 3′-UTR VNTR polymorphism of the dopamine transporter gene. *J. Psychiatry Neurosci.* **2004**, *29*, 134–137. [PubMed]
14. Frieling, H.; Römer, K.D.; Scholz, S.; Mittelbach, F.; Wilhelm, J.; De Zwaan, M.; Jacoby, G.E.; Kornhuber, J.; Hillemacher, T.; Bleich, S. Epigenetic Dysregulation of Dopaminergic Genes in Eating Disorders. *Int. J. Eat. Disord.* **2010**, *43*, 577–583. [CrossRef] [PubMed]
15. Leventakou, V.; Micali, N.; Georgiou, V.; Sarri, K.; Koutra, K.; Koinaki, S.; Vassilaki, M.; Kogevinas, M.; Chatzi, L. Is There an Association between Eating Behaviour and Attention-Deficit/Hyperactivity Disorder Symptoms in Preschool Children? *J. Child Psychol. Psychiatry* **2016**, *57*, 676–684. [CrossRef] [PubMed]
16. Ding, K.; Yang, J.; Reynolds, G.P.; Chen, B.; Shao, J.; Liu, R.; Qian, Q.; Liu, H.; Yang, R.; Wen, J.; et al. DAT1 methylation is associated with methylphenidate response on oppositional and hyperactive-impulsive symptoms in children and adolescents with ADHD. *World J. Biol. Psychiatry* **2017**, *18*, 291–299. [CrossRef]
17. Adriani, W.; Romano, E.; Pucci, M.; Pascale, E.; Cerniglia, L.; Cimino, S.; Tambelli, R.; Curatolo, P.; Granstrem, O.; Maccarrone, M.; et al. Potential for diagnosis versus therapy monitoring of attention deficit hyperactivity disorder: A new epigenetic biomarker interacting with both genotype and auto-immunity. *Eur. Child Adolesc. Psychiatry* **2018**, *27*, 241–252. [CrossRef]
18. Cimino, S.; Cerniglia, L.; Ballarotto, G.; Marzilli, E.; Pascale, E.; D'Addario, C.; Adriani, W.; Tambelli, R. DNA Methylation at the DAT Promoter and Risk for Psychopathology: Intergenerational Transmission between School-Age Youths and Their Parents in a Community Sample. *Front. Psychiatry* **2018**, *8*, 303. [CrossRef]
19. Cimino, S.; Cerniglia, L.; Ballarotto, G.; Marzilli, E.; Pascale, E.; D'Addario, C.; Adriani, W.; Maremmani, A.; Tambelli, R. Children's DAT1 polymorphism moderates the relationship between parents' psychological profiles, children's DAT methylation, and their emotional/behavioral functioning in a normative sample. *Int. J. Environ. Res. Public Health* **2019**, *16*, 2567. [CrossRef]
20. Heijmans, B.T.; Tobi, E.W.; Stein, A.D.; Putter, H.; Blauw, G.J.; Susser, E.S.; Slagboom, P.E.; Lumey, L.H. Persistent epigenetic differences associated with prenatal exposure to famine in humans. *Proc. Natl. Acad. Sci. USA* **2008**, *105*, 17046–17049. [CrossRef]
21. Peter, C.J.; Fischer, L.K.; Kundakovic, M.; Garg, P.; Jakovcevski, M.; Dincer, A.; Amaral, A.C.; Ginns, E.I.; Galdzicka, M.; Bryce, C.P.; et al. DNA methylation signatures of early childhood malnutrition associated with impairments in attention and cognition. *Biol. Psychiatry* **2016**, *80*, 765–774. [CrossRef] [PubMed]
22. Davies, P.T.; Cicchetti, D. Toward an integration of family systems and developmental psychopathology approaches. *Dev. Psychopathol.* **2004**, *16*, 477–481. [CrossRef] [PubMed]
23. Calkins, S.D.; Dollar, J.M. Emotion: Commentary. A biopsychosocial perspective on maternal psychopathology and the development of child emotion regulation. *J. Pers. Disord.* **2014**, *28*, 70–77. [CrossRef] [PubMed]
24. Golds, L.; de Kruiff, K.; MacBeth, A. Disentangling genes, attachment, and environment: A systematic review of the developmental psychopathology literature on gene-environment interactions and attachment. *Dev. Psychopathol.* **2020**, *32*, 357–381. [CrossRef]
25. Weaver, I.C.; Cervoni, N.; Champagne, F.A.; D'Alessio, A.C.; Sharma, S.; Seckl, J.R.; Dymov, S.; Szyf, M.; Meaney, M.J. Epigenetic programming by maternal behavior. *Nat. Neurosci.* **2004**, *7*, 847–854. [CrossRef]
26. American Psychiatric Association. *Diagnostic and Statistical Manual of Mental Disorders (DSM-5 (R))*, 5th ed.; American Psychiatric Association Publishing: Arlington, TX, USA, 2013.
27. Three, Z.T. *Diagnostic Classification of Mental Health and Developmental Disorders of Infancy and Early Childhood*, 2nd ed.; ZERO TO THREE, National Center for Infants, Toddlers, & Families: Washington, DC, USA, 2005.
28. Lucarelli, L.; Cimino, S.; D'Olimpio, F.; Ammaniti, M. Feeding Disorders of Early Childhood: An Empirical Study of Diagnostic Subtypes. *Int. J. Eat. Disord.* **2013**, *46*, 147–155. [CrossRef]
29. Norris, M.L.; Spettigue, W.; Hammond, N.G.; Katzman, D.K.; Zucker, N.; Yelle, K.; Santos, A.; Gray, M.; Obeid, N. Building evidence for the use of descriptive subtypes In youth with avoidant restrictive food intake disorder. *Int. J. Eat. Disord.* **2018**, *51*, 170–173. [CrossRef]

30. Chatoor, I.; Lucarelli, L. Feeding development and disorders. In *Encyclopedia of Infant and Early Childhood Development*, 2nd ed.; Benson, J.B., Ed.; Elsevier: Amsterdam, The Netherlands, 2020; pp. 621–632.
31. Cerniglia, L.; Marzilli, E.; Cimino, S. Emotional-Behavioral Functioning, Maternal Psychopathologic Risk and Quality of Mother-Child Feeding Interactions in Children with Avoidant/Restrictive Food Intake Disorder. *Int. J. Environ. Res. Public Health* **2020**, *17*, 3811. [CrossRef]
32. Chatoor, I. *Diagnosis and Treatment of Feeding Disorders in Infants, Toddlers, and Young Children*; Zero to Three Press: Washington, DC, USA, 2009.
33. American Psychiatric Association. *Feeding and Eating Disorders: DSM-5 (R) Selections*; American Psychiatric Association Publishing: Arlington, TX, USA, 2015.
34. Dahl, M.; Sundelin, C. Feeding problems in an affluent society. Follow-up at four years of age in children with early refusal to eat. *Acta. Paediatr.* **1992**, *81*, 575–579. [CrossRef]
35. Pennell, A.; Couturier, J.; Grant, C.; Johnson, N. Severe Avoidant/Restrictive Food Intake Disorder and Coexisting Stimulant Treated Attention Deficit Hyperactivity Disorder: Severe ARFID and Coexisting ADHD. *Int. J. Eat. Disord.* **2016**, *49*, 1036–1039. [CrossRef]
36. Ammaniti, M.; Lucarelli, L.; Cimino, S.; D'Olimpio, F.; Chatoor, I. Feeding Disorders of Infancy: A Longitudinal Study to Middle Childhood. *Int. J. Eat. Disord.* **2012**, *45*, 272–280. [CrossRef] [PubMed]
37. Lavender, J.M.; Wonderlich, S.A.; Engel, S.G.; Gordon, K.H.; Kaye, W.H.; Mitchell, J.M. Dimensions of Emotion Dysregulation in Anorexia Nervosa and Bulimia Nervosa: A Conceptual Review of the Empirical Literature. *Clin. Psychol. Rev.* **2015**, *40*, 111–122. [CrossRef] [PubMed]
38. Lieberman, M.; Houser, M.E.; Voyer, A.P.; Grady, S.; Katzman, D.K. Children with avoidant/restrictive food intake disorder and anorexia nervosa in a tertiary care pediatric eating disorder program: A comparative study. *Int. J. Eat. Disord.* **2019**, *52*, 239–245. [CrossRef] [PubMed]
39. Lucarelli, L.; Sechi, C.; Cimino, S.; Chatoor, I. Avoidant/Restrictive Food Intake Disorder: A Longitudinal Study of Malnutrition and Psychopathological Risk Factors from 2 to 11 Years of Age. *Front. Psychol.* **2018**, *9*, 1608. [CrossRef] [PubMed]
40. Ammaniti, M.; Lucarelli, L.; Cimino, S.; D'Olimpio, F.; Chatoor, I. Maternal psychopathology and child risk factors in infantile anorexia. *Int. J. Eat. Disord.* **2010**, *43*, 233–240. [CrossRef]
41. Champagne, F.A.; Curley, J.P. Epigenetic Mechanisms Mediating the Long-Term Effects of Maternal Care on Development. *Neurosci. Biobehav. Rev.* **2009**, *33*, 593–600. [CrossRef]
42. Barker, E.D.; Walton, E.; Cecil, C.A.M. Annual Research Review: DNA methylation as a mediator in the association between risk exposure and child and adolescent psychopathology. *J. Child Psychol. Psychiatry* **2018**, *59*, 303–322. [CrossRef]
43. Norrholm, S.D.; Jovanovic, T.; Smith, A.K.; Binder, E.; Klengel, T.; Conneely, K.; Mercer, K.B.; Davis, J.S.; Kerley, K.; Winkler, J.; et al. Differential genetic and epigenetic regulation of catechol-O-methyltransferase is associated with impaired fear inhibition in posttraumatic stress disorder. *Front. Behav. Neurosci.* **2013**, *7*, 30. [CrossRef]
44. Duman, E.A.; Canli, T. Influence of Life Stress, 5-HTTLPR Genotype, and SLC6A4 Methylation on Gene Expression and Stress Response in Healthy Caucasian Males. *Biol. Mood Anxiety Disord.* **2015**, *5*, 1. [CrossRef]
45. Achenbach, T.M. *Manual for the Aseba Preschool Forms & Profiles: An Integrated System of Multi-Informant Assessment*; Research Center for Children, Youth, & Families: Burlington, VT, USA, 2000.
46. Frigerio, A.; Cattaneo, C.; Cataldo, M.; Schiatti, A.; Molteni, M.; Battaglia, M. Behavioral and emotional problems among Italian children and adolescents aged 4 to 18 years as reported by parents and teachers. *Eur. J. Psychol. Assess.* **2004**, *20*, 124–133. [CrossRef]
47. Geeraerts, S.B.; Deutz, M.H.; Deković, M.; Bunte, T.; Schoemaker, K.; Espy, K.A.; Prinzie, P.; van Baar, A.; Matthys, W. The Child Behavior Checklist Dysregulation Profile in Preschool Children: A Broad Dysregulation Syndrome. *J. Am. Acad. Child Adolesc. Psychiatry* **2015**, *54*, 595–602. [CrossRef] [PubMed]
48. Derogatis, L.R. *SCL-90-R Symptom Checklist-90-R Administration, Scoring, and Procedures Manual*; National Computer Systems: Minneapolis, MN, USA, 1994.
49. Prunas, A.; Sarno, I.; Preti, E.; Madeddu, F.; Perugini, M. Psychometric Properties of the Italian Version of the SCL-90-R: A Study on a Large Community Sample. *Eur. Psychiatry* **2012**, *27*, 591–597. [CrossRef] [PubMed]
50. Cerniglia, L.; Cimino, S.; Bevilacqua, A.; Ballarotto, G.; Marzilli, E.; Adriani, W.; Tambelli, R. Patterns of DNA methylation at specific loci of the dopamine transporter 1 gene and psychopathological risk in trios of mothers, fathers and children. *Eur. J. Dev. Psychol.* **2020**, 1–28. [CrossRef]
51. Hayden, E.P.; Hanna, B.; Sheikh, H.I.; Laptook, R.S.; Kim, J.; Singh, S.M.; Klein, D.N. Child dopamine active transporter 1 genotype and parenting: Evidence for evocative gene-environment correlations. *Dev. Psychopathol.* **2013**, *25*, 163–173. [CrossRef] [PubMed]
52. Hirata, T.; Uemura, T.; Shinohara, M.; Hirano, M. Association between Dopamine Transporter Gene (DAT1) Polymorphisms and Eating Disorders with Binge Eating Behavior. *Open J. Psychiatr.* **2017**, *7*, 329–343. [CrossRef]
53. Hayes, A.F. *Introduction to Mediation, Moderation, and Conditional Process Analysis, Second Edition: A Regression-Based Approach*, 2nd ed.; Guilford Publications: New York, NY, USA, 2018.
54. Jaenisch, R.; Bird, A. Epigenetic regulation of gene expression: How the genome integrates intrinsic and environmental signals. *Nat. Genet.* **2003**, *33*, 245–254. [CrossRef]

55. Jones, P.A. Functions of DNA methylation: Islands, start sites, gene bodies and beyond. *Nat. Rev. Genet.* **2012**, *13*, 484–492. [CrossRef]
56. Seo, D.; Patrick, C.J.; Kennealy, P.J. Role of Serotonin and Dopamine System Interactions in the Neurobiology of Impulsive Aggression and Its Comorbidity with Other Clinical Disorders. *Aggress. Violent Behav.* **2008**, *13*, 383–395. [CrossRef]
57. Volkow, N.D.; Wang, G.J.; Maynard, L.; Jayne, M.; Fowler, J.S.; Zhu, W.; Logan, J.; Gatley, S.J.; Ding, Y.S.; Wong, C.; et al. Brain dopamine is associated with eating behaviors in humans. *Int. J. Eat. Disord.* **2003**, *33*, 136–142. [CrossRef]
58. Tauscher, J.; Pirker, W.; Willeit, M.; de Zwaan, M.; Bailer, U.; Neumeister, A.; Asenbaum, S.; Lennkh, C.; Praschak-Rieder, N.; Brücke, T.; et al. [123I] beta-CIT and single photon emission computed tomography reveal reduced brain serotonin transporter availability in bulimia nervosa. *Biol. Psychiatry* **2001**, *49*, 326–332. [CrossRef]
59. Peyre, H.; Speranza, M.; Cortese, S.; Wohl, M.; Purper-Ouakil, D. Do ADHD Children with and without Child Behavior Checklist-Dysregulation Profile Have Different Clinical Characteristics, Cognitive Features, and Treatment Outcomes? *J. Atten. Disord.* **2015**, *19*, 63–71. [CrossRef] [PubMed]
60. Katsuki, D.; Yamashita, H.; Yamane, K.; Kanba, S.; Yoshida, K. Clinical Subtypes in Children with Attention-Deficit Hyperactivity Disorder According to Their Child Behavior Checklist Profile. *Child Psychiatry Hum. Dev.* **2020**. [CrossRef]
61. Faraone, S.V.; Bonvicini, C.; Scassellati, C. Biomarkers in the Diagnosis of ADHD—Promising Directions. *Curr. Psychiatry Rep.* **2014**, *16*, 11. [CrossRef]
62. Lahey, B.B.; Rathouz, P.J.; Lee, S.S.; Chronis-Tuscano, A.; Pelham, W.E.; Waldman, I.D.; Cook, E.H. Interactions between early parenting and a polymorphism of the child's dopamine transporter gene in predicting future child conduct disorder symptoms. *J. Abnorm. Psychol.* **2011**, *120*, 33–45. [CrossRef]
63. Drury, S.S.; Theall, K.P.; Keats, B.J.B.; Scheeringa, M. The role of the dopamine transporter (DAT) in the development of PTSD in preschool children. *J. Trauma Stress.* **2009**, *22*, 534–539. [CrossRef] [PubMed]
64. Gervasini, G.; Gordillo, I.; García-Herráiz, A.; Flores, I.; Jiménez, M.; Monge, M.; Carrillo, J.A. Influence of dopamine polymorphisms on the risk for anorexia nervosa and associated psychopathological features. *J. Clin. Psychopharmacol.* **2013**, *33*, 551–555. [CrossRef]
65. Anreiter, I.; Sokolowski, H.M.; Sokolowski, M.B. Gene–environment interplay and individual differences in behavior: Gene-environment interplay. *Mind Brain Educ.* **2018**, *12*, 200–211. [CrossRef]
66. Belsky, J.; Pluess, M. Beyond diathesis stress: Differential susceptibility to environmental influences. *Psychol. Bull.* **2009**, *135*, 885–908. [CrossRef]
67. Hoexter, M.Q.; Fadel, G.; Felício, A.C.; Calzavara, M.B.; Batista, I.R.; Reis, M.A.; Shih, M.C.; Pitman, R.K.; Andreoli, S.B.; Mello, M.F.; et al. Higher striatal dopamine transporter density in PTSD: An in vivo SPECT study with [(99m)Tc]TRODAT-1. *Psychopharmacology* **2012**, *224*, 337–345. [CrossRef]
68. Mongillo, E.A.; Briggs-Gowan, M.; Ford, J.D.; Carter, A.S. Impact of traumatic life events in a community sample of toddlers. *J. Abnorm. Child Psychol.* **2009**, *37*, 455–468. [CrossRef]
69. Maguire, S.A.; Williams, B.; Naughton, A.M.; Cowley, L.E.; Tempest, V.; Mann, M.K.; Teague, M.; Kemp, A.M. A systematic review of the emotional, behavioural and cognitive features exhibited by school-aged children experiencing neglect or emotional abuse: Systematic review of school-aged neglect/emotional abuse. *Child Care Health Dev.* **2015**, *41*, 641–653. [CrossRef]
70. Basten, M.M.; Althoff, R.R.; Tiemeier, H.; Jaddoe, V.W.; Hofman, A.; Hudziak, J.J.; Verhulst, F.C.; van der Ende, J. The dysregulation profile in young children: Empirically defined classes in the Generation R study. *J. Am. Acad. Child Adolesc. Psychiatry* **2013**, *52*, 841–850.e2. [CrossRef] [PubMed]
71. Cimino, S.; Cerniglia, L.; Porreca, A.; Ballarotto, G.; Marzilli, E.; Simonelli, A. Impact of parental binge eating disorder: Exploring children's emotional/behavioral problems and the quality of parent-child feeding interactions. *Infant Ment. Health J.* **2018**, *39*, 552–568. [CrossRef] [PubMed]
72. Cerniglia, L.; Muratori, P.; Milone, A.; Paciello, M.; Ruglioni, L.; Cimino, S.; Levantini, V.; Tambelli, R. Paternal psychopathological risk and psychological functioning in children with eating disorders and Disruptive Behavior Disorder. *Psychiatry Res.* **2017**, *254*, 60–66. [CrossRef] [PubMed]
73. Parkes, A.; Sweeting, H. Direct, indirect, and buffering effects of support for mothers on children's socioemotional adjustment. *J. Fam. Psychol.* **2018**, *32*, 894–903. [CrossRef] [PubMed]
74. Rollè, L.; Prino, L.E.; Sechi, C.; Vismara, L.; Neri, E.; Polizzi, C.; Trovato, A.; Volpi, B.; Molgora, S.; Fenaroli, V.; et al. Parenting stress, mental health, dyadic adjustment: A structural equation model. *Front. Psychol.* **2017**, *8*, 839. [CrossRef] [PubMed]
75. Cimino, S.; Marzilli, E.; Tafà, M.; Cerniglia, L. Emotional-Behavioral Regulation, Temperament and Parent–Child Interactions Are Associated with Dopamine Transporter Allelic Polymorphism in Early Childhood: A Pilot Study. *Int. J. Environ. Res. Public Health* **2020**, *17*, 8564. [CrossRef]
76. Paschall, K.W.; Mastergeorge, A.M. A review of 25 years of research in bidirectionality in parent–child relationships: An examination of methodological approaches. *Int. J. Behav. Dev.* **2016**, *40*, 442–451. [CrossRef]
77. Lee, S.S.; Chronis-Tuscano, A.; Keenan, K.; Pelham, W.E.; Loney, J.; Van Hulle, C.A.; Cook, E.H.; Lahey, B.B. Association of maternal dopamine transporter genotype with negative parenting: Evidence for gene x environment interaction with child disruptive behavior. *Mol. Psychiatry* **2010**, *15*, 548–558. [CrossRef]

78. Auerbach, J.G.; Zilberman-Hayun, Y.; Atzaba-Poria, N.; Berger, A. The contribution of maternal ADHD symptomatology, maternal DAT1, and home atmosphere to child ADHD symptomatology at 7 years of age. *J. Abnorm. Child Psychol.* **2017**, *45*, 415–427. [CrossRef]
79. Cicchetti, D.; Blender, J.A. A multiple-levels-of-analysis perspective on resilience: Implications for the developing brain, neural plasticity, and preventive interventions. *Ann. N. Y. Acad. Sci.* **2006**, *1094*, 248–258. [CrossRef] [PubMed]
80. Lavigne, J.V.; Herzing, L.B.; Cook, E.H.; Gouze, K.R.; Hopkins, J.; Bryant, F.B. Gene × environment effects of serotonin transporter, dopamine receptor D4, and monoamine oxidase A genes with contextual and parenting risk factors on symptoms of oppositional defiant disorder, anxiety, and depression in a community sample of 4-year-old children. *Dev. Psychopathol.* **2013**, *25*, 555–575. [CrossRef] [PubMed]
81. McKay, J.A.; Groom, A.; Potter, C.; Coneyworth, L.J.; Ford, D.; Mathers, J.C.; Relton, C.L. Genetic and non-genetic influences during pregnancy on infant global and site specific DNA methylation: Role for folate gene variants and vitamin B12. *PLoS ONE* **2012**, *7*, e33290. [CrossRef] [PubMed]
82. Maestro, S.; Cordella, M.R.; Intorcia, C.; Roversi, C.; Scardigli, S.; Silvestri, V.; Sara Calderoni, M.D. Parent-child interaction treatment for preschoolers with feeding disorders. *Isr. J. Psychiatry Relat. Sci.* **2016**, *53*, 63–72. [PubMed]

behavioral sciences

MDPI

Review

Traditional Chinese Medicine Body Constitutions as Predictors for Depression: A Systematic Review and Meta-Analysis

Sin Yee Yap [1], Foong Leng Ng [1,2], Menaga Subramaniam [1], Yang Mooi Lim [1,3] and Chai Nien Foo [1,4,*]

1 Centre for Cancer Research, M. Kandiah Faculty of Medicine and Health Sciences, Universiti Tunku Abdul Rahman, PT21144, Jalan Sungai Long, Bandar Sungai Long, Kajang 43000, Selangor, Malaysia
2 Department of Traditional Chinese Medicine, M. Kandiah Faculty of Medicine and Health Sciences, Universiti Tunku Abdul Rahman, PT21144, Jalan Sungai Long, Bandar Sungai Long, Kajang 43000, Selangor, Malaysia
3 Department of Pre-Clinical Science, M. Kandiah Faculty of Medicine and Health Sciences, Universiti Tunku Abdul Rahman, Lot PT21144, Jalan Sungai Long, Bandar Sungai Long, Kajang 43000, Selangor, Malaysia
4 Department of Population Medicine, M. Kandiah Faculty of Medicine and Health Sciences, Universiti Tunku Abdul Rahman, PT21144, Jalan Sungai Long, Bandar Sungai Long, Kajang 43000, Selangor, Malaysia
* Correspondence: foocn@utar.edu.my

Abstract: Traditional Chinese medicine body constitution (TCMBC) reflects a person's vulnerability to diseases. Thus, identifying body constitutions prone to depression can help prevent and treat depression. The review aimed to assess and summarize the existing evidence that explores the relationship between TCMBC and depression. Psychology and Behavioral Sciences Collection, MEDLINE, PubMed, CNKI, Wanfang, SinoMed, Embase, VIP, CINAHL, and CMJ were searched from inception to April 2021. Observational studies assessing the association between TCMBC and depression were selected. The quality of the included studies were assessed using the Newcastle–Ottawa Scale (NOS). Eighteen studies were included in the systematic review and thirteen in the meta-analysis. The pooled odd ratios of developing depression for Qi-stagnation, Qi-deficiency, Yang-deficiency, Yin-deficiency, and Balanced constitutions were 3.12 (95% CI, 1.80–5.40; I^2 = 94%), 2.15 (95% CI, 1.54–3.01; I^2 = 89%), 1.89 (95% CI, 0.71–5.03; I^2 = 81%), 1.41 (95% CI, 0.91–2.20; I^2 = 57%), and 0.60 (95% CI, 0.40–0.90; I^2 = 94%), respectively. The findings suggest that the evaluation of a person's TCMBC could be useful the in prevention and treatment of depression. However, more case-control and cohort studies are required to further confirm the association between TCMBC and depression.

Keywords: traditional Chinese medicine; body constitution; depression; predictor; systematic review; meta-analysis

1. Introduction

Depression is the cancer of the 21st century. It is one of the leading causes of the overall global burden of disease [1]. As of 2017, about 264 million people suffered from depression globally, with a higher prevalence in women (4.1%) than men (2.7%) [1]. Depression often develops at a young age and is constantly recurring [2]. Depression is not merely excessive sadness, but rather, a combination of factors related to negative thoughts, other symptoms and the bodily impact that lead to significant impairments in how an individual functions in daily life. Depressed individuals are shown to be vulnerable to heart diseases [3], diabetes [4], stroke [5] and infectious diseases [6]. Depression is a significant cause of mortality [7] and an important risk factor for suicide. According to the World Health Organization (WHO), nearly 800,000 people die due to suicide each year, which means that every 40 s, a person kills him/herself. Globally, suicide is the second leading cause of death in children, adolescents and young adults [8].

There are variations in the types of depression and their severities. The most common type of depression is major depressive disorder (MDD), also known as clinical depression. It is characterized by depressed mood and loss of interest or pleasure [9]. According to the fifth edition of the Diagnostic and Statistical Manual of Mental Disorders (DSM-5), at least one of these two symptoms must be present along with another five or more symptoms for at least two weeks for a person to be diagnosed with MDD. Several other symptoms include sleeping problems, changes in appetite, constant fatigue, difficulty concentrating, agitation or slowed movement, feeling guilty or worthlessness, unexplainable pains and suicidal thoughts [9]. Dysthymia, also known as a persistent depressive disorder, is an ongoing and chronic form of depression. Its symptoms are often less severe than MDD but longer lasting. The essential feature of this disorder is the presence of a sad mood on most days for at least two years [9]. Besides, some people may experience seasonal affective disorder (SAD) during fall or winter due to reduced daylight [9]. SAD usually wears off during Spring and Summer. The main symptoms include social withdrawal, oversleeping, low energy and weight gain [9]. Another subtype of depression is bipolar disorder, which also called manic depression. People who suffer from bipolar disorder can have extreme mood swings from emotional highs to lows [9]. During the low phases, they will experience symptoms of MDD.

Depression is often caused by a combination of various factors, rather than just one cause. There is a range of contributing factors that can lead to depression. The genes and traits that one inherits from their parents make them prone to depression [10]. Lack of social support, troubled relationships or loss of loved ones can also induce suicidal thoughts and feelings of worthlessness, increasing depression risk [10]. Other risk factors for depression include stressful life events, childhood trauma, substance use, poor nutrition and lack of exercise [10]. This is consistent with past reviews and meta-analyses that found social support [11–13], substance use [14], diet [15], physical activity [16] and exposure to early life stress, such as childhood trauma and loss of loved ones [17], were associated with depression risk. In addition, depression is also a common complication of other chronic illnesses. For instance, a recent Danish study showed that people who suffered from heart diseases and stroke were more likely to have subsequent depression [18].

Currently, the screening and diagnosis of depression is mainly based on symptoms. Psychiatrists diagnose depression according to patients' descriptions of symptoms, questionnaires and clinical behaviour observations, and subsequently categorize the patients according to the DSM-5 [9] and the eleventh revision of International Statistical Classification of Diseases and Related Health Problems (ICD-11) [19]. There is no laboratory test to identify depression due to its heterogeneous nature. The complex interaction of genetic, biological, psychological and environmental factors that contribute to depression affects the accuracy of diagnosis, our understanding towards its pathophysiology, and our ability to develop effective treatments.

Depression is treatable; however, many depressed individuals fail to receive adequate treatment, especially those in low- and middle-income countries [20]. Barriers to effective care include inaccurate diagnosis, lack of facilities and trained personnel, social discrimination and high treatment costs [21]. Treatments of depression usually include medications and psychotherapies. There are several types of antidepressants available, such as selective serotonin reuptake inhibitors (SSRIs), tricyclic antidepressants (TCAs) and monoamine oxidase inhibitors (MAOIs) [9,22]. However, these drugs may induce a range of side effects, such as dry mouth, vision problems, dizziness, irritability, bleeding abnormalities, seizure and constipation [9,22,23]. Psychotherapies are also known as talk therapies. Examples of psychotherapies are cognitive-behavioral therapy (CBT), interpersonal therapy (IPT) and problem-solving therapy [9,24]. Past meta-analyses demonstrated that pharmacotherapy [25,26] and psychotherapy [25,27,28] were associated with reduced risk of relapse and recurrence in depression.

Traditional Chinese medicine (TCM) is one of the oldest medical systems globally. An important aspect of TCM is the prevention of diseases by maintaining or restoring the harmony and equilibrium of Yin-Yang within the human body [29,30]. Illness often occurs due to the imbalance of Yin-Yang. According to TCM theories, the five fundamental substances (essence, Qi, blood, body fluids and spirit) and the five viscera (liver, spleen, lung, heart and kidney) are closely related to each other and the formation of body constitution [31]. Biased body constitutions result from the impaired viscera function and dysregulation of fundamental substances [31]. The concept of Traditional Chinese medicine body constitution (TCMBC) reflects a person's unique physical, physiological and psychological functions [32]. It is determined by hereditary and acquired factors in the process of human life [32]. Pathologically, TCMBC also influences a person's susceptibility to certain pathogenic factors and diseases, as well as their reaction to treatment [32]. It is the foundation for TCM practitioners to diagnose, treat and prevent diseases [33]. TCMBC is alterable due to its relative stability and dynamic variability [34]. A biased constitution can be modified towards a neutral type through acquired factors such as exercise and diet. An appropriate amount of physical activity can produce strong muscles and bones, promote the blood circulation and Qi dynamic and enhance visceral function [32]. This can then prevent the formation of biased constitutions, such as Blood-stasis (BSC) and Qi-stagnation (QSC). On the contrary, lack of exercise will result in flabby muscles, restricted flow of Qi and blood and impaired spleen and stomach function, which can contribute to the formation of a Phlegm-dampness constitution (PDC) [32]. Furthermore, a healthy diet and sufficient nutrients can produce a strong physique and good constitution, while an unbalanced diet and malnutrition could lead to a weaker constitution [32]. Very often, biased and unbalanced constitutions are detected among depressed populations [35–37]. For example, Chen et al. found that women with Yang- and Yin-deficient constitutions had a higher risk of depression [35], while Xiong et al. found that college students with Qi-stagnation and Qi-deficiency constitutions were more prone to depression [38].

The China Association for Traditional Chinese Medicine classified TCMBC into nine types, namely the Balanced constitution (BC), Qi-stagnation constitution (QSC), Blood stasis constitution (BSC), Qi-deficiency constitution (QDC), Yin-deficiency constitution (YIDC), Yang-deficiency constitution (YADC), Phlegm-dampness (PDC), Damp-heat constitution (DHC) and Inherited special constitution (ISC) [34]. Among them, BC is a neutral type, while the rest are biased and unbalanced types. BC is a harmonious constitution, with a balance of Yin-Yang [32,39]. People with this constitution display common features, such as a normal body shape, strong physique, optimistic personality, good adaptability, energetic nature and strong immune system [31,32,40]. People with BC seldom get sick, and if they do, they recover from sickness easily [32]. Generally, people with QSC often cope poorly with stressful situations. People with this constitution exhibit a thin physique, mood swings, suspiciousness, overthinking and excessive worrying [31,32,40]. People with BSC usually have dull skin and dark lips, get bruises easily, are forgetful and are averse to cold environments and weather [31,32,40]. Additionally, they are prone to body pain and bleeding [31,32]. Next, people with QDC are easily exhausted due to weak immunity [31,32,40]. They are prone to panting and colds, and are easily affected by sudden climate changes. These people require a longer time to recover from sickness [31,32]. People with YIDC have warm palms and soles, are impatient and exhibit an extroverted nature [40]. These people are always thirsty, prefer cold drinks and dislike hot and dry weather [31,32]. In contrast, people with YADC are usually introverted, quiet, shy and have cold limbs [40]. They prefer hot meals and summer over winter [31,32]. The main characteristics of PDC include excessive phlegm production, overweightedness, chest tightness and a mild-mannered and patient nature [31,32,40]. These people like high sugar and high fat food and dislike damp environments [31,32]. People with DHC usually have oily skin, are prone to acne outbreaks, have a bitter taste in their mouths, and experience difficult and sticky bowel movements [31,32,40]. They are irritable and averse to hot and humid climates [32]. Lastly, people with ISC often have an inherent sensitivity to certain allergens, such as pollen, odors, food and medicines [40]. They tend to have conditions like asthma and are sensitive to environmental changes [31,32].

Conventionally, TCM practitioners describe the etiologies and symptoms of depression caused by extreme emotional changes using "yu" or "yuzheng", which means blockage, stagnation, not flowing, clogging, or obstruction [41]. In TCM, the deficiency of Qi (vital energy) is believed to be the main cause of depression [42,43]. Qi deficiency could be due to physiological dysfunctions in the human body, which include inflammation, abnormal blood circulation, formation of dampness or phlegm [43]. Hence, strengthening the Qi and fixing imbalances of the physiological systems are the principles for healing depression [44]. In TCM, the liver is in charge of dispersion and dredging to regulate digestion, absorption and emotions, as well as the circulation of Qi, blood and body fluids [31,45]. Normally, the liver-Qi is the first to be affected directly during an emotional change, followed by disharmony of the Qi among the five viscera, which can then lead to the dysregulation of the Qi and blood [43]. A dysfunction of liver dispersion and dredging can also lead to the repression of spleen function, followed by the dysregulation of heart-Qi, then leading to the "shen" (spirit) becoming restless, which can result in an unstable and depressed mood [43]. This is because our spirit resides in the heart, and heart-Qi is in charge of pumping blood and the regulation of blood flow within the human body [31]. Past studies have confirmed this theory, where the abnormal dispersion of liver-Qi causes depression [46–51].

Currently, application and research on TCMBCs are mainly performed in Asian countries, such as China [35–38], Japan [52,53], Hong Kong [54,55], the Philippines [56] and Malaysia [57]. Identification of TCMBCs that are vulnerable to depression can allow us to modify them towards harmony and balance. TCMBC has clinical significance in preventing depression as it can be applied to indicate a person's overall health conditions and help prevent depression in the early phase. With the extensive application of TCMBC in the past decade, a number of studies have revealed that depression is correlated to TCMBC [58–62]. However, the findings of the associations are inconsistent and lack a systematic review to clarify the strength of these associations. Only a narrative review reporting the potential role of TCMBC in the development of depression was published [63]. Hence, there is a need for a comprehensive review to evaluate the association between TCMBC and depression. To date, and to our knowledge, this is the first systematic review and meta-analysis investigating the association between TCMBC and depression. This systematic review and meta-analysis aims to assess and to summarize the existing empirical data that explored the relationship between TCMBC and depression. The key objectives are as follows: (1) to report whether TCMBC is associated with depression; and (2) to assess whether TCMBC predicts depression. The findings of this review will provide knowledge and references for developing measures to manage depression.

2. Materials and Methods

The conduct and reporting of this systematic review and meta-analysis were strictly based on the Preferred Reporting Items for Systematic reviews, and Meta-Analyses (PRISMA) [64] and Meta-analysis of Observational Studies in Epidemiology (MOOSE) [65] guidelines, following an a priori protocol. The study protocol was registered and published at the International Prospective Register of Systematic Reviews (PROSPERO) with a registration number of CRD42021267651, and is under review for publication.

2.1. Data Sources and Search Strategy

Comprehensive literature searches were conducted in the following databases: Psychology and Behavioral Sciences Collection, MEDLINE, PubMed, Chinese National Knowledge Infrastructure (CNKI), Wanfang, SinoMed, Embase, Chinese Scientific Journal Database (VIP), Cumulated Indexed to Nursing and Allied Health Literature (CINAHL) and Chinese Medical Journal Database (CMJ). No restriction was set on the publication date. The database searches were limited to journal articles written in the English and Chinese languages only. The database searches were conducted from December 2020 to April 2021. The search terms used are presented in Table 1. Additionally, the references of the included studies were manually searched to identify other relevant studies.

Table 1. Search terms.

Concept	Search Terms
Depression	depression OR depressive disorder OR *yuzheng*
TCMBC	traditional Chinese medicine constitution OR traditional Chinese medicine body constitution

Note: *yuzheng* refers to depression in traditional Chinese medicine.

2.2. Eligibility Criteria

The main inclusion criteria were related to: (1) study type: observational studies including cohort, case-control and cross-sectional studies that investigate the association between TCMBC and depression; (2) participant: all subjects and populations were considered; if there was a control group, the subjects should be from the general population and without depression; (3) outcome: the correlation between TCMBC and depression were reported; (4) measurement of TCMBC and depression: the identification of TCMBC and depression through validated instruments. Only articles published in English and Chinese were included.

The exclusion criteria were as follows: (1) was not a journal article (e.g., conference abstract, dissertations and reports); (2) was not primary research (e.g., systematic review and meta-analysis); (3) lacked sufficient information to determine eligibility; (4) involved non-human subjects; (5) did not explicitly focus on the association between TCMBC and depression.

2.3. Study Selection

For English databases (Psychology and Behavioral Sciences Collection, MEDLINE, PubMed, and Embase), two reviewers (SYY and MS) independently conducted the searches and screened the titles and abstracts of all retrieved articles, followed by the full text screening of potentially eligible studies. For Chinese databases (CNKI, Wanfang, SinoMed, VIP, CINAHL, and CMJ), two reviewers (SYY and FLN) independently conducted the searches and screened the titles and abstracts of all retrieved articles, followed by the full text screening of potentially eligible studies. The full texts were reviewed according to predefined inclusion criteria. Disagreements at both screening levels (title/abstract and full text) were resolved through discussion and consultation with other authors (YML and CNF).

2.4. Data Extraction

Three reviewers (SYY, FLN and MS) independently extracted the data from the included studies using a standardized data extraction spreadsheet. Disagreements were resolved through discussion with other authors (YML and CNF). The following data were extracted: first author, year of publication, study design, study subjects, sampling method, study location, sample size, age, gender, ethnicity, depression measurement, TCMBC measurement, type of constitutions studied, main results (e.g., p value, odd ratio (OR) and 95% confidence interval (CI)). The primary outcome was the association between TCMBC and depression.

2.5. Missing Data

When encountering missing data, the corresponding authors of the potentially eligible studies were contacted by E-mail to retrieve further data or clarifications. The studies were excluded and the data synthesis was conducted using available data when the authors did not respond or failed to provide the relevant data requested within a month.

2.6. Assessment of Risk of Bias and Certainty of Evidence

Three reviewers (SYY, FLN and MS) independently performed risk of bias assessment using the Newcastle–Ottawa Scale (NOS) [66,67]. The NOS evaluates the quality of the included studies regarding three main aspects: (1) selection; (2) comparability; (3) exposure. The maximum scores for case-control and cohort studies are 9 and for cross-sectional studies are 10. Regarding the quality of the included case-control and cohort studies, they were considered as poor if the score was 0 to 5 and good if the score was 6 to 9. For the quality of cross-sectional studies, they were rated as poor if the score was 0 to 4, medium if the score was 5 to 6, good if the score was 7 to 8 and very good if the score was 9 to 10. Disagreements in the quality assessment were adjudicated by discussion with other authors (YML and CNF).

The quality of evidence and the strength of recommendation of this review were evaluated using the Grading of Recommendations Assessment, Development and Evaluation (GRADE) guidelines [68]. Five criteria were considered when decreasing the level of certainty, including risk of bias, imprecision, inconsistency, indirectness and publication bias. Whereas, three additional criteria, which included large magnitude of effect, dose-response gradient, and when residual confounders would decrease the magnitude of effect (when an effect is observed), were considered when upgrading the level of certainty. The overall quality can be rated as very low, low, moderate and high. The lowest quality of evidence for any of the outcomes determine the overall quality of evidence.

2.7. Data Synthesis and Analysis

Data from the eligible studies were summarized descriptively in tabular format and narrative text. The characteristics of the studies were reported and grouped in the table based on population types (diseased and general populations). Cochrane Software Review Manager (RevMan), version 5.3 (The Cochrane Collaboration, 2020) was used to perform statistical analysis if a meta-analysis was allowed. Meta-analyses were performed if there was sufficient number of studies ($n \geq 2$), adequate quality of studies (moderate and good quality) and similarity in the study design. Inverse variance analysis was used in the meta-analyses. The extracted ORs and 95% CIs were converted to log ORs and standard errors (SE) using the RevMan calculator. The Chi-square test and I^2 test were used to evaluate the statistical heterogeneity among the included studies. In the presence of statistical heterogeneity ($p < 0.05$ or $I^2 > 50\%$) [69], a random effect model was used, otherwise, a fixed-effect model was adopted [70]. For constitution types with sufficient data and adequate quality, pooled effect sizes (OR and 95% CI) were reported. Publication bias was assessed using funnel plots if the minimum number of studies was reached ($n \geq 10$) [71]. The symmetry of the plots was examined to evaluate potential publication bias.

3. Results

3.1. Study Selection

A total of 1629 records were retrieved based on the search strategy. After removing duplicated records and reviewing titles and abstracts, 84 potentially relevant articles were identified for further full-text screening. Sixty-six studies were excluded because the authors failed to provide relevant data, or the studies measured different outcomes, and did not meet the inclusion criteria, respectively. Overall, eighteen studies were eligible for inclusion in this systematic review and thirteen studies were eligible for meta-analysis. The study selection process and the rationale for study exclusion is reported in Figure 1.

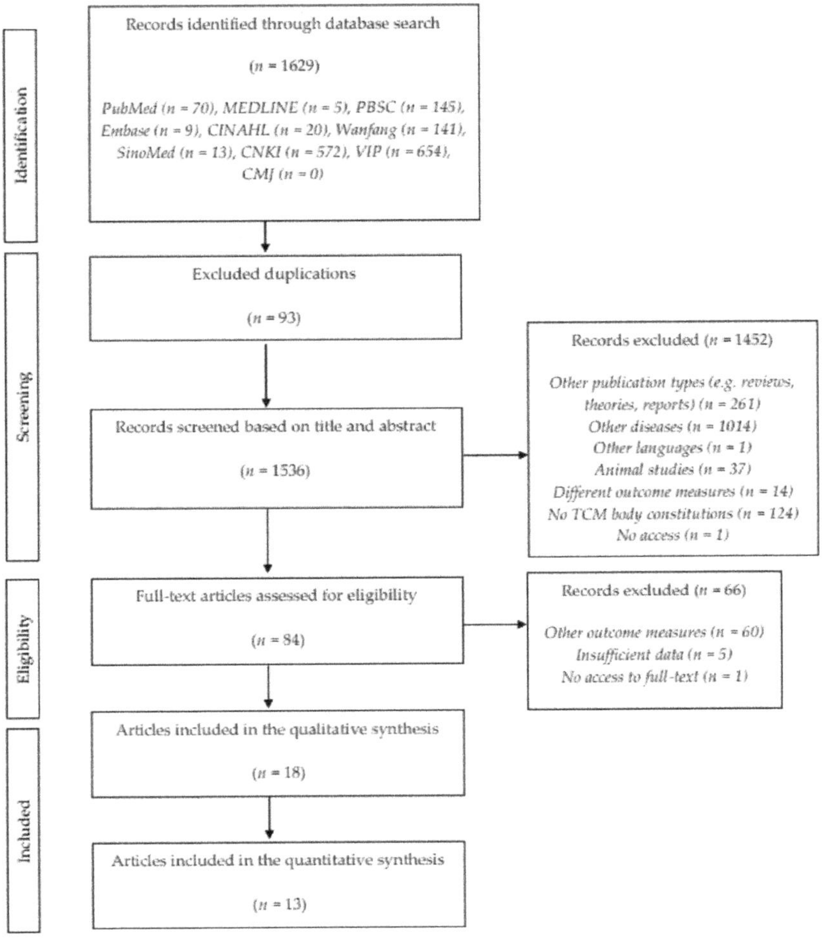

Figure 1. PRISMA flowchart.

3.2. Characteristics of Included Studies

Details of the included studies are summarized in Table 2. Eleven out of eighteen studies were conducted among diseased populations, which included hospital outpatients and inpatients. Whereas another seven were focused on healthy populations, which included samples from biobank, community or institutional groups. The included studies were published in the past decade, between 2010 and 2021. Five were case-control studies and thirteen were cross-sectional studies. The total sample size was 14,799, with an average sample size of 822. The age of the subjects ranged between eighteen and seventy-five years old. Two studies were focused on female subjects only and the rest were focused on both males and females. All of the studies were conducted in China ($n = 18$). Sixteen studies were written in Chinese and the other two were written in English. The method for depression and TCMBC measurement was based on validated self-reported questionnaires. Four instruments were used to identify depression: Hamilton Depression Rating Scale (HAMD) (Cronbach's alpha = 0.8 [72]) contributing the most studies ($n = 6$), followed by the Self-Rating Depression Scale (SDS) (Cronbach's alpha = 0.73) [73] ($n = 5$), Beck Depression Inventory II (BDI-II) (Cronbach's alpha 0.946 [74]) ($n = 5$) and Chinese Classification of Mental Disorders (CCMD-3) ($n = 1$). For studies using identical depression scales, there were variations for the cut-off points used among the studies. For example, the cut-off points for SDS ranged between 50 and 52. Two instruments used to identify TCMBC included the Chinese Medicine Constitution Questionnaire (CMCQ) (n = 17) (Cronbach's alphas in each subscale = 0.72~0.80 [75,76]) and the Body Constitution Questionnaire (BCQ) (*n* = 1) (Cronbach's alpha = 0.8 [55]). Both instruments consist of different subscales to categorize each type of constitution. Participants were categorized according to their highest score among the subscales. Most of the studies (*n* = 16) focused on all nine types of TCMBC while the rest (*n* = 2) focused on specific constitution types.

Table 2. Characteristics of included studies.

Author, Year	Study Design	Study Subjects	Sample Size	Age Range	Sex	Study Area	Depression Measurement	Body Constitution Measurement	Constitution (Specific/All Nine)	Main Findings	Effect Sizes OR [95% CI]
Diseased populations											
Deng et al., 2019 [77]	CS	Neurological patients	132	42.51 ± 6.03	U	China	SDS	CMCQ	All	YADC and QSC were independently correlated with depression state.	**YADC**: 3.021 [0.264–5.619]; **QSC**: 2.053 [1.256–3.251]
Ke et al., 2019 [78]	CC	Cervical cancer patients	289	56.84 ± 14.47	F	China	SDS	CMCQ	All	BSC, QSC and QDC were risk factors of depression in patients with cervical cancer.	**BSC**: 2.923 [1.986–3.864]; **QSC**: 4.158 [1.014–9.869]; **QDC**: 1.875 [1.067–2.024]
Liao et al., 2017 [79]	CS	Chronic hemodialysis patients.	467	63 ± 12	U	China	BDI-II	CCMQ	All	QDC is associated with depression in chronic HD patients	**QDC**: 4.05 [1.69–9.72]
Liu & Li, 2010 [80]	CC	Post-stroke depressed patients	90	40–67	U	China	HAMD	CMCQ	QSC, BSC, BC	PSD patients with QSC have a higher depression tendency compared to BSC and BC.	**QSC**: 34.544 [10.325–117.219]; **BCS**: 0.192 [0.056–0.682]; **BC**: 0.234 [0.086–0.632]
Liu et al., 2019 [81]	CC	Patients with post-cerebral infarction	252	18–75	U	China	HAMD	CMCQ	All	For post-cerebral infarction, QSC and QDC are the major body constitutions which can lead to depression.	**QSC**: 3.865 [2.124–4.385]; **QDC**: 2.127 [1.985–3.654]
Pang et al., 2018 [82]	CC	Post-first ischemic stroke patient	207	61.94 ± 13.54	U	China	HAMD	CMCQ	All	Post-first ischemic stroke depression is closely related to constitution types of QSC, PDC and YIDC.	**QSC**: 4.58 [1.500–14.001]; **PDC**: 2.98 [1.010–8.605]; **YIDC**: 0.317 [0.122–0.826]
Sun et al., 2012 [83]	CC	Post stroke patients	353	61.4 ± 9.00	U	China	CCMD-3	CMCQ	All	QSC, YADC and QDC were risk factors for depression among post stroke patients	**QSC**: 2.794 [1.137–7.171]; **YADC**: 3.757 [1.137–12.118]; **QDC**: 3.840 [1.357–12.808]
Tang et al., 2020 [84]	CS	Irritable bowel syndrome patient	147	≥18	U	China	HAMD	CMCQ	All	There is a certain correlation between TCMBC and depression in IBS patients, in which QDC and QSC are more likely to produce depression.	**QDC**: 4.195 [1.385–12.708]; **QSC**: 9.607 [2.09–44.157]
Wu et al., 2019 [85]	CS	Diabetic patients	214	52.31 ± 12.25	U	China	HAMD	CMCQ	All	There exists a correlation between depression after T2DM and Chinese medicine constitution to some extent.	**YIDC**: 1.793 [1.027–2.125]; **QSC**: 1.534 [0.124–0.863]; **QDC**: 1.219 [0.847–2.121]
Zhao et al., 2020 [62]	CS	Patients with coronary heart disease	160	58.41 ± 6.81	U	China	SDS	CMCQ	All	QDC and QSC were independent risk factors for depression in patients with CHD.	**QDC**: 2.491 [1.324–4.731]; **QSC**: 3.543 [1.175–10.638]
Zhang et al., 2015 [86]	CS	Adult patients with epilepsy	209	18–70	U	China	HAMD	CMCQ	All	QDC and QSC are prone to depression in adult patients with epilepsy, while BC is the protective factor.	**QDC**: 5.549 [2.194–14.039]; **QSC**: 4.068 [1.678–9.861]; **BC**: 0.439 [0.250–0.771]
Healthy populations											
Chen et al., 2021 [35]	CS	Women from Taiwan Biobank	1423	30–70	F	China	NS	BCQ	YADC, YIDC, PDC	Women who have YADC or YIDC were more prone to depression.	**YADC**: 1.047 [1.007–1.089]; **YIDC**: 1.049 [1.009–1.090]
Deng & Chen, 2011 [58]	CS	General population	7506	≥18	U	China	SDS	CMCQ	ALL	People with QDC, DHC and QSC had high tendency of depression, while people with BC had a lower tendency of depression.	**BC**: 0.601 [0.525–0.689]; **QDC**: 1.556 [1.305–1.855]; **DHC**: 2.140 [1.705–2.686]; **QSC**: 2.154 [1.720–2.697]

Table 2. *Cont.*

Author, Year	Study Design	Study Subjects	Sample Size	Age Range	Sex	Study Area	Depression Measurement	Body Constitution Measurement	Constitution (Specific/All Nine)	Main Findings	Effect Sizes OR [95% CI]
Jiang et al., 2018 [59]	CS	Beijing Railway crews	281	20–35	U	China	SDS	CMCQ	ALL	QDC was significantly correlated to depression among railway crews.	**QDC**: 2.03 [1.05–3.94]
Qiu & Xu, 2015 [60]	CS	University students	764	NS	U	China	BDI	CMCQ	ALL	BC is the protective factor for depression among the students, while QDC and QSC are the risk factors.	**BC**: 0.976 [0.978–1.001]; **QDC**: 1.019 [0.987–1.015]; **QSC**: 1.042 [0.989–1.016]
Qiu & Xu, 2016 [87]	CS	University students	684	NS	U	China	BDI	CMCQ	ALL	QDC, YADC, YIDC, QSC, BC, and BSC were the predictors for depression.	**BC**: 1.013 [−0.026, −0.001]; **QDC**: 1.649 [0.039–0.061]; **YADC**: 1.234 [−0.031, −0.011]; **YIDC**: 1.185 [0.005–0.029]; **QSC**: 1.878 [0.051–0.075]; **BSC**: 1.174 [−0.030, −0.003]
Xiong et al., 2019 [38]	CS	University students	950	NS	U	China	BDI-II	CMCQ	ALL	BC is the protective factor while QDC and QSC are the risk factors for depression among university students.	**BC**: 0.380 [0.236–0.610]; **QDC**: 1.693 [1.111–2.578]; **QSC**: 2.994 [1.965–4.561]
Zhang et al., 2019 [61]	CS	University students	671	20.40 ± 1.48	U	China	BDI-II	CMCQ	ALL	Results showed that YADC, YIDC, QDC, PDC, ISC and QSC were risk factors of depression.	**YADC**: 3.486 [1.902–6.389]; **YIDC**: 2.085 [1.018–4.267]; **QDC**: 6.015 [3.142–11.514]; **PDC**: 2.556 [1.145–5.707]; **ISC**: 8.888 [4.406–17.929]; **QSC**: 16.049 [7.919–32.525]

Note: TCMBC, Traditional Chinese medicine body constitution; CS, cross-sectional study; CC, case-control study; NS, not specify or report in the article; U, unisex; F, female; SDS, Self-Rating Depression Scale; BDI-II, Beck Depression Inventory II; HAMD, Hamilton Depression Rating Scale; CCMD-3, Chinese Classification of Mental Disorders; CMCQ, Chinese Medicine Constitution Questionnaire; BCQ, Body Constitution Questionnaire; QSC, Qi-stagnation constitution; BSC, Blood-stasis constitution; BC, Balanced constitution; YADC, Yang-deficiency constitution; YIDC, Yin-deficiency constitution; PDC, Phlegm-damp constitution; HD, hemodialysis; PSD, Post-stroke depression; IBS, Irritable bowel syndrome; T2DM, Type 2 diabetes mellitus; CHD, coronary heart disease.

3.3. Quality Appraisal

The quality assessment of the included studies is reported in Table 3. Seven studies were rated as good quality, seven were medium quality and four were poor quality. The NOS scores of all included studies ranged between 5 and 8. The average score for case control studies was 5.2 and for cross-sectional studies was 6.5. Poor quality studies were excluded from the meta-analyses. The inter-rater reliability for this review was 94%.

Table 3. Quality assessment of the included studies by the Newcastle–Ottawa Scale (NOS).

Author, Year	Selection	Comparability	Outcome	Total Score
Chen et al., 2021 [35]	★★	★★	★★★	7
Deng & Chen, 2011 [58]	★	★	★★★	5
Deng et al., 2019 [77]	★	★★	★★★	5
Jiang et al., 2018 [59]	★★	★	★★★	6
Ke et al., 2019 [78] cc	★★★	★	★	5
Liao et al., 2017 [79]	★★★	★★	★★★	8
Liu & Li, 2010 [80] cc	★★★	★	★	5
Liu et al., 2019 [81] cc	★★★	★	★★	6
Pang et al., 2018 [82] cc	★★★	★	★	5
Qiu & Xu, 2015 [60]	★★	★	★★★	6
Qiu & Xu, 2016 [87]	★	★	★★★	6
Sun et al., 2012 [83] cc	★★★	★	★	5
Tang et al., 2020 [84]	★★	★	★★★	6
Zhang et al., 2015 [86]	★★	★	★★★	6

Table 3. *Cont.*

Author, Year	Selection	Comparability	Outcome	Total Score
Wu et al., 2019 [85]	★★	★	★★★	7
Xiong et al., 2019 [38]	★★	★	★★★	7
Zhang et al., 2019 [61]	★★	★	★★★	7
Zhao et al., 2020 [62]	★★★	★	★★★	7

Note: [cc], case control study. A maximum of one star can be awarded for each numbered item within the selection and exposure section. A maximum of two stars can be given for the comparability section. The maximum scores for case-control studies and cross-sectional studies are 9 and 10, respectively. For the quality of case-control studies, it was considered as poor if the score was 0 to 5 and good if the score was 6 to 9. For the quality of cross-sectional studies, it was considered as poor if the score was 0 to 4, medium if the score was 5 to 6, good if the score was 7 to 8, and very good if the score was 9 to 10.

3.4. Systematic Review of Associations between TCMBC and Depression

All nine types of TCMBC were showed to be associated with depression, with QSC contributing the most (n = 15), followed by QDC (n = 14), BC (n = 6), YADC (n = 5), YIDC (n = 5), BSC (n = 3), PDC (n = 2), DHC (n = 1), and ISC (n = 1).

3.4.1. Qi-Stagnation Constitution

Among the studies that revealed a link between QSC and depression, diseased populations were more frequently observed, with a higher prevalence among post-stroke patients [80–82,84], followed by cervical cancer patients [78], diabetic patients [86], epileptic patients [87], heart disease patients [62], irritable bowel syndrome (IBS) patients [85] and neurological patients [77]. In addition, the other five studies were carried out among general populations, which included university students [38,60,61,83], and young adults [58]. These studies showed consistent results where QSC significantly predicted depression. Four studies were excluded from the meta-analysis due to poor quality [78,80,82,84] and the other one was excluded due to differences in the study design [81].

3.4.2. Qi-Deficiency Constitution

Among the studies that found a correlation between QDC and depression, eight were conducted on diseased populations, including cervical cancer patients [78], chronic hemodialysis patients [79], diabetic patients [86], epileptic patients [87], heart disease patients [62], IBS patients [85] and post-stroke patients [81,84], Whereas in general populations, most studies focused on university students [38,60,61,83], followed by railway crews [59] and young adults [58]. All studies suggest that QDC is a significant risk factor for depression. Three studies were excluded from the meta-analysis due to poor quality [78,84] and differences in the study design [81].

3.4.3. Yang-Deficiency Constitution

Of the five studies indicating a link between YADC and depression, two were from diseased populations, which included neurological patients [77] and post-stroke patients [84]. The rest were from university students [61,83] and women [35]. The consistent findings suggest that YADC is a risk factor for depression. One study was excluded from the meta-analysis due to poor quality [84].

3.4.4. Yin-Deficiency Constitution

Five studies showing that YIDC is significantly related to depression were conducted among diabetic patients [86], post-stroke patients [82], women [35] and university students [61,83]. There were inconsistent findings among the studies, in which Pang et al. showed that YIDC was negatively associated with depression. While the rest showed that YIDC was positively associated with depression [35,61,83,86]. One study was excluded from the meta-analysis due to poor quality [82].

3.4.5. Blood-Stasis Constitution

Three out of eighteen included studies indicated that BSC was correlated with depression among cervical cancer patients [78], post-stroke patients [80], and university students [83]. Inconsistent findings were observed among the included studies. Two studies found that BSC was negatively correlated to depression [80,83]. In contrast, Ke et al. [78] found that BSC was positively correlated with depression. No meta-analysis was performed for this constitution type because there was only a single study of sufficient quality [83].

3.4.6. Phlegm-Dampness Constitution

Only two studies demonstrated a link between PDC and depression. One was conducted among post-stroke patients [82] and the other among university students [61]. Both studies showed consistent results, suggesting that PDC was a risk factor for depression. No meta-analysis was performed for this constitution type because there was only a single study of sufficient quality [61].

3.4.7. Damp-Heat Constitution

There was one study conducted among young adults which revealed that DHC was correlated with depression [58]. The findings showed that DHC was a risk factor for depression. No meta-analysis was performed for this constitution type due to the insufficient number of studies.

3.4.8. Inherited Special Constitution

Only one study focused on university students found that ISC was related to depression [61]. Their findings suggested that ISC was a risk factor for depression. No meta-analysis was performed for this constitution type due to the insufficient number of studies.

3.4.9. Balanced Constitution

Six out of eighteen included studies demonstrated a relationship between balanced constitution and depression. The majority of the studies were focused on general populations, such as university students [38,60,83] and young adults [58]. The rest were focused on epileptic patients [87] and post-stroke patients [80]. All studies showed consistent results, in which BC was found to be a protective factor for depression. One study was excluded from meta-analysis because of differences in the study design [80].

3.5. Meta-Analyses of Association between TCM Body Constitution and Depression

For the association between each type of TCMBC and depression, a meta-analysis was conducted only when there was sufficient data ($n \geq 2$ and with adequate quality).

3.5.1. Qi-Stagnation Constitution

Among eighteen included studies, ten studies involving 11,437 subjects reported an association between QSC and depression. The random effects model was used because the statistical heterogeneity of the included studies was significant ($I^2 = 94\%$). The results showed that the association between QSC and depression was significant, with a pooled OR and 95% CI of 3.12 [1.80–5.40] (see Figure 2).

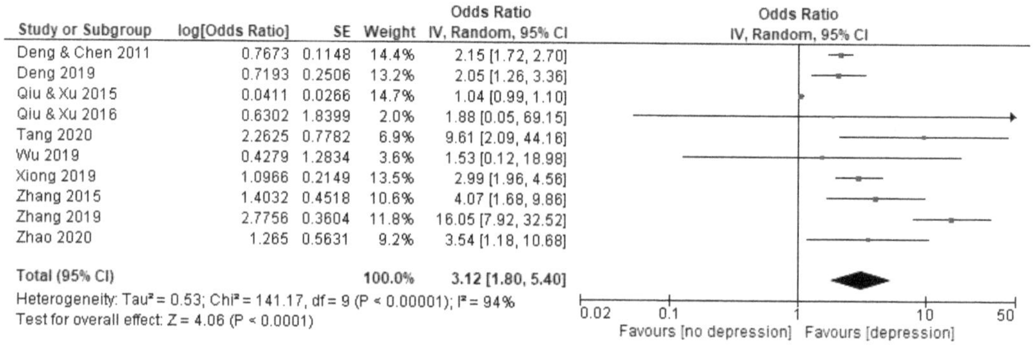

Figure 2. Forest plot of studies on association between QSC and depression. Note: red square represents the result of each study; line represents the 95% CI of the results; diamond represents the pooled results.

3.5.2. Qi-Deficiency Constitution

Eleven studies with a total of 12,053 subjects reported an association between QDC and depression. The random effects model was used because the statistical heterogeneity of the included studies was significant (I^2 = 89%). The results showed that the association between QDC and depression was significant, with a pooled OR and 95% CI of 2.15 [1.54–3.01] (see Figure 3).

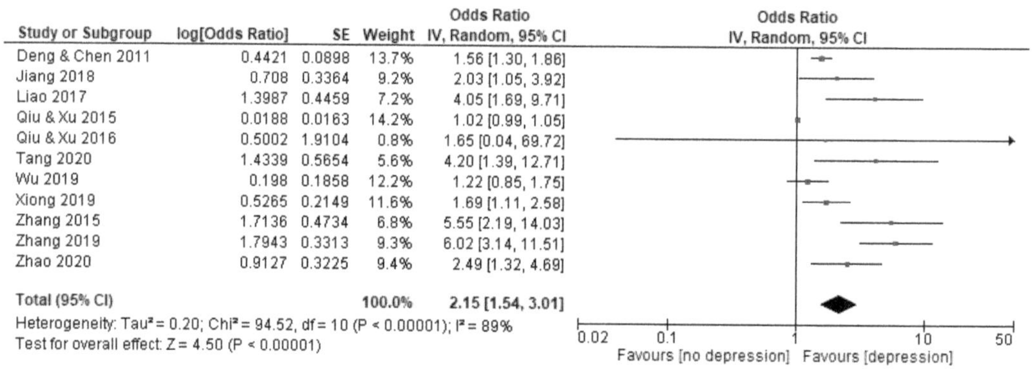

Figure 3. Forest plot of studies on association between QDC and depression. Note: red square represents the result of each study; line represents the 95% CI of the results; diamond represents the pooled results.

3.5.3. Yang-Deficiency Constitution

Four studies with a total of 2910 subjects reported an association between YADC and depression. The random effects model was used because the statistical heterogeneity of the included studies was significant (I^2 = 81%). The results showed that the association between YADC and depression was significant, with a pooled OR and 95% CI of 1.89 [0.71–5.03] (see Figure 4).

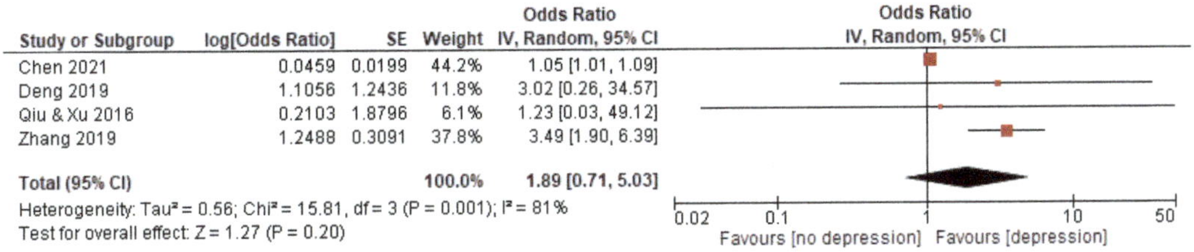

Figure 4. Forest plot of studies on association between YADC and depression. Note: red square represents the result of each study; line represents the 95% CI of the results; diamond represents the pooled results.

3.5.4. Yin-Deficiency Constitution

Four studies with a total of 2992 subjects reported an association between YIDC and depression. The random effects model was used because the statistical heterogeneity of the included studies was significant (I^2 = 57%). The results showed that the association between YIDC and depression was significant, with a pooled OR and 95% CI of 1.41 [0.91–2.20] (see Figure 5).

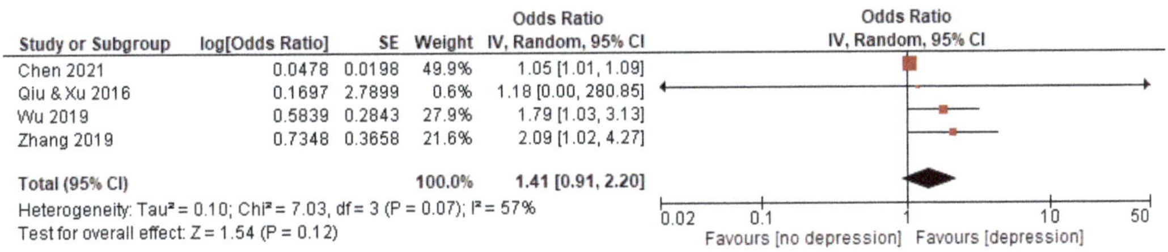

Figure 5. Forest plot of studies on association between YIDC and depression. Note: red square represents the result of each study; line represents the 95% CI of the results; diamond represents the pooled results.

3.5.5. Balanced Constitution

Five studies with a total of 10,113 subjects reported an association between BC and depression. The random effects model was used because the statistical heterogeneity of the included studies was significant (I^2 = 94%). The results showed that the association between BC and depression was significant, with a pooled OR and 95% CI of 0.60 [0.40–0.90] (see Figure 6).

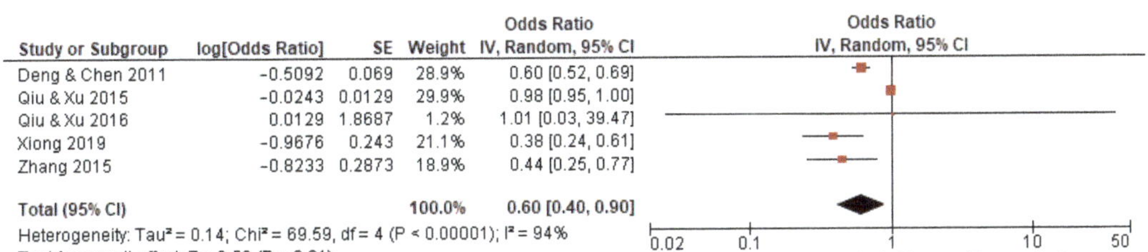

Figure 6. Forest plot of studies on association between BC and depression. Note: red square represents the result of each study; line represents the 95% CI of the results; diamond represents the pooled results.

3.6. Risk of Bias

A visualization of the funnel plots suggests no clear evidence of publication bias (see Figures 7 and 8). For other constitution types, we were unable to perform a publication bias analysis due to the small number of studies [71].

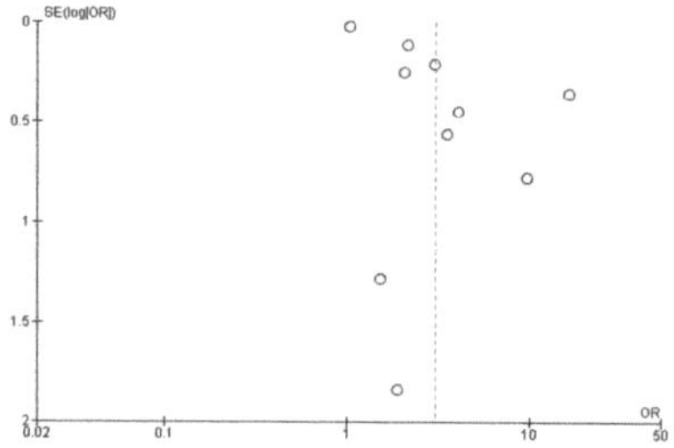

Figure 7. Funnel plot of studies on association between QSC and depression. Note: dot represents individual studies; blue dotted line represents the overall effect.

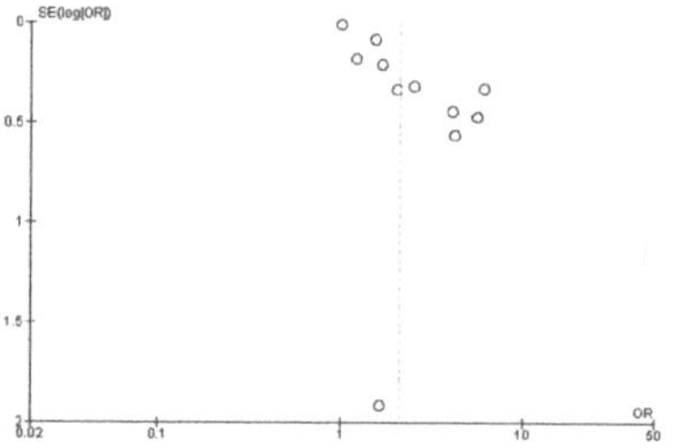

Figure 8. Funnel plot of studies on association between QDC and depression. Note: dot represents individual studies; blue dotted line represents the overall effect.

3.7. Certainty of Evidence

The detailed GRADE ratings for each meta-analysis are reported in Table 4. As all the included studies in these meta-analyses were observational studies, the level of certainty was initially rated as low. One point was deducted for all meta-analyses due to inconsistency (due to the presence of statistical heterogeneity). However, for the associations of QSC and QDC with depression, the quality of evidence was increased by one point due to the large magnitude of effect. The overall quality of evidence of was rated as very low.

Table 4. GRADE assessment of all meta-analyses.

Number of Studies	Study Design	Risk of Bias	Inconsistency	Imprecision	Indirectness	Publication Bias	Other Considerations	Number of Subjects	Effect Sizes [95% CI]	Overall Quality of Evidence
QSC										
10	Observational studies	Not serious	Serious [a]	Not serious	Not serious	Not detected	Very strong association [c]	11,437	3.12 [1.80, 5.40]	Low
QDC										
11	Observational studies	Not serious	Serious [a]	Not serious	Not serious	Not detected	Very strong association [c]	12,053	2.15 [1.54, 3.01]	Low
YADC										
4	Observational studies	Not serious	Serious [a]	Not serious	Not serious	Not detected [b]	None	2910	1.89 [0.71, 5.03]	Very low
YIDC										
4	Observational studies	Not serious	Serious [a]	Not serious	Not serious	Not detected [b]	None	2992	1.41 [0.91, 2.20]	Very low

Table 4. *Cont.*

Number of Studies	Study Design	Risk of Bias	Inconsistency	Imprecision	Indirectness	Publication Bias	Other Considerations	Number of Subjects	Effect Sizes [95% CI]	Overall Quality of Evidence
BC										
5	Observational studies	Not serious	Serious [a]	Not serious	Not serious	Not detected [b]	None	10,113	0.60 [0.40, 0.90]	Very low

Note: [a] significant heterogeneity was detected ($I^2 > 50\%$); [b] unable to perform publication bias assessment due to small number of studies; [c] magnitude of the effect was large (OR > 2); Low quality indicated that the authors' confidence in the effect estimate is limited; Very low quality indicated that the authors have very little confidence in the estimated effect.

4. Discussion

Traditional Chinese medicine body constitutions (TCMBC) are classified based on the harmony and balance of Yin-Yang, Qi and blood within the human body. There are nine types of TCMBC, where Balanced constitution (BC) is a neutral constitution, and the rest are the biased constitutions, namely Qi-stagnation (QSC), Blood-stasis (BSC), Qi-deficiency constitution (QDC), Yin-deficiency constitution (YIDC), Yang-deficiency constitution (YADC), Phlegm-dampness (PDC), Damp-heat constitution (DHC) and Inherited special constitution (ISC) [34]. This review shows that all nine types of TCMBC were associated with depression. Of the nine constitutions, QSC, QDC, BC, YADC, YIDC, BSC and PDC showed significant relationships with depression among both diseased and general populations. QSC, QDC, YADC and YIDC were independent risk factors for depression. When compared to other biased constitutions, people with QSC and QDC were 3.12 and 2.15 times more likely to be depressed, respectively. The strong positive associations between biased TCMBC (e.g., QSC, QDC, YADC and YIDC) and depression could be explained by the interactions between fundamental substances (essence, Qi, blood, body fluids and spirit) and viscera (liver, spleen, lung, heart and kidney). Generally, the blockage of Qi and blood and the abnormal liver functions are considered correlated to depression in TCM.

According to TCM, Qi plays an essential role in propelling, warming and transforming [31,32]. There are variations in the functions of Qi in different viscera. The propelling effect of Qi is responsible for stimulating and maintaining the normal function of internal organs [88]. For example, heart-Qi is responsible for promoting blood circulation [89], whereas liver-Qi regulates the smooth movement of Qi [43,90]. The impaired propelling function of Qi can cause hypofunction of the viscera and subsequent deficiency problems [91]. Furthermore, Qi with a warming effect is called Yang-Qi. In TCM, Yang-Qi in the heart warms and dredges our blood vessels to promote blood circulation [92], while Yang-Qi in the spleen warms and transforms food and water [93,94], ensuring good digestion and absorption [94]. If the warming effect of Qi is weakened, it will result in restricted circulation of Qi and blood, as well as the devitalization of the visceral functions. Additionally, Qi-transformation is vital in maintaining the balance of fundamental substances within our body [32]. For example, Qi is involved in producing and transforming other fundamental substances, such as blood, essence and body fluid. If the transforming function of Qi is weakened, physiological functions will be affected, resulting in various diseases. Overall, a lack or deficiency of Qi will lead to the development of weak immunity. In TCM, the liver plays important roles in regulating emotions and the maintenance of the movement of Qi and blood [31,43,45]. When the liver functions normally, free flow of Qi and blood is maintained, ensuring the transport of essential nutrients to other viscera, which results in good physical and mental health [45]. If the liver's function of dispersion and dredging is abnormal, the flow of Qi and blood in the body may be obstructed, which can result in various problems, such as insomnia, melancholy, sentimentality, mood swings and even depression [31,43,48,51]. Disruptions of Qi and blood in viscera will affect a person's mental activities, and abnormal mental activities can affect the Qi and blood in viscera, as well. For example, excessive emotions like panic, stress and sadness can cause dysfunctions of Qi, blood and viscera, and eventually lead to the development of depression [43].

On the contrary, BC is shown to be a significant protective factor against depression. This result was expected, because BC is defined as a neutral and harmonious constitution type, with a balance of Yin-Yang, Qi and blood in the body. People with this constitution usually have an optimistic personality and good adaptability. High optimism helps reduce the incidence of depression because optimistic people often think positively and are more resistant to stress. Moreover, change induces negative emotions, such as stress, anxiety and even depression. People with good adaptability can handle and adapt to changes quickly; their ability to cope with changed or changing situations can subsequently minimize their risk of depression. Besides, people with BC tend to practice healthier lifestyles compared to people with biased TCMBCs. Heathy lifestyles characterized by balanced diet and sufficient exercise are shown to be beneficial for mental health [95].

The strength of this review is that its findings can contribute to the prevention and treatment of depression through the modification of TCMBC. Since this review identified those with QSC and QDC as populations at high risk for depression, we suggest that screening of TCMBC be added to depression screening protocols. When a person is identified as either QSC or QDC, they should be considered at high risk for depression. Since TCMBC is modifiable, depression can actually be prevented before it even develops in people with QSC and QDC. In order to modify these biased constitutions towards a balanced constitution, moderate amount of exercise, such as yoga and cardio, is highly recommended for people with QSC and QDC, as it can help promote the circulation of Qi and blood in the body [31]. Moreover, sleeping at regular times and getting adequate sleep is vital for nourishing the Qi [31]. As for diet, these people should eat a greater variety of foods that can nourish the blood and help with Qi movement, such as dark leafy greens, bean sprouts, berries and red meats [31].

This review has several limitations. First, the application of TCMBC is still in infancy in countries other than China, and the sources of the included studies were all from China. The majority of the included studies were written in Chinese, even though we searched four English databases and six other Chinese databases. This could be due to the lack of application of TCMBC in countries other than China. Currently, there is only one previous study related to TCMBC and depression among non-Chinese populations, conducted among African students studying in China [96]. However, the study is not included in our review due to different outcome measures. Thus, the findings of this review cannot be generalized to other populations. Secondly, the study design of the included studies were mostly cross-sectional studies, followed by case-control studies. No case-control studies were included in the meta-analysis. Hence, the temporal relationship and the causal link between TCMBC and depression is unknown. Third, all the included studies were observational studies using self-reported questionnaires as the measurement tool; therefore, recall bias may be present. Fourth, there was presence of high heterogeneity. This could be due to the variations in sample sizes, sample populations and measurement tools. Fifth, the validation of TCMBC-related questionnaires are limited to the Chinese and English languages only. This could explain why TCMBC is not widely applicable in other countries. Further research is likely to significantly impact our confidence regarding the estimated effects, as the levels of certainty of the current review measured by GRADE were rated as low and very low, respectively.

5. Conclusions

This review demonstrated that Qi-stagnation, Qi-deficiency, Yang-deficiency, Yin-deficiency and Balanced constitutions are significant predictors for depression, of which, Balanced constitution is the protective factor. Because most of the included studies were cross-sectional, we suggest that more case-control and cohort studies be analyzed to confirm the association between TCMBC and depression.

Author Contributions: Conceptualization: C.N.F., Y.M.L. and F.L.N.; Data curation: S.Y.Y., M.S. and F.L.N.; Formal analysis: S.Y.Y., M.S. and F.L.N.; Funding acquisition: C.N.F., Y.M.L. and F.L.N.; Investigation: S.Y.Y., M.S., F.L.N., C.N.F. and Y.M.L.; Methodology: C.N.F., Y.M.L., F.L.N., M.S. and S.Y.Y.; Project administration: C.N.F., Y.M.L., F.L.N., M.S. and S.Y.Y.; Supervision: C.N.F., Y.M.L. and F.L.N.; Validation: C.N.F., Y.M.L., F.L.N., M.S. and S.Y.Y.; Writing—original draft: S.Y.Y. and C.N.F.; Writing—review & editing: C.N.F., Y.M.L., F.L.N., M.S. and S.Y.Y. All authors have read and agreed to the published version of the manuscript.

Funding: This study was supported by the Universiti Tunku Abdul Rahman Research Fund (UTARRF), (Project number IPSR/RMC/UTARRF/2019-C2/F01 and IPSR/RMC/UTARRF/2022-C1/F02).

Institutional Review Board Statement: Not applicable.

Informed Consent Statement: Not applicable.

Data Availability Statement: Not applicable.

Conflicts of Interest: The authors declare no conflict of interest. The funders had no role in the design of the study; in the collection, analyses, or interpretation of data; in the writing of the manuscript; or in the decision to publish the results.

References

1. James, S.L.; Abate, D.; Abate, K.H.; Abay, S.M.; Abbafati, C.; Abbasi, N.; Abbastabar, H.; Abd-Allah, F.; Abdela, J.; Abdelalim, A.; et al. Global, Regional, and National Incidence, Prevalence, and Years Lived with Disability for 354 Diseases and Injuries for 195 Countries and Territories, 1990–2017: A Systematic Analysis for the Global Burden of Disease Study 2017. *Lancet* **2018**, *392*, 1789–1858. [CrossRef]
2. Who Health Organization (WHO). Adolescent Mental Health. Available online: https://www.who.int/news-room/fact-sheets/detail/adolescent-mental-health (accessed on 20 August 2021).
3. Rajan, S.; McKee, M.; Rangarajan, S.; Bangdiwala, S.; Rosengren, A.; Gupta, R.; Kutty, V.R.; Wielgosz, A.; Lear, S.; AlHabib, K.F.; et al. Association of Symptoms of Depression With Cardiovascular Disease and Mortality in Low-, Middle-, and High-Income Countries. *JAMA Psychiatry* **2020**, *77*, 1052–1063. [CrossRef]
4. Deleskog, A.; Ljung, R.; Forsell, Y.; Nevriana, A.; Almas, A.; Möller, J. Severity of Depression, Anxious Distress and the Risk of Type 2 Diabetes—A Population-Based Cohort Study in Sweden. *BMC Public Health* **2019**, *19*, 1174. [CrossRef]
5. Tsai, T.-Y.; Lu, M.-C.; Livneh, H.; Chiu, S.-Y.; Lai, N.-S.; Guo, H.-R. Does Depression Increase the Risk of Stroke in Patients with Rheumatoid Arthritis? A Population-Based Cohort Study. *BMJ Open* **2017**, *7*, e014233. [CrossRef]
6. Andersson, N.W.; Goodwin, R.D.; Okkels, N.; Gustafsson, L.N.; Taha, F.; Cole, S.W.; Munk-Jørgensen, P. Depression and the Risk of Severe Infections: Prospective Analyses on a Nationwide Representative Sample. *Int. J. Epidemiol.* **2016**, *45*, 131–139. [CrossRef]
7. Cuijpers, P.; Vogelzangs, N.; Twisk, J.; Kleiboer, A.; Li, J.; Penninx, B.W. Comprehensive Meta-Analysis of Excess Mortality in Depression in the General Community versus Patients with Specific Illnesses. *Am. J. Psychiatry* **2014**, *171*, 453–462. [CrossRef]
8. WHO Suicide. Available online: https://www.who.int/news-room/fact-sheets/detail/suicide (accessed on 14 August 2021).
9. American Psychiatric Association. *Diagnostic and Statistical Manual of Mental Disorders*, 5th ed.; American Psychiatric Association: Washington, DC, USA, 2013; ISBN 978-0-89042-555-8.
10. NIH NIMH. Depression. Available online: https://www.nimh.nih.gov/health/topics/depression#part_145399 (accessed on 14 August 2021).
11. Wang, J.; Mann, F.; Lloyd-Evans, B.; Ma, R.; Johnson, S. Associations between Loneliness and Perceived Social Support and Outcomes of Mental Health Problems: A Systematic Review. *BMC Psychiatry* **2018**, *18*, 156. [CrossRef] [PubMed]
12. Labrague, L.J. Psychological Resilience, Coping Behaviours and Social Support among Health Care Workers during the COVID-19 Pandemic: A Systematic Review of Quantitative Studies. *J. Nurs. Manag.* **2021**, *29*, 1893–1905. [CrossRef]
13. Du, L.; Shi, H.-Y.; Qian, Y.; Jin, X.-H.; Li, Y.; Yu, H.-R.; Liu, X.-M.; Fu, X.-L.; Chen, H.-L. Association between Social Support and Suicidal Ideation in Patients with Cancer: A Systematic Review and Meta-Analysis. *Eur. J. Cancer Care* **2021**, *30*, e13382. [CrossRef]
14. Esmaeelzadeh, S.; Moraros, J.; Thorpe, L.; Bird, Y. Examining the Association and Directionality between Mental Health Disorders and Substance Use among Adolescents and Young Adults in the U.S. and Canada—A Systematic Review and Meta-Analysis. *J. Clin. Med.* **2018**, *7*, 543. [CrossRef]
15. Lassale, C.; Batty, G.D.; Baghdadli, A.; Jacka, F.; Sánchez-Villegas, A.; Kivimäki, M.; Akbaraly, T. Healthy Dietary Indices and Risk of Depressive Outcomes: A Systematic Review and Meta-Analysis of Observational Studies. *Mol. Psychiatry* **2019**, *24*, 965–986. [CrossRef] [PubMed]
16. Schuch, F.B.; Vancampfort, D.; Firth, J.; Rosenbaum, S.; Ward, P.B.; Silva, E.S.; Hallgren, M.; Ponce De Leon, A.; Dunn, A.L.; Deslandes, A.C.; et al. Physical Activity and Incident Depression: A Meta-Analysis of Prospective Cohort Studies. *AJP* **2018**, *175*, 631–648. [CrossRef] [PubMed]

17. LeMoult, J.; Humphreys, K.L.; Tracy, A.; Hoffmeister, J.-A.; Ip, E.; Gotlib, I.H. Meta-Analysis: Exposure to Early Life Stress and Risk for Depression in Childhood and Adolescence. *J. Am. Acad. Child Adolesc. Psychiatry* **2020**, *59*, 842–855. [CrossRef] [PubMed]
18. Wium-Andersen, M.K.; Wium-Andersen, I.K.; Prescott, E.I.B.; Overvad, K.; Jørgensen, M.B.; Osler, M. An Attempt to Explain the Bidirectional Association between Ischaemic Heart Disease, Stroke and Depression: A Cohort and Meta-Analytic Approach. *Br. J. Psychiatry* **2020**, *217*, 434–441. [CrossRef]
19. WHO. *International Statistical Classification of Diseases and Related Health Problems*, 11th ed.; World Health Organization: Geneva, Switzerland, 2019.
20. Semrau, M.; Evans-Lacko, S.; Alem, A.; Ayuso-Mateos, J.L.; Chisholm, D.; Gureje, O.; Hanlon, C.; Jordans, M.; Kigozi, F.; Lempp, H.; et al. Strengthening Mental Health Systems in Low- and Middle-Income Countries: The Emerald Programme. *BMC Med.* **2015**, *13*, 79. [CrossRef]
21. Institute of Medicine (US) Committee on Pathophysiology and Prevention of Adolescent and Adult Suicide Chapter: 9 Barriers to Effective Treatment and Intervention. In *Reducing Suicide: A National Imperative*; Goldsmith, S.K.; Pellmar, T.C.; Kleinman, A.M.; Bunney, W.E. (Eds.) National Academies Press: Washington, DC, USA, 2002; ISBN 978-0-309-08321-8.
22. Jafferany, M.; Stamu-O'Brien, C.; Mkhoyan, R.; Patel, A. Psychotropic Drugs in Dermatology: A Dermatologist's Approach and Choice of Medications. *Dermatol. Ther.* **2020**, *33*, e13385. [CrossRef]
23. Wang, S.-M.; Han, C.; Bahk, W.-M.; Lee, S.-J.; Patkar, A.A.; Masand, P.S.; Pae, C.-U. Addressing the Side Effects of Contemporary Antidepressant Drugs: A Comprehensive Review. *Chonnam Med. J.* **2018**, *54*, 101–112. [CrossRef]
24. Ng, M.Y.; DiVasto, K.A.; Cootner, S.; Gonzalez, N.; Weisz, J.R. What Do 30 Years of Randomized Trials Tell Us about How Psychotherapy Improves Youth Depression? A Systematic Review of Candidate Mediators. *Clin. Psychol. Sci. Pract.* **2020**, e12367. [CrossRef]
25. Guidi, J.; Fava, G.A. Sequential Combination of Pharmacotherapy and Psychotherapy in Major Depressive Disorder: A Systematic Review and Meta-Analysis. *JAMA Psychiatry* **2021**, *78*, 261–269. [CrossRef]
26. Bahji, A.; Ermacora, D.; Stephenson, C.; Hawken, E.R.; Vazquez, G. Comparative Efficacy and Tolerability of Adjunctive Pharmacotherapies for Acute Bipolar Depression: A Systematic Review and Network Meta-Analysis. *Can. J. Psychiatry* **2021**, *66*, 274–288. [CrossRef]
27. Cuijpers, P.; Quero, S.; Noma, H.; Ciharova, M.; Miguel, C.; Karyotaki, E.; Cipriani, A.; Cristea, I.A.; Furukawa, T.A. Psychotherapies for Depression: A Network Meta-Analysis Covering Efficacy, Acceptability and Long-Term Outcomes of All Main Treatment Types. *World Psychiatry* **2021**, *20*, 283–293. [CrossRef] [PubMed]
28. Van Bronswijk, S.; Moopen, N.; Beijers, L.; Ruhe, H.G.; Peeters, F. Effectiveness of Psychotherapy for Treatment-Resistant Depression: A Meta-Analysis and Meta-Regression. *Psychol. Med.* **2019**, *49*, 366–379. [CrossRef] [PubMed]
29. Marshall, A.C. Traditional Chinese Medicine and Clinical Pharmacology. *Drug Discov. Eval. Methods Clin. Pharmacol.* **2020**, 455–482. [CrossRef]
30. Lu, A.-P.; Jia, H.-W.; Xiao, C.; Lu, Q.-P. Theory of Traditional Chinese Medicine and Therapeutic Method of Diseases. *World J. Gastroenterol.* **2004**, *10*, 1854–1856. [CrossRef]
31. Xing, Y.R.; Zhang, X.D.; Huang, G.P.; Sun, L.J.; Qiao, W.B. *Basic Theory of Chinese Medicine*; Shaanxi Science and Technology Press: Xianyang, China, 2016.
32. Hu, D. 6 Concept of Constitutional Theory. In *Traditional Chinese Medicine: Theory and Principles*; Walter de Gruyter GmbH & Co KG: Beijing, China, 2015; ISBN 978-3-11-041766-1.
33. Li, L.; Yao, H.; Wang, J.; Li, Y.; Wang, Q. The Role of Chinese Medicine in Health Maintenance and Disease Prevention: Application of Constitution Theory. *Am. J. Chin. Med.* **2019**, *47*, 495–506. [CrossRef]
34. Wang, Q. Classification and Diagnosis Basis of Nine Basic Constitutions in Chinese Medicine. *J. Beijing Univ. Tradit. Chin. Med.* **2005**, *28*, 1–8.
35. Chen, S.; Liu, Y.; Hsueh, K.; Tang, P. Body Constitution of Traditional Chinese Medicine Caused a Significant Effect on Depression in Adult Women. *Complementary Ther. Clin. Pract.* **2021**, *42*, 101288. [CrossRef]
36. Cheng, H. The Relationship between Individual TCM Constitution Types and Young and Middle-Aged Depression. *Smart Healthcare* **2020**, *11*, 61–63. [CrossRef]
37. Liu, M.; Jiang, Y.; Wang, X.; Liu, Q.; Wu, H. The Role of Rumination and Stressful Life Events in the Relationship between the Qi Stagnation Constitution and Depression in Women: A Moderated Mediation Model. *Evid.-Based Complementary Altern. Med.* **2017**, *2017*, e7605893. [CrossRef]
38. Xiong, L.; Wan, F.; Huang, M.; Lin, H.; Xiong, G.; Peng, Y.; Zhao, S. Correlation between Nine Types of Traditional Chinese Medicine Constitution and Depression of Students in Vocational and Technical Colleges. *Kexue Zixun (Keji Guanli)* **2019**, *38*, 69–70.
39. Ruan, F.F. The Harmony of Yin and Yang. In *Sex in China: Studies in Sexology in Chinese Culture*; Perspectives in Sexuality; Ruan, F.F., Ed.; Springer: Boston, MA, USA, 1991; pp. 11–28. ISBN 978-1-4899-0609-0.
40. Sun, Y.; Zhao, Y.; Xue, S.A.; Chen, J. The Theory Development of Traditional Chinese Medicine Constitution: A Review. *J. Tradit. Chin. Med. Sci.* **2018**, *5*, 16–28. [CrossRef]
41. Ou, M. *Chinese-English Dictionary of Traditional Chinese Medicine*; Joint Publishing Co. Ltd.: Hong Kong, China, 1988.
42. Li, C.; Huang, J.; Cheng, Y.-C.; Zhang, Y.-W. Traditional Chinese Medicine in Depression Treatment: From Molecules to Systems. *Front. Pharmacol.* **2020**, *11*, 586. [CrossRef]

43. Ye, J.; Cai, S.; Cheung, W.M.; Tsang, H.W.H. An East Meets West Approach to the Understanding of Emotion Dysregulation in Depression: From Perspective to Scientific Evidence. *Front. Psychol.* **2019**, *10*, 574. [CrossRef]
44. Feng, D.; Tang, T.; Lin, X.; Yang, Z.; Yang, S.; Xia, Z.; Wang, Y.; Zheng, P.; Wang, Y.; Zhang, C. Nine Traditional Chinese Herbal Formulas for the Treatment of Depression: An Ethnopharmacology, Phytochemistry, and Pharmacology Review. *NDT* **2016**, *12*, 2387–2402. [CrossRef]
45. Liu, Z.-W.; Shu, J.; Tu, J.-Y.; Zhang, C.-H.; Hong, J. Liver in the Chinese and Western Medicine. *IMI* **2017**, *4*, 39–45. [CrossRef]
46. Zhao, J. Jieyu Decoction for Depression. *J. Sichuan Tradit. Chin. Med.* **1992**, *8*, 31.
47. Jin, G.; Liang, Y. Seasonal Pathogenesis of Depression and Its Enlightenment. *J. Beijing Univ. Tradit. Chin. Med.* **1997**, *20*, 15–16.
48. Guo, Y.; Liu, C. Wang Yanheng's Experience in the Treatment of Depression. *Hebei Chin. Med.* **2002**, *24*, 100–101.
49. Liu, B. Experience of Jieyu Decoction in the Treatment of 31 Cases of Latent Depression. *Tianjin Tradit. Chin. Med.* **1991**, *8*, 326.
50. Zhao, Z.; Zhao, M. Clinical Observation on 180 Cases of Depression Treated with Kang Wei Kang. *J. Shandong Tradit. Chin. Med.* **1999**, *18*, 110–111.
51. Park, J. Acupuncture in the Treatment of Depression: A Manual for Practice and Research. *Focus Altern. Complementary Ther.* **2002**, *7*, 69. [CrossRef]
52. Kanezawa, S.; Zhu, Y.-B.; Wang, Q. Correlation between Chinese Medicine Constitution and Skin Types: A Study on 187 Japanese Women. *Chin. J. Integr. Med.* **2020**, *26*, 174–179. [CrossRef] [PubMed]
53. Shi, G.; Kyo, H.; Kawasaki, T.; Kanaya, S.; Sato, M.; Tokuda-Kakutani, S.; Watanabe, H.; Murayama, N.; Ohashi, M.; Altaf-Ul-Amin, M.; et al. Evaluation and Interpretation of 9 Body Constitution Scores of CCMQ-J by Seven Independent Questionnaires. *Jpn. J. Complementary Altern. Med.* **2019**, *16*, 79–93. [CrossRef]
54. Wong, W.; Lam, C.L.K.; Wong, V.T.; Yang, Z.M.; Ziea, E.T.C.; Kwan, A.K.L. Validation of the Constitution in Chinese Medicine Questionnaire: Does the Traditional Chinese Medicine Concept of Body Constitution Exist? *Evid.-Based Complementary Altern. Med.* **2013**, *2013*, e481491. [CrossRef]
55. Wong, W.; Lam, C.L.K.; Su, Y.-C.; Lin, S.J.-S.; Ziea, E.T.-C.; Wong, V.T.; Wai, L.K.; Kwan, A.K.L. Measuring Body Constitution: Validation of the Body Constitution Questionnaire (BCQ) in Hong Kong. *Complementary Ther. Med.* **2014**, *22*, 670–682. [CrossRef]
56. Meriam, B.M. Association between the Traditional Chinese Medicine Nine Body Constitution Types and the Western Medicine Complications of Hypertension among Adult Filipino Hypertensive Patients. *Health Sci. J.* **2021**, *10*, 105–114.
57. Yap, S.Y.; Foo, C.N.; Lim, Y.M.; Ng, F.L.; Mohd-Sidik, S.; Tang, P.Y.; Najar Singh, J.K.; Pheh, K.-S. Traditional Chinese Medicine Body Constitutions and Psychological Determinants of Depression among University Students in Malaysia: A Pilot Study. *Int. J. Environ. Res. Public Health* **2021**, *18*, 5366. [CrossRef]
58. Deng, H.; Chen, Y. Study of the relation between Body Constitution and incidence tendency of depression or anxiety. *Hainan Med. J.* **2011**, *22*, 141–144.
59. Jiang, M.; Ding, J.; Song, Q.; Wu, X. TCM constitutions and depression-anxiety status in crew of high-speed rail trains of Beijing Railway: A survey and a correlation study. *J. Beijing Univ. Tradit. Chin. Med.* **2018**, *41*, 248–252.
60. Qiu, N.; Xu, Y. A Research of the Relationship between College Students' Depression and Traditional Chinese Medicine Constitution, Five Personality. *Med. Philos.* **2015**, *36*, 89–91.
61. Zhang, X.; Zhang, X.; Yang, T.; Zhanh, H. Relationship Between Chinese Medicine Constitution and Depression of 671 College Students in Nanjing. *J. Nanjing Univ. Tradit. Chin. Med. (Soc. Sci. Ed.)* **2019**, *20*, 245–249.
62. Zhao, L.; Chang, N.; Liu, X.; Wang, L.; Qiao, D. Study on the Correlation between Anxiety and Depression of Coronary Heart Disease and Constitution of Traditional Chinese Medicine. *J. Liaoning Univ. Tradit. Chin. Med.* **2020**, *22*, 59–62. [CrossRef]
63. Liang, X.; Wang, Q.; Jiang, Z.; Li, Z.; Zhang, M.; Yang, P.; Wang, X.; Wang, Y.; Qin, Y.; Li, T.; et al. Clinical Research Linking Traditional Chinese Medicine Constitution Types with Diseases: A Literature Review of 1639 Observational Studies. *J. Tradit. Chin. Med.* **2020**, *40*, 690–702. [CrossRef]
64. Page, M.J.; McKenzie, J.E.; Bossuyt, P.M.; Boutron, I.; Hoffmann, T.C.; Mulrow, C.D.; Shamseer, L.; Tetzlaff, J.M.; Akl, E.A.; Brennan, S.E.; et al. The PRISMA 2020 Statement: An Updated Guideline for Reporting Systematic Reviews. *BMJ* **2021**, *372*, n71. [CrossRef] [PubMed]
65. Stroup, D.F.; Berlin, J.A.; Morton, S.C.; Olkin, I.; Williamson, G.D.; Rennie, D.; Moher, D.; Becker, B.J.; Sipe, T.A.; Thacker, S.B. Meta-Analysis of Observational Studies in Epidemiology: A Proposal for Reporting. Meta-Analysis Of Observational Studies in Epidemiology (MOOSE) Group. *JAMA* **2000**, *283*, 2008–2012. [CrossRef] [PubMed]
66. Herzog, R.; Álvarez-Pasquin, M.J.; Díaz, C.; Del Barrio, J.L.; Estrada, J.M.; Gil, Á. Are Healthcare Workers' Intentions to Vaccinate Related to Their Knowledge, Beliefs and Attitudes? A Systematic Review. *BMC Public Health* **2013**, *13*, 154. [CrossRef]
67. Wells, G.; Shea, B.; O'Connell, D.; Peterson, J.; Welch, V.; Losos, M.; Tugwell, P. *The Newcastle-Ottawa Scale (NOS) for Assessing the Quality of Nonrandomised Studies in Meta-Analyses*; Ottawa Hospital Research Institute: Ottawa, ON, Canada, 2014.
68. Guyatt, G.H.; Oxman, A.D.; Vist, G.E.; Kunz, R.; Falck-Ytter, Y.; Alonso-Coello, P.; Schünemann, H.J. GRADE: An Emerging Consensus on Rating Quality of Evidence and Strength of Recommendations. *BMJ* **2008**, *336*, 924–926. [CrossRef] [PubMed]
69. Higgins, J.P.T.; Thompson, S.G.; Deeks, J.J.; Altman, D.G. Measuring Inconsistency in Meta-Analyses. *BMJ* **2003**, *327*, 557–560. [CrossRef]
70. Nikolakopoulou, A.; Mavridis, D.; Salanti, G. How to Interpret Meta-Analysis Models: Fixed Effect and Random Effects Meta-Analyses. *Evid.-Based Ment. Health* **2014**, *17*, 64. [CrossRef]

71. Higgins, J.; Thomas, J.; Chandler, J.; Cumpston, M.; Li, T.; Page, M.; Welch, V. *Cochrane Handbook for Systematic Reviews of Interventions Version 6.2*; The Cochrane Collaboration: London, UK, 2021.
72. Raimo, S.; Trojano, L.; Spitaleri, D.; Petretta, V.; Grossi, D.; Santangelo, G. Psychometric Properties of the Hamilton Depression Rating Scale in Multiple Sclerosis. *Qual. Life Res.* **2015**, *24*, 1973–1980. [CrossRef]
73. Sedighi, S.; Najarzadegan, M.R.; Ghasemzadeh, H.; Khodabandeh, M.; Khazaei, M.; Mirzadeh, M.; Babakhanian, M.; Rokni, A.; Ghazanfarpour, M. Factor Structure and Psychometric Properties of Zung Self-Rating Depression Scale in Women with a Sick Child. *Int. J. Pediatrics* **2020**, *8*, 11581–11586. [CrossRef]
74. Park, K.; Jaekal, E.; Yoon, S.; Lee, S.-H.; Choi, K.-H. Diagnostic Utility and Psychometric Properties of the Beck Depression Inventory-II Among Korean Adults. *Front. Psychol.* **2020**, *10*, 2934. [CrossRef] [PubMed]
75. Medicine CAFTC Traditional Chinese Medicine Constitution Classsification and Decision (ZYYXH/T157-2009). *World J. Integr. Tradit. West Med.* **2009**, *4*, 3–4.
76. Zhu, Y.; Wang, Q.; Hideki, O. Evaluation on Reliability and Validity of the Constitution in Chinese Medicine Questionnaire (CMCQ). *Chin. J. Behav. Med. Sci.* **2007**, *16*, 651–654.
77. Deng, W.; Peng, Y.; Ouyang, J. Study on the Relation between Anxiety, Depression and Constitution of Traditional Chinese Medicine. *J. Sichuan Tradit. Chin. Med.* **2019**, *37*, 66–69.
78. Ke, Y.; Yu, M.; Mai, W.; Liu, C. Analysis of Risk Factors of Depression in Patients with Cervical Cancer and Its Correlation with TCM Constitution. *Shandong J. Tradit. Chin. Med.* **2019**, *38*, 766–769. [CrossRef]
79. Liao, Y.; Chou, C.; Chang, C.; Li, T.; Sun, M.-F.; Chang, H.; Tsai, F.; Yen, H. Qi Deficiency Is Associated with Depression in Chronic Hemodialysis Patients. *Complement. Ther. Med.* **2017**, *30*, 102–106. [CrossRef]
80. Liu, B.; Li, H. Syndrome Relationship Between TCM Qi-Stagnation Constitution and Post-Stroke Depression. *Henan Tradit. Chin. Med.* **2010**, *11*, 1068–1070. [CrossRef]
81. Liu, X.; Liao, Z.; Lu, S.; Zeng, Y.; Zhou, J.; Zhang, Y.; Cao, J.; Hu, C. Analysis of Risk Factors of Post-cerebral Infarction Depression and Its Correlation with Body Constitution. *Shandong J. Tradit. Chin. Med.* **2019**, *38*, 952–956.
82. Pang, J.; Liu, J.; Tian, J. Study on Traditional Chinese Medicine Constitution Types, Syndrome Types and Serum Homocysteine Level of Patients with Post-First Ischemic Stroke Depression. *Shandong J. Tradit. Chin. Med.* **2018**, *37*, 814–846. [CrossRef]
83. Sun, S.; Qi, X.; Xie, C.; Dong, Q.; Yang, Q.; Liang, R. Correlation between Post-Stroke Depression and TCM Body Constitution. *Chin. J. Integr. Med. Cardio-Cerebrovasc. Dis.* **2012**, *10*, 368–369.
84. Tang, X.; Yang, X.; Huang, Y.; Sun, Z.; Li, F.; Fan, Q.; Chen, Y.; Song, M.; Ouyang, F.; Wang, R. The correlation-analysis between TCM constitution and anxiety or depression-related irritable bowel syndrome. *Chin. J. Integr. Tradit. West. Med. Dig.* **2020**, *28*, 940–943.
85. Wu, L.; Huang, F.; Wang, Q.; Liu, Z. Study on the Correlation between Depression after Type 2 Diabetes and Chinese Medicine Constitution. *J. New Chin. Med.* **2019**, *51*, 319–322. [CrossRef]
86. Zhang, Q.; Nie, L.; Sun, J.; Wang, X.; Zhang, Y.; Ding, C.; Liu, J. Research on the correlation of depression and constitution in adult patients with epilepsy. *China J. Tradit. Chin. Med. Pharm.* **2015**, *30*, 1680–1683.
87. Qiu, N.; Xu, Y. The Relationship Betwen Traditional Chinese Medicine University Students' Depresion and Traditional Chinese Medicine (TCM) Constitution. *China J. Health Psychol.* **2016**, *24*, 614–618.
88. Al-Shura, A.N. *Advanced Hematology in Integrated Cardiovascular Chinese Medicine*; Academic Press: Cambridge, MA, USA, 2019; Volume 3, ISBN 978-0-12-817573-6.
89. Shi, J.; Luo, L.; Chen, J.; Wang, J.; Zhao, H.; Wang, W. Study on the Differences between Traditional Chinese Medicine Syndromes in NYHA I-IV Classification of Chronic Heart Failure. *Evid.-Based Complement. Altern. Med.* **2019**, *2019*, 2543413. [CrossRef] [PubMed]
90. Zhijie, Z.; Shaoming, L.; Yueyang, Z.; Jingzhe, Y.; Tao, K.; Chengli, W.; Peng, N.; Xiaochao, C.; Xuesong, L.; Yusen, J.; et al. Traditional Chinese Medicine Syndrome Elements of Male Infertility Revealed by Latent Tree Model Analysis. *J. Tradit. Chin. Med.* **2018**, *38*, 926–935. [CrossRef]
91. Zhaoguo, L.; Qing, W.; Yurui, X. *Key Concepts in Traditional Chinese Medicine II*; Zhaoguo, L., Qing, W., Yurui, X., Eds.; Springer: Singapore, 2021; pp. 1–121; ISBN 9789811623981.
92. Han, F.; Zhang, H. Summary of Zhang Hongxing's Experience in Treating Refractory Angina Pectoris with Traditional Chinese Medicine. *J. Clin. Nurs. Res.* **2021**, *5*, 115–119. [CrossRef]
93. Chen, Y.; Chen, Z.; Zhang, P. Discussion on the Application of Warm Yang to Promote Qi Transformation in Acne Mastitis from "Yang Promotes Qi Transformation and Yin Promotes Forming". *J. Clin. Nurs. Res.* **2021**, *5*, 155–158. [CrossRef]
94. Zhu, J.; Liu, S.; Guo, Y.; Hou, L.; Su, X.; Li, Y.; Han, B.; Liu, D.; Wang, Q.; Chen, J.J.; et al. A New Model of Diarrhea with Spleen-Kidney Yang Deficiency Syndrome. *Evid.-Based Complementary Altern. Med.* **2018**, *2018*, 4280343. [CrossRef]
95. Dale, H.; Brassington, L.; King, K. The Impact of Healthy Lifestyle Interventions on Mental Health and Wellbeing: A Systematic Review | Emerald Insight. *Ment. Health Rev. J.* **2014**, *19*, 1–26. [CrossRef]
96. Zhu, Q.; Chen, M.; Fang, F.; Zhou, Y.; Huang, F.; Gu, W.; Li, B. On Influencing Factors of Depression in Foreign Students. *West. J. Tradit. Chin. Med.* **2013**, *26*, 45–47.

MDPI AG
Grosspeteranlage 5
4052 Basel
Switzerland
Tel.: +41 61 683 77 34

Behavioral Sciences Editorial Office
E-mail: behavsci@mdpi.com
www.mdpi.com/journal/behavsci

www.ingramcontent.com/pod-product-compliance
Lightning Source LLC
Chambersburg PA
CBHW061600210926
51850CB00009B/2169
* 9 7 8 3 7 2 5 8 5 4 9 7 4 *